Counselling in Primary Health Care

Second Edition

Editorial Advisors in Primary Care

Yvonne Carter, David Mant, Duncan Keeley, Ancy Chivers, Tina Ambury

Other related titles published by Oxford University Press

Women's health (fourth edition), *Edited by Ann McPherson and Deborah Waller*

Infection, *Lesley Southgate, Cameron Lockie, Shelley Heard, and Martin Wood*

Men's health, *Edited by Tom O'Dowd and David Jewell*

Prescribing in primary care, *Edited by Richard Hobbs and Colin Bradley*

Community-based maternity care, *Edited by Geoffrey Marsh and Mary Renfrew*

Primary care for older people, *Steve Iliffe and Vari Drennan*

Practical genetics in primary care, *Peter Rose and Anneke Lucassen*

Research methods and audit in general practice (third edition),
David Armstrong and John Grace

Counselling in Primary Health Care

Second Edition

Edited by

Jane Keithley

Department of Sociology and Social Policy
University of Durham
UK

Tim Bond

Graduate School of Education
University of Bristol
UK

Geoffrey Marsh

General Practitioner (formerly)
Stockton-on-Tees
UK

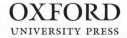
OXFORD
UNIVERSITY PRESS

MT

OXFORD
UNIVERSITY PRESS

Great Clarendon Street, Oxford OX2 6DP

Oxford University Press is a department of the University of Oxford.
It furthers the University's objective of excellence in research, scholarship,
and education by publishing worldwide in

Oxford New York

Athens Auckland Bangkok Bogotá Buenos Aires Calcutta
Cape Town Chennai Dar es Salaam Delhi Florence Hong Kong Istanbul
Karachi Kuala Lumpur Madrid Melbourne Mexico City Mumbai
Nairobi Paris São Paulo Shanghai Singapore Taipei Tokyo Toronto Warsaw
and associated companies in Berlin Ibadan

Oxford is a registered trade mark of Oxford University Press
in the UK and in certain other countries

Published in the United States
by Oxford University Press Inc., New York

British Library Cataloguing in Publication Data

Data available

Library of Congress Cataloguing in Publication Data

ISBN 0 19 263156 X (Pbk)

10 9 8 7 6 5 4 3 2 1

Typeset in Minion
by Cepha Imaging Pvt Ltd, India
Printed in Great Britain
on acid-free paper by
Biddles Ltd, Guildford & King's Lynn

12/22/04

Preface

In the mid-1990s, the first edition of this book referred to the 'rise and rise of counselling' in primary care. Counselling had become an accepted part of the range of services provided by many primary health care teams and counsellors were employed in around one-third of practices (Sibbald *et al.* 1993). Subsequently, expansion continued: by the late 1990s the proportion of practices with a counsellor was around 50% (Mellor-Clark *et al.*, 2001). It has been suggested that the National Health Service (NHS) is now the largest employer of counsellors in the UK (Eatock 2000). Alongside this continuing growth, the context within which counselling services are provided has been transformed. Hence the need for a second edition.

Our objectives remain broadly the same. We aim to provide a comprehensive and accessible discussion of what counselling in primary care entails, who provides it and who might be helped; and of the issues that need to be considered if counsellors are to be part of the primary care team. However, changes in the NHS and in the debates around counselling have radically challenged primary care counselling on a number of fronts.

In the NHS, the 1990s witnessed a shift in the balance of power and resources towards a 'primary-care-led' health service. More and more services were to be provided in local, community-based settings rather than in acute hospitals. General practitioners (GPs), initially through fundholding and then, after 1997, through primary care groups and primary care trusts (referred to as primary care organisations, or PCOs throughout this book), were also given more responsibility in deciding how health service resources were to be allocated and what secondary services were to be commissioned. At the same time, governments and the public have demanded more regulation and transparency from those providing health services. The latter are to be held more clearly accountable for their professional practice and increasingly required to demonstrate that decisions about the provision of services are 'evidence-based'.

These changes have had important repercussions for counselling in primary care. They have offered the potential for growth alongside other elements of primary care. However, this growth is in the form of a more 'managed' service, organized at PCO level, as opposed to the *ad hoc* arrangements with individual practices that were common in 1995, when this book was first published. In addition, counsellors are now more likely to find themselves challenged to demonstrate their credentials and justify their practice in ways acceptable to the health service. These changes (sometimes seen as threats) in primary care counselling have taken place in the context of a growing body of challenges to the validity and efficacy of counselling more generally.

Many of the chapters in this book reflect these changes and challenges. We have contributors who are strong supporters of counselling and others who are more sceptical, either about certain forms of counselling or about counselling as a whole. In the conclusion we draw the issues together and discuss their implications more fully. In the rest of this introduction, however, we return to similar questions as those we raised in the preface to the first edition—questions that are still relevant, but that, given the changes noted above, evoke a somewhat different response.

What exactly is counselling?

This book was first published at a time when counselling was only provided in a minority of practices. The proportion is now around half, meaning that more of those working in primary care have some familiarity with counselling services and counsellors. However, we would suggest that many remain unsure of what counselling actually is. They still wonder what goes on in the counsellor's room, in those 50-minute or hour-long sessions. What is it that distinguishes a 'talking *therapy*' from talking? More GPs and nurses working in primary care will have been introduced to 'counselling skills' as an important element in their interaction with patients. What is the difference, if any, between practising counselling skills and providing counselling?

Counsellors come from many disciplinary and professional backgrounds. They have undergone a variety of types, levels and amounts of training. Counselling is therefore unlikely to be a standard product, simple to describe. This is reflected in the range of our contributors, many of them practising counsellors, coming from nursing, medicine, social work, psychology, sociology, social policy and economics, as well as those whose primary professional affiliation is to counselling itself. Nevertheless, all of them—even those who are critical of the enterprise—would assert that counselling is a distinctive activity, with a common core.

The nature of counselling is most fully described by Tim Bond, in Chapter 1, but is also explored in a number of other chapters, especially those addressing specific problem areas. Some of our contributors have also used scenarios and case histories to illustrate the ways they work with their clients.

Who should counsel?

The research by Sibbald *et al.* (1993) showed that, in the early 1990s, practices reported a variety of different types of individuals to be providing counselling in primary care. This ranged from GPs and practice nurses with an interest in the field (but sometimes little extra training), practising counselling alongside their original role, to social workers, psychologists and individuals specifically appointed as counsellors. The distinction between 'counselling' and 'counselling skills' is important here and there seems to be far more agreement that primary care workers should acquire and practise counselling skills in their interactions with patients, than that nurses and GPs should themselves also be primary care counsellors (see Chapters 1–3).

Within counselling itself, two major trends in the 1990s have relevance to the question of who should counsel in primary care. Firstly, the moves towards standardized accreditation through the British Association of Counselling and Psychotherapy (BACP) make it easier for GPs and PCOs to judge the qualifications and experience of counsellors. However, as in the early days of medicine, there are competing professional bodies, including the Division of Counselling Psychology in the British Psychological Society (BPS) and the United Kingdom Council for Psychotherapy (UKCP). There has also been the emergence of a new and very energetic professional group with a particular interest in this area of work, namely the Association of

Counsellors and Psychotherapists in Primary Care. This is indicative of a second major trend in counselling that follows the pattern of development of many professions. Counselling has become increasingly differentiated into 'specialisms'. One of these specialisms is primary care counselling itself. However, as counselling, like medicine, develops more specialist practitioners, this raises the question—addressed by a number of our contributors—of when counselling support can be provided in what is for many the *generic* setting of primary care and when specialist referral is appropriate.

Who should be counselled?

The continuing high proportion of GP consultations which include a psychosocial element suggests the demand for counselling, as for health care more generally, could be a bottomless pit. At the same time, the voice of sceptics, arguing that counselling is of little proven value and may even be harmful, has grown stronger, suggesting that we should look critically at the apparent high level of need and demand.

Our first edition included discussion of a number of the problem areas in which it was most frequently suggested that counselling might have a role to play. The wider range of such problem areas included in this edition reflects the developments in the field that have, paradoxically, run alongside growing challenges to the counselling movement; hence there are chapters on physical and sexual abuse (Chapter 15) and on trauma (Chapter 14), for example. We have also added discussions on counselling young people (Chatper 9) and on counselling across social, sexual and ethnic differences (Chapter 7). We still do not claim, however, to have produced an exhaustive list!

Does counselling offer value for money?

PCOs have an explicit responsibility to use the health care resources available to them in ways that will most benefit the health of their local populations. More than ever, therefore, the supporters and providers of counselling services must be prepared to produce evidence of the effectiveness and cost-effectiveness of such services. The amount of such evidence has grown rapidly in recent years. It paints a mixed picture and we have included an extended review from two researchers with substantial experience in this field (Rowland and Goss in Chapter 5) as well as a critical perspective (Chapter 6). In addition, many of our other contributors discuss the evidence base relating to the particular aspects of counselling on which they focus. It will be apparent from these that the debate about outcomes is about both the substantive question of whether it works and the methodological question of how we can tell. Randomized controlled trials of the outcomes of counselling have often produced mixed or negative results, but the supporters of counselling have criticized these as inappropriate for use in counselling evaluations. On the other hand, some of the most favourable evaluations of counselling have depended heavily on client views and, partly as a result, such studies have been seen as lacking 'objectivity' and as 'unscientific'. The chapter by Keithley *et al.* (Chapter 8) reviews their usefulness, as well as containing a descriptive account of the experience of counselling from the client's perspective.

All those involved in decisions about primary care, and the counsellors themselves, need to be aware of the range of research evidence, of its strengths and its limitations. Used with a critical eye, research makes a valuable contribution to debate about the allocation of resources to counselling services, and can assist in the audit and evaluation of such services where they are provided.

How to go about it

This edition devotes less attention to the practicalities of establishing, operating and recruiting counsellors to a counselling service in primary care than its predecessor. The efforts of organizations such as the Counselling in Primary Care Trust (CPCT) and the BACP have ensured that guidelines are readily available, and contact details for these organizations are given on p. 00. However, written guidelines cannot adequately cover some of the less tangible issues that may be important in the success or failure of such services. Integration into the primary care team, confidentiality, referral and communication, the impact of counselling on the primary care team itself and the relationship between medical models and counselling models of care are key factors discussed, for example, in the chapters by Dammers and Wiener (Chapter 2), Cocksedge (Chapter 3) and Foster (Chapter 4)—all individuals with long-standing, 'hands-on' experience of such work.

So who will find this book useful?

This book aims to be an informative and useful resource for those responsible for commissioning, working with and providing counselling services in primary care. It is for all those who are seeking a better understanding of the nature and aims of counselling and of the state of the debate about its value, costs and effectiveness, especially as a part of primary care. Although most of our contributors believe strongly in the benefits that counselling can produce for health, we have also sought to represent the views of those who are more sceptical, either of counselling as a whole (Harris in Chapter 6) or of some models of counselling (Gournay in Chapter 10). Decisions about whether to provide counselling and, if so, of what kind and to whom, need to be made in the knowledge of the contemporary debate and the range of opinions that exist. Where such services are provided, we hope that all members of the primary care team (including counsellors) will find this book helps them to understand what counselling—primary care and specialist counselling—can contribute to the care of patients and how such services can be best integrated into the overall efforts of the team to promote the health of their practice population.

J.K., T.B., G.N.M.
November 2001

References

Eatock, J. (2000) Counselling in primary care: past, present and future. *British Journal of Guidance and Counselling*, **28**, 161–173.

Mellor-Clark, J., Simms-Ellis, S. and Burton, M. (2001) National survey of counsellors working in general practice: evidence for growing professionalisation? (Occasional Paper 79) Royal College of General Practitioners, London.

Sibbald, B., Addington-Hall, J., Brenneman, D. and Freeling, P. (1993) Counsellors in English and Welsh general practices. *British Medical Journal*, **306**, 29–33.

Contents

Contributors

Tim Bond is a reader in counselling and professional ethics at the University of Bristol. He is a former chair of the British Association for Counselling and Psychotherapy and currently a member of their Professional Conduct Committee. He has researched and written extensively about ethics for the talking therapies, including reports for the Department of Health. He is author of *Standards and Ethics for Counselling in Action* (Sage, 2000).

Simon Cocksedge is a general practitioner in Chapel-en-le-Frith, Derbyshire, a course organizer for vocational training in general practice and a lecturer in the School of Primary Care, University of Manchester. He has a particular interest in counselling (he has trained and worked as a counsellor), palliative care (he is medical adviser to High Peak Hospicecare) and research into aspects of doctor–patient relationships.

Jane Dammers is a general practitioner, undergraduate teaching associate and group leader for the vocational training scheme at the University of Newcastle; she is also joint co-ordinator of a programme with a multidisciplinary approach to develop mentoring and other forms of support for those working in primary care. She has been interested in developing 'psychological mindedness' in general practice, and in exploring the full potential of bringing counsellors and therapists into the work of primary care. She has helped to convene national and local conferences for counsellors and general practitioners over the past 11 years.

John Eatock is an Anglican priest who has worked for the past 12 years primarily as a counsellor in primary care. He is a former chair of the Counselling in Medical Settings Division and was founding chair of the Faculty of Healthcare Counsellors and Psychotherapists of the British Association for Counselling and Psychotherapy (BACP). He trained in counselling at the University of Manchester and in counselling supervision at Ripon and York St John. Currently he is a senior counsellor with Salford Mental Health Trust, lecturer in counselling at the University of Salford and healthcare programme consultant to BACP. John has contributed widely to counselling in primary care via articles, training and contributions to research. He is a fellow of BACP.

Kim Etherington is a lecturer at the University of Bristol, and is a BACP accredited counsellor and supervisor in private practice. She has previously worked as an occupational therapist NHS general and psychiatric hospitals, social services and charitable organization, including a child guidance clinic and a community for people with autism.

Joan Foster is chair of the Association of Counsellors and Psychotherapists in Primary Care (CPC). She has held the position from the founding of CPC in 1998. She is a practising primary care counsellor. Joan is a director of PriMHE (Primary Care Mental Health Education). She acts as a consultant on behalf of CPC to a number of primary care groups, advising them on the setting up of managed counselling services. She has been a provider of a managed primary care counselling service herself.

Stephen Goss is Research Development Manager with the British Association for Counselling and Psychotherapy and Hon. Research Fellow at the University of Strathclyde Counselling Unit. His recent published works include the edited text, with Nancy Rowland, *Evidence Based Counselling and Psychological Therapies* (Routledge, London). As counsellor, psychotherapist and clinical supervisor he has worked in primary medical care, private practice and higher education settings. Now a full-time researcher he has interests in evaluation, the development of pluralist methodologies and related issues in the philosophy of science. He also has an interest in the development of innovative means of service delivery.

Kevin Gournay is a chartered psychologist and a registered nurse who spent many years in full-time practice as a cognitive behaviour therapist. For the last decade he has devoted most of his time to research and training. He has completed eight large randomized controlled trials, two (community psychiatric nurses and practice nurses) in primary care, as well as studies of epidemiology, treatment interventions and evaluations of training. He is deputy head of the Health Services Research Department at the Institute of Psychiatry, London. He was appointed CBE in 1998 and a fellow of the Academy of Medical Sciences in 2000.

Myles Harris is a London doctor, writer and journalist. He has practised medicine in London, Canada, Papua New Guinea, Australia, Africa and the West Indies. In 1987, he published *Breakfast in Hell* (Picador, London and Simon & Schuster, New York), an account of working with the Red Cross during the Ethiopian famine in 1984. He has written on science, politics and medicine for the *Spectator,* the *Daily Telegraph,* the *Sunday Telegraph,* the London *Evening Standard,* the *Daily Mail* and the *Nursing Times.*

Glyn Hudson-Allez is a psychologist and psychosexual therapist who worked for 8 years in primary health care. She has authored many articles and chapters on counselling, and in 1997 she published *Time Limited Therapy in a General Practice Setting* (Sage, London). She is currently in private practice and is Deputy Chair of the Association of Counsellors and Psychotherapists in Primary Care (CPC).

Sue Jennings is a pioneer in using creative methods with people with a range of physical and psychological disorders. One of her specialisms is in working with people with fertility disorders, particularly 'unexplained' infertility. She is a trainer for many professional groups, including counsellors, psychotherapists and creative arts therapists, as well as medical students. She has 15 books currently in print, including *Creative Drama in Groupwork* and *Introduction to Developmental Playtherapy.* She is a professional actor on television and in the theatre and lives in Glastonbury, Somerset, where she runs the Rowan Studio.

Jane Keithley is a lecturer in social policy at Durham University. She has a background in nursing and has been the chair of two NHS trusts and of a branch of Relate. Her PhD thesis was a study of counselling in primary care. Her research interests are in health and health policy and her most recent publications are about the relationships between crime and health.

Geoffrey Marsh was a general practitioner in Stockton-on-Tees for over 35 years. During that time, he developed a comprehensive primary health care team and carried out a number of research studies into teamworking. Counsellors have been members of that team for approximately 35 years. In 1974 he was a visiting associate professor at the University of Iowa, USA, and from 1978 to 1980 he was RCGP Wolfson Visiting Professor to Canada. He has a special interest in general practice obstetrics. In his retirement, he has acted as a medicolegal expert.

Pip Mason is a registered nurse trained in counselling. She has over 20 years' experience in the field of alcohol and drug problems and a special interest in promoting early intervention in a primary care setting. She has researched the impact of placing alcohol counsellors into primary health care teams and developed ways of delivering counselling appropriate to this setting. With Steve Rollnick (a psychologist) and Chris Butler (a general practitioner) she authored *Health Behavior Change: a Guide for Practitioners* (1999). Currently Pip is self-employed, training health and social care professionals in addictions counselling, and is honorary lecturer in the School of Psychology at the University of Birmingham.

Joan McSloy is a community education co-ordinator for Hexham Queen Elizabeth High School. Her work within education, youth and community and counselling has always centred around the needs and rights of young people. She is particularly interested in the ethical issues surrounding the management of confidentiality with under-16s in team and multiagency settings.

Simon Parritt is a chartered counselling psychologist, director of the Association to Aid the Sexual and Personal Relationships of People with a Disability (SPOD)[*] and senior lecturer at the Institute of Sexuality and Human Relations.[†] He is a psychosexual and relationship counsellor and has a clinical and research interest in the issues surrounding sexuality, disability and chronic illness. He also offers consultancy and supervision for counsellors and health professionals working with disabled people. His most recent published research was a study of therapists' work with sexuality, relationships and disability published in 2000 in *Sexual and Relationship Therapy*.

Dorothy Poingdestre has been in the Methodist Diaconal Order since 1971, into which she was ordained in 1977. She gained her Certificate of Qualification in Social Work in 1985. As part of her diaconal work she conducted funerals and visited the dying, which led to her special interest of working with the dying and bereaved. After 6 years as a social worker in a busy general hospital, she was a Senior Social Worker in St. Joseph's Hospice in Hackney, London for 8 years.

....

[*] SPOD (the Association to Aid the Sexual and Personal Relationships of People with a Disability), 286 Camden Road, London N7 0BJ. Telephone: 020 7607 8851; fax: 020 7700 0236.

[†] The Institute of Sexuality and Human Relations, 131 Sunny Garden Road, London NW4 1SH. Telephone: 020 8203 5376.

Nancy Rowland is Head of Communication/Dissemination at the NHS Centre for Research and Dissemination, based at the University of York. Her main area of interest is in disseminating research findings to the NHS and in getting evidence into practice. She has a long-standing interest in counselling in primary care and has researched and written about the evidence base for counselling in this setting.

Sheila Thompson is a psychiatric social worker and group psychotherapist who was formerly a principal social worker at St Joseph's Hospice in Hackney. She has written a number of books about psychotherapy and counselling, the most recent being *The Group Context* (Jessica Kingsley, 1999).

Gillian Turner is a consultant community paediatrician with a special interest in young people's health. She managed the Northumberland Young People's Health Project from 1996 to 1998, working with young people to develop and evaluate a network of multidisciplinary drop-in health sessions for this group.

Jan Wiener is a training analyst and supervisor for the Society of Analytical Psychology and the British Association of Psychotherapists. She works in the NHS as an adult psychotherapist at Thorpe Coombe Hospital, Walthamstow (formerly Claybury), in an inner London general practice surgery and in private practice. She is joint chair with Dr Andrew Elder of the Primary Care Section of the Association of Psychoanalytic Psychotherapy (APP) in the NHS. She has written several papers and chapters on different aspects of psychotherapy in primary care and her book, *Counselling and Psychotherapy in Primary Health Care: a Psychodynamic Approach*, co-authored with Mannie Sher, was published by Macmillan in 1998.

Michael Wright is a Registered Counsellor of the British Association for Counselling and Psychotherapy, and has a private practice as a counsellor and trainer in Middlesbrough, with a specialist interest in post-trauma work. He was Occupational Health Co-ordinator for Cleveland County Council where he was responsible for planning the counselling response in the event of major incidents in the county. He is a former Chair of the Association for Pastoral and Spiritual Care and Counselling. An Anglican priest for 37 years, and he is now a Quaker.

Ali Zarbafi is an Anglo-Iranian psychotherapist. He completed his training at the Institute of Psychotherapy and Social Studies in 1994. He has worked in general practitioner's surgeries in London for over nine years. He has also worked extensively with refugees over the last 15 years. He is a founder member of the Imago Multilingual Psychotherapy Centre and has given papers on working multilingually and on trauma. He has a private practice in West London.

Part 1

Counselling and primary care

Chapter 1

The nature and the role of counselling in primary care

Tim Bond

Introduction

The development of counselling services in primary health care is at a critical and fairly unpredictable phase. By 2000, it was estimated that over half the practices in Britain had counsellors as members of the primary care team (Mellor-Clark *et al.*, 2001). The introduction of primary care group purchasing has created a period of uncertainty and change, with some practices losing counselling services either temporarily or in the longer term. Equally, in some areas, there has been a growth in provision with counselling being made available to more practices. The management of counselling services also appears to be changing with a trend towards delivering counselling within psychological therapy teams through mental health trusts. Coincidental with all these changes are strong indications that government is determined to introduce statutory regulations for the psychological therapies. This has inevitably sharpened the competition for territory and status between the different professional bodies brought together under this broad title in ways reminiscent of the regulation of medicine in the nineteenth century. At the time of writing (2001) it is difficult to see how this combination of circumstances will unfold, other than to say that the provision of counselling may look very different in five years' time. One of the immediate effects is to sharpen attention on the relationship between counselling, counselling psychology and psychotherapy. The providers of counselling in primary care are rapidly becoming more attentive to professional requirements determined by one or more of the relevant national bodies, namely the British Association for Counselling and Psychotherapy (BACP), the British Psychological Society (BPS) and the United Kingdom Council for Psychotherapy (UKCP).

In this chapter, I will be seeking to cast some light on what frequently seems to those outside, and often to those inside, the field to be rather abstruse and arcane differences between counselling, counselling psychology and psychotherapy. One further trend is noteworthy. Counselling in primary care and in health settings in general is becoming a specialism within its own right. Arguably, large professional bodies covering a full range of counselling in a wide variety of settings have struggled to keep pace with the rapidity of developments in this sector. BACP has developed a Faculty of Healthcare Counsellors and Psychotherapists to address this need. A parallel organization has grown out of the Counselling in Primary Care Trust—the Association of

Counsellors and Psychotherapists in Primary Care. Both bodies have been active in monitoring and responding to the rapidly changing circumstances of their members.

My experience of talking to GPs, primary care staff and the providers of services that are the subject of this book suggests that 'counselling' will remain the popular generic title for the provision of systematic consultations in primary care for addressing emotional, psychological and social issues that influence a person's health and well-being. Although I am not aware of any research on the subject, it appears that counselling is perceived by patients and some staff as less stigmatizing or pathologizing than referral to psychology, psychotherapy and, especially, psychiatry. This is in part due to the stigma and fear of mental illness. Perhaps more significantly, counselling is a term that is more wide ranging and includes assistance with difficulties arising in everyday life which do not necessarily imply any deficiency in the person affected. The potential for a wide range of applications of a generally popular term can become a source of confusion. Although there are numerous different meanings given to counselling in medical settings, I think most of the confusion around 'counselling' arises from three different usages, which are mutually incompatible. Because the same term is used for each of these different activities, it is very easy for two people to assume they are talking about the same thing when this is not the case. I have heard health workers talking about 'the desirability of a patient receiving counselling' and for the conversation to go on for some minutes before it becomes apparent that one person is advocating a series of sessions of psychosocial support to help with a general mood of anxiety and depression, in contrast to the other person who is thinking in terms of some practical advice about the patient's child-care problems. These misunderstandings often become apparent if the conversation continues for some time. However, in the hurried exchanges between people working in a busy practice, differences in meaning can go unnoticed. This can be confusing for staff. What is expected when someone is asked to counsel someone? It is even more confusing for patients. I have had some say to me that 'Dr … has been giving me counselling, but it was rather different from what you are doing'. The patient's perplexity could be the result of the doctor and myself having trained in different methods of counselling. However, more often the confusion seems to arise from the different meanings of counselling currently in use in medical settings.

Current usage of 'counselling'

There are wider and narrower usages of the term 'counselling'. Some of the narrower ones are mutually exclusive.

Generic use

There are some considered reasons why some people prefer to avoid using 'counselling' in more precisely defined ways and advocate a more inclusive or wider meaning. One of the reasons for retaining a generic approach to counselling is a concern that the exclusive use of 'counselling' by a select few working in specialized roles, who are trained, certificated and members of professional bodies, has the effect of restricting the wide availability of counselling in the community (Murgatroyd 1985). From this perspective, counselling and helping are synonymous and complementary ways of offering assistance in everyday life that ought not to be colonized as the basis for forming a new profession. This seemingly antiprofessionalization argument may be a form of professional protectionism by other mental health professions against the intrusion of a new service. However, this argument cannot be simply dismissed as thinly disguised self-interest. The development of the distinction between formal counselling and counselling skills (see later) is arguably an attempt to disseminate and foster aspects of counselling within general society whilst enabling the accumulation of knowledge and expertise by a profession of counsellors.

Philip Burnard's views (Burnard 1999) are of particular interest because his preference for the wider usage of 'counselling' is based on his experience of working in health care settings and a concern to ensure the dissemination of aspects of counselling more widely across services. As a nurse tutor, he was concerned to discover that nurses are reluctant to use facilitative skills with patients. This is not merely a matter of skills, but of an attitude and a belief that the nurse knows best, or at least better than the patient. This is contrary to the growing practice of involving patients in decisions about their own care. Therefore, Burnard is interested in extending nurses' skills to include more facilitative interventions which involve the patients in making decisions for themselves about their treatment. He draws on John Heron's six categories of therapeutic intervention as the underpinning model. Heron (1990) divided the possible interventions into authoritative and facilitative. Authoritative interventions include: prescriptive (offering advice), informative (offering information) and confronting (challenging). Facilitative interventions include: cathartic (enabling expression of pent-up emotions), catalytic (drawing out) and supportive (confirming or encouraging). Burnard concluded that it is desirable for nurses to use the full range of interventions, and, therefore, defines counselling as the effective use of verbal interventions involving 'both client-centred *and* more prescriptive counselling' [his emphasis]. He is, therefore, taking a strongly generic view of counselling.

In contrast to this wider definition of counselling, there are two narrower definitions in popular use which are mutually exclusive.

Counselling as advice

The first of these regards counselling as the same as giving advice. This view has had a long tradition which reaches back to at least the seventeenth century. In 1625 Francis Bacon, the essayist, wrote 'The greatest Trust, betweene Man and Man is the Trust of Giving Counsell'. It is a reasonable inference that he is thinking of advice because as he develops his argument he identifies the 'Inconveniences of Counsell'. These include 'the Danger of being unfaithfully counselled, and more for the good of them that counsell than of him that is counselled'. He also states that only people with expertise are suitable to provide 'counsell'. In modern dictionaries, both 'counsel' and 'counselling' retain the general meaning of 'advise' (Pearsall 1998). This usage is still commonplace in legal and medical circles. When I was working on a report about HIV counselling, a doctor was so committed to the use of 'counselling' to mean 'advising' that he wrote to me to express exasperation at all the fuss being made about counselling which he regarded as merely a 'popular term for giving advice to people' (Bond 1992).

However, modern dictionaries also acknowledge the existence of a more specialized use of 'counselling' as a method used by trained professionals to help someone resolve personal, social or psychological problems (Pearsall 1998). This more specialized usage has a shorter history of at least 70 years, which I will consider next.

Counselling in psychological and social care

The use of the word 'counselling' in its narrowest meaning first became popular in the 1920s in the USA. The term emerged in reaction against the exclusivity of psycho-analysis and psychotherapy. When Carl Rogers started working as a psychologist in America, he was not permitted to practise psychotherapy, which was restricted to medical practitioners. Therefore, he called his work 'counseling' (US spelling) (Thorne 1990). It seems probable that Rogers took the term from vocational counselling that had been developed as part of a radical community action programme by Frank Parsons (1854–1908) when he established a counselling centre in the North End of Boston, a deprived city area. Rogers also had a radical agenda. The person-centred nature of his method meant that counselling itself was part of a movement to democratize talking therapies by emphasizing the importance of the client's contribution. This has remained an important influence, even though as counselling has developed many new models for practice have developed. In all of these, there is an emphasis on counselling as the principled use of relationship, with the aim of enabling the client to achieve his or her own improved well-being. Two major ethical principles are closely associated with this way of counselling: respect for the client's capacity for self-determination and the importance of confidentiality. This is the use of the term 'counselling' espoused by the BACP. The definition used within the *Code of Ethics and Practice for Counsellors* (British Association for Counselling 1997) makes specific reference to the client's capacity for self-determination.

> The overall aim of counselling is to provide an opportunity for the client to work towards living in a way that he or she experiences as more satisfying and resourceful ... The counsellor's role is to facilitate the client's work in ways which respect the client's values, personal resources, and capacity for choice within his or her cultural context.

Sometimes self-determination is referred to as 'autonomy' or 'independence'. Although the suitability of some of these terms is increasingly questioned from feminist and multicultural perspectives, these disagreements tend to be about the best way of representing respect for the client's sense of self and self in relation to society. The ethical importance of respecting the client as a person, accepting differences between people in how they conceive of and respond to issues presented in counselling, and building on clients' existing resourcefulness are shared values that most counsellors would regard as informing their professional ethic.

Nearly a decade ago, the Counselling in General Practice Working Party of the Royal College of General Practitioners adopted the use of the term 'counselling' in this narrower usage of a professionally distinctive service. They used 'counselling' to refer to an activity undertaken by a trained counsellor working in accordance with the role as defined by the British Association for Counselling with its distinctive ethic and philosophy (Sheldon 1992).

Counselling and advice

In comparison to most other professions, counsellors are diffident about making claims to give advice. For nearly a decade successive codes for counsellors have included a statement that 'Counsellors do not normally give advice' (British Association for Counselling 1997, B.13.6).

It is doubtful whether this statement is any longer accurate. It may once have been a convenient way of challenging preconceptions about counsellors as being primarily advisors and asserting a more facilitative style of working. However, there is some empirical evidence that the prohibition on giving advice sometimes resulted in thinly disguised advice-giving (Silverman 1996). Some approaches to counselling have also found the prohibition to be problematic, especially those working in a cognitive behavioural tradition. After all what is the ethical value of withholding advice without good reason if that advice could contribute to the well-being of the client? It is probably more accurate to say that counsellors are judicious in their use of advice. To offer authoritative advice too readily could be counterproductive. It could induce dependence and passivity in a relationship that depends on the client's active involvement to be effective. The aim of counselling is to enable the client to discover and build on his/her own wisdom rather than have wisdom imparted to them from the counsellor. Perhaps because of the growing body of knowledge available to counsellors, they are more willing to offer information that is considered helpful and even to express opinions as to the best way of acting on that information. However, the way that this is done is likely to be intended to elicit the client's reactions and to work towards a solution to which the client is personally committed. The increasing use of short-term and time-limited work has contributed to a change in practice over advice-giving. Sometimes, in primary care, the counsellor's role is assisting clients in deciding how to respond to information and opinions provided by clinicians.

Counselling and psychotherapy

There is no universally accepted distinction between the terms 'counselling' and 'psychotherapy'. They have developed out of different historical traditions, which has led some practitioners to suggest a clear distinction between them in purpose and level of expertise required. One view seeks to differentiate them on the basis that counselling is primarily concerned with current environmental and social issues, in contrast to psychotherapy which is more concerned with personal psychology and neurosis. Some support for the differentiation of counselling and psychotherapy would be found amongst those working in psychodynamic and cognitive behavioural approaches. However, practitioners working within the humanistic approaches tend to regard the distinction as relatively insignificant as counsellors and psychotherapists tend to work in the same way. Comprehensive considerations of the issue in Britain concluded that there was little evidence of counselling and psychotherapy being distinguishable in terms of training, function or methods of working (Feltham 1995; James & Palmer 1996). Differentiation may be more concerned with claims to social status and territory. Memorably, Windy Dryden (1996) suggested that the only

Table 1.1 Characteristics of counselling and psychotherapy

Counselling	Psychotherapy
Educational	Reconstructive
Situational	Issues arising from personality
Problem-solving	Analytic
Conscious awareness	Preconscious and unconscious
Emphasis on working with people who do not have severe or persistent emotional problems	Emphasis on 'neurotics' or working with persistent and/or severe emotional problems
Focus on present	Focus on past
Shorter length of contract	Longer length of contract

significant difference is the hourly rate of pay, with psychotherapists charging substantially more. The situation is fluid at the moment. It is probably the case that the UKCP will seek to maintain a hierarchical distinction of roles in which counselling is concerned with current problem-solving whereas psychotherapy addresses personally 'deeper' issues rooted in the personality. In contrast the British Association for Counselling has changed its name to the British Association for Counselling and Psychotherapy (BACP) with effect from September 2000. This association has members supportive of the kinds of distinctions epitomized in Table 1.1 as well as members who view the terms 'counselling' and 'psychotherapy' as no more than different labels for the same activity.

Counselling and counselling skills

One of the most important distinctions to emerge in recent years is that between counselling and counselling skills. It is also a distinction with considerable implications for medical practice. Unfortunately, it is also one which has been subject to considerable misunderstandings.

The most obvious misunderstanding is based on the idea that 'counselling skills' is a label for a set of activities unique to counselling. Although the term 'counselling skills' is sometimes used on this basis, it is quickly discredited because any attempt to list specific 'counselling skills', for example active listening, paraphrasing, using open questions, reflective responses, etc., quickly looks indistinguishable from lists labelled social skills, communication skills, interpersonal skills, etc.

In order to understand what is meant by 'counselling skills', it is useful to examine the two words separately. Here the use of the word 'counselling' is an indication of the historical source of the concept. It serves to indicate that whilst these skills are not unique to counselling, it is the way they have been articulated in counselling that has been useful to other roles which employ counselling skills. For example, advice-giving has a much longer history than counselling skills, but the tendency has been to concentrate on the content of the advice rather than the way it is delivered. However, the methods which advisers use to communicate with clients can be adapted to improve the way advice is given and hence maximize the client's involvement in the decision-making. 'Counselling' in this context is acknowledging the source of the concept and

Table 1.2 Detection of counselling skills in the pattern of communication

Style	Pattern of flow	Time ratio (I : R)
Imparting expertise	Interactor → Recipient	80 : 20
Conversation	Interactor ↔ Recipient	50 : 50
Counselling skills	Interactor ← Recipient	20 : 80

I, interactor; R, recipient.

method of communication. Similarly, nurses, tutors, personnel managers, social workers and many others have all recognized that there are advantages in adopting the methods of communication used in counselling to aspects of their own role. One way in which an outside observer might detect that counselling skills are being used is in the pattern of communication (Table 1.2).

Imparting expertise involves the expert in communicating his/her knowledge and expertise to the recipient which takes up most of the consultation time available. This contrasts with conversation where both participants tend to contribute for equal lengths of time and in a pattern which flows backwards and forwards. The use of counselling skills will usually change the pattern of communication in favour of the recipient, who speaks for most of the available time. Part of the expertise in using counselling skills is learning how to communicate briefly in ways which do not interrupt the flow of the speaker, but at the same time help the speaker to address more effectively the issues which concern them. When counselling skills are being used, an outside observer might notice that the recipient is encouraged to take greater control of the agenda of the dialogue than in other styles of communication. In other words, the values implicit in the use of counselling skills are similar to those of counselling, placing an emphasis on the client's capacity for self-determination in how help is sought as well as for any decisions or actions that may result (Bond 1989).

Other things which might be apparent to an outside observer include the way the recipient is encouraged or enabled to participate in deciding the agenda for the total transaction. In other words, the values implicit in the interactions are similar to those of counselling, with an emphasis on the client's capacity for self-determination.

The term 'skills' in 'counselling skills' is sometimes taken very literally to mean 'discrete behaviours' but this is not the way 'skills' is understood in the social sciences. Skills which are used to enhance relationships can be distinguished from 'physical skills', as in sport or work, and 'mental' and 'intellectual skills', not merely on the basis of observable behaviours. They are inextricably linked to the goal of the person using them. For instance, Michael Argyle (1981) defines 'socially skilled behaviour' as 'behaviour effective in realising the goals of the interactor'. In the context of counselling skills, these goals are to implement the values of counselling by assisting the self-expression and autonomy of the recipient.

One of the ways in which an independent observer might be able to distinguish between counselling skills and counselling is by whether the contracting is explicit between the two people. This is highlighted in one of the alternative definitions for counselling which is still in popular use:

> People become engaged in counselling when a person, occupying regularly or temporarily the role of counsellor, offers or agrees explicitly to offer time, attention or respect to another person or persons temporarily in the role of client. (British Association for Counselling 1984)

This definition was originally devised to distinguish between spontaneous or *ad hoc* counselling and formal counselling. The overt nature of the latter involving 'offers' and explicit agreements was seen as 'the dividing line between the counselling task and the *ad hoc* counselling, and is the major safe-guard of the rights of the consumer' (British Association for Counselling 1985). In primary care the distinction between counselling and using counselling skills provides a way of valuing situations in which clinicians offer *ad hoc* counselling as an integral part of their work without necessarily presenting it as though it is the same as a formal session with a counsellor. Recent changes in the curriculum for the training of doctors and nurses have tended to incorporate training in counselling and communication skills (Smith & Norton 1999). Where this occurs it increases the potential for mutual understanding between clinicians and counsellors in primary care as well as greater consistency and coherence between the range of services offered in the practice as experienced by the patient. There are three frequent misconceptions that I encounter in discussions about counselling skills. These are:

1 *Using counselling skills is always a lower order activity than counselling.* This need not be the case. Arguably the user of counselling skills may be working under more demanding circumstances than the counsellor who usually has the benefit of more extended periods of time, which have already been agreed in advance. In comparison, the user of counselling skills may be working more opportunistically with much less certainty about the duration of the encounter. Users of counselling skills can be more or less skilled, just like counsellors. However, using counselling skills is not a role in itself but something important used to enhance the performance of another role. This means that the capacity to use counselling skills effectively will depend not only on being skilled in their use but also on someone's competence in their primary role, for example the nurse, tutor, etc. For all these reasons, using counselling skills can be more skilled than counselling. It certainly cannot be assumed that using counselling skills is a lower order activity.

2 *People in occupational roles, other than counsellor, cannot counsel.* This would mean that doctors, nurses, youth workers, etc., cannot counsel but can only use counselling skills. This is not the case. With appropriate training, counselling supervision, and clear contracting with the client in ways consistent with counselling, it seems to me anyone can change roles to that of 'counsellor'. There are important issues about keeping the boundaries between different roles clear and managing overlapping roles or dual relationships, but these are separate issues (Herlihy & Corey 1992). In 1998 the Medical Defence Union noted an increase in the number of practice nurses who offered counselling. It was willing to offer assistance to them but expected them to be properly trained and supervised (Medical Defence Union 1998). It seems reasonable to me that not every doctor wants to become a counsellor. It is a

specialized activity which appeals to relatively small numbers of health workers and, realistically, probably only a few of these have the time to devote to it. On the other hand, my experience is that most doctors who have been trained in the use of counselling skills have found them useful in consultations with patients. They provide a way of responding immediately to the large number of emotional difficulties presented by patients in primary care that do not in themselves justify referral on to counselling or other types of assistance.

3 *Anyone with the occupational title 'counsellor' is always counselling.* This is not the case. As the concept of counselling has narrowed down into a specifically contracted role, there is a need for counsellors to distinguish between when they are counselling and when they are performing other roles, including training, supervision, managing, etc. In each of these other roles a counsellor is likely to be using counselling skills.

I opened this section by suggesting that the distinction between counselling and counselling skills is one of the most important to have emerged. It is a distinction that has enabled counsellors to continue to develop a range of knowledge and expertise without necessarily making exclusive claims to everyday helping skills, a claim that would be manifestly absurd. Instead the opportunity for systematic reflection provided by a professional context has led to a degree of refinement in understanding and practice that can be offered back to people with caring roles in the community and other professions. One of the contributions that many counsellors can offer to multidisciplinary health teams is training in more effective listening and counselling skills.

Background of counsellors working in primary health care

The background of counsellors working in primary health care settings is quite varied. Many have been trained by Relate, formerly known as the National Marriage Guidance Council. This training consists of over 150 hours of formal training and between 170 and 220 hours of closely supervised counselling practice. The use of Relate-trained counsellors in primary health care has a long and successful history (Marsh & Barr 1975; Corney 1986). Alternatively, others have been accredited by the British Association for Counselling (BAC), which requires 450 hours of training and 450 hours of supervised practice and having received personal counselling. Accredited status by BAC or a number of other professional organisations with comparable requirements is the main way of achieving registration with the United Kingdom Register of Counsellors. Many counsellors working in primary health care are also members of either the Faculty of Healthcare Counsellors and Psychotherapists, a section of BAC, or the recently formed Association of Counsellors and Psychotherapists in Primary Care, a development initiated by the Counselling in Primary Care Trust. Many are members of both. In addition some counsellors may acquire their professional standing through the Counselling Psychology Section of the British Psychological Society or the United Kingdom Council for Psychotherapy. All these organizations and their schemes are widely accepted as reputable although the proliferation of bodies with an interest in this area of work is a potential source of confusion.

Table 1.3 What is essential and desirable in a counsellor in primary care

Criteria	Essential	Desirable
Education and professional qualifications	450 hours training	BACP accreditation or equivalent
Knowledge	One theoretical approach to counselling	Variety of counselling theories and methods
	Psychosomatic disease and psychology of chronic or terminal illness	Psychotropic drugs and their side effects
	BACP code of ethics— particularly about confidentiality	Psychopathology by visiting admission unit of psychiatric hospital
Experience	250 hours *supervised* counselling over 2 years	At least 300 hours gained over at least 3 years
Personality	Dependable	Aware of boundaries around punctuality
	Considered approachable by a wide range of patients?	Friendly
Physical attributes	Good enough health and sufficient sight and hearing not to make special demands on clients	Able to work under pressure and to monitor and manage own stress level
Special circumstances	A constructive member of a multidisciplinary team	Understanding of culture of medical settings and willingness to develop appropriate counselling skills among team members

The Counselling in Primary Health Care Trust (1992) was one of the first organizations to consider what is the essential background for a counsellor working in this setting and to make suggestions for what is desirable. I have updated their recommendations in Table 1.3.

Ethics and standards of practice for counsellors

Counsellors have developed reasonably comprehensive ethics and standards of practice. Inevitably, because counselling is such a new role, the standards are still evolving. However, it is useful to be aware of a number of key issues.

Confidentiality

For medical staff and counsellors alike, confidentiality is both an ethical and legal requirement. However, the implementation of confidentiality is different. Medical services are provided on the basis that the treatment needs to continue even if the person providing it changes due to rotas, or for other reasons. Information about patients is, therefore, not usually confidential to a single person, but is shared across a team on a confidential basis in order to ensure continuity of treatment. In contrast, the counselling relationship depends on the client's trust in a particular individual and there is no assumption that the counsellor is interchangeable with others. This is reflected in the caution required of counsellors in how they manage personally sensitive information disclosed in confidence. Whereas it is probably common practice for members of the primary care team to rely on implicit consent for disclosures to other members of the team, counsellors are more likely to require explicit consent unless there substantial reasons in favour of disclosure. This has implications for record-keeping. The code of practice which accompanied the Human Fertilisation and Embryology Act (HFEA) 1990 provides a useful example of how counsellors and team members can manage confidentiality about personal information relating to patients, whilst ensuring that essential information can be communicated. The code states:

> 6.24 A record should be kept of all counselling offered and whether or not the offer is accepted.
> 6.25 All information obtained in the course of counselling should be kept confidential subject to 3.24.
> 3.24 If a member of the team has a cause for concern as a result of information given to him or her in confidence, he or she should obtain the consent of the person concerned before discussing it with the rest of the team. If a member of the team receives information which is of such gravity that confidentiality *cannot* be maintained, he or she should use his or her own discretion, based on good professional practice, in what circumstances it should be discussed with the rest of the team.

This code of practice assumes a slightly more rigorous separation of records and practice over confidentiality than the procedures advocated by Dr June McLeod (1992) in her contribution to the Counselling in General Practice Working Party. The HFEA code would simply require that an entry of whether a patient was offered counselling and whether the offer was accepted or rejected was entered on the medical records. In contrast, McLeod recommends that counsellors complete a card with a brief record of dates, progress and outcome of counselling to be kept with the medical records. The counsellor's working notes would be kept separately and would be confidential to the counsellor. Whatever method is adopted, it is important that the patient is informed about the limits of confidentiality.

After misunderstandings about what constitutes counselling, tensions arising from differences about the practice of confidentiality are the second major source of difficulty which can frustrate the most effective use of counsellors in primary care.

Counselling supervision

In most professions, supervision is mandatory for trainees and for those in a probationary period after training. In contrast, counsellors are required to have regular and continuing counselling supervision. The code for ethics requires that 'counsellors must have appropriate, regular and on-going supervision' (British Association for Counselling 1997, A.6).

Counselling supervision is not in any way a managerial relationship. Managerial issues should be dealt with between the counsellor and the medical practice. The counselling supervisor is someone who is experienced as a counsellor and independent of the situation in which the counselling is provided. The supervisor's role is directed towards helping the counsellor to develop his/her own standards of practice and to foster an 'internalized supervisor'. The tasks of supervision can be categorized thus:

1 Formative: learning new methods and insights.

2 Restorative: getting personal support and relief from the consequences of being exposed to others' emotional pain as well as that of the counsellor's.

3 Normative: ensuring adequate standards of ethics and practice are maintained.

These three tasks were first described by Francesca Inskipp and Brigid Proctor (1989). As a result of my study of good practice in HIV counselling, I have added a fourth:

4 Perspective: stepping back to take an overview of the total pattern of work with clients and to review the interface between counselling and other methods of helping or treating clients, including interprofessional relationships.

These tasks have to be held in balance with each other so that one does not predominate over the others. For example, if the restorative were to dominate over the others, counselling supervision would become indistinguishable from personal counselling. The counsellor's 'internalized supervisor' needs to be an all rounder.

Discussions in supervision are anonymous. The identity of individual clients is protected in the interests of preserving confidentiality.

A minimum frequency of supervision recommended by the British Association for Counselling is one and a half hours per month, but some counsellors have more frequent supervision because of the difficulty of their cases, volume of work or because they find it increases their efficacy.

Prohibition of sex with clients

Unfortunately, a small number of counsellors abuse their position of trust by entering into sexual relationships with clients. This phenomenon is shared with all the caring professions. So far as I am aware, no such accusations have been made against counsellors in primary care. However, the belief that counsellors have sex with clients is sufficiently commonplace to be worthy of consideration.

There is no doubt that any sexual activity between a counsellor and a current client is regarded as unethical by the BACP. Sex with former clients is also considered unethical in many circumstances, particularly if the subject matter of the counselling concerns relationship or sexual difficulties.

Counsellors who are members of BACP view sexual intimacy with clients in ways which parallel health care workers' relationships with patients. Counselling inevitably involves psychological intimacy rather than physical exposure and, therefore, requires comparable levels of trust. Clients also sometimes imbue counsellors with power, or experience a sense of dependency. For all these reasons, counsellors need to be scrupulous about maintaining personal boundaries between themselves and clients. When a complaint of sexual misconduct has been upheld, counsellors have been expelled not only from BACP, but also from other professional bodies. This does not stop someone continuing to practise as a counsellor, for it is currently an unregulated occupation, and anyone can set up as a counsellor. However, it illustrates the importance of ensuring that a counsellor adheres to an appropriate code of ethics and practice for the protection of clients and the primary health care team in which the counsellor is working.

Counselling in practice

What does counselling look like in actual practice? Many counsellors are restricted in the number of sessions that can be offered to individual patients in the first instance. Six to 10 sessions of 50 minutes appears to be usual (Rowland 1992). Clients with exceptional needs who are showing significant progress may be offered more sessions depending on the resources available.

The counselling relationship is probably most widely thought of in terms of stages. In the initial stage, the emphasis is on trust-building and enabling the client to describe the situation which is causing the difficulty. With some clients this may remain the major activity, because the client regains a sense of control and order in the process of exploring the issue which causes them concern. In parallel with this initial phase, the counsellor may be conducting a systematic assessment. For some clients merely identifying and voicing the nature of the problem is sufficient for them to progress without any further assistance. With most clients, however, it is necessary to move on to a second stage which is primarily directed at creating a change which will give the client additional resources to assist with the problem. This may involve gaining new insight, learning new skills, redefining personal goals or reassessing important relationships. A third stage involves considering alternative ways of applying the new resources and then putting them into action.

All counsellors probably use rather similar approaches in the initial stage. The aim is to provide an enabling relationship characterized by warmth, genuineness and empathy. These are qualities which are widely considered essential to the effectiveness of counselling (Truax & Carkhuff 1967) and certainly to the stage of trust-building. The counsellor may also attempt to negotiate a contract with the client about the practical arrangements, confidentiality and the therapeutic goal of the client. These negotiations help to increase the client's sense of control and also to identify the focus of the counselling. In this way the client is encouraged to focus on what he/she is really concerned about. Many other strategies and techniques may be used to this end. The counsellor's task is to notice what a client experiences as significant, and to build up a picture of what is said, what is implied and what is left unsaid. Gradually a picture of the client's perception emerges and this forms the foundation upon which the counsellor builds.

The next stage in the counselling relationship will vary according to the theoretical model of the counsellor. There are probably over 200 different published models of counselling. I will describe three of the most widely used. Psychodynamic counselling has developed from the work of Sigmund Freud but is often considerably modified. The counsellor's concern is the client's internal relationships with people who have been significant in that person's development. These internalized relationships and associated feelings may have their origins in early childhood and may no longer rely on the promptings of an external person to evoke them. The aim of successful counselling in this model is to enable a person to balance the potentially conflicting demands of basic psychological needs, the demands of conscience and the external realities of the situation (Jacobs 1999).

Person-centred counselling was developed by Carl Rogers and is superficially quite different from a psychodynamic approach. In contrast with psychodynamic counselling, which emphasizes the counsellor's ability to understand the effect of past influences on the client's present experience, a person-centred counsellor seeks to use the current relationship between client and counsellor as the source of new personal development and emphasizes the role of the client as the expert in selecting what is important and healing to him or her. The quality of the relationship is extremely important and is sometimes described as '*trying to put the loving into helping*' (Mearns & Thorne 1999).

In contrast, again, cognitive behavioural counselling is primarily directed towards changing the way someone 'self-talks' in order to achieve beneficial changes (Trower *et al.* 1988).

Some counsellors are purists and work exclusively with one model. Others are committed to drawing on a range of models in order to find the method best suited to a particular client. It is generally considered better to be systematically rather than randomly eclectic as this reduces the risk of presenting the client with mixed messages and potentially confusing the client's problem further (Culley 1990).

Who will benefit from counselling?

A wide range of people appear to benefit from counselling. Anyone who is capable of expressing themselves verbally and who has usually been quite resourceful in the way they have coped with life until they become troubled by a particular issue will almost certainly benefit. Sometimes counselling can be useful to people who have a long history of not coping, but this is much less certain.

There are certain issues which are generally considered as being suitable for counselling:

◆ Bereavement
◆ Recovery from trauma due to accident, major disaster, major medical treatment, diagnosis of serious illness or physical/sexual abuse (post-traumatic stress syndrome)
◆ Terminal illness
◆ Coping with anxiety associated with major transitions in life, for example adolescence to young adulthood, changes in occupation, moving out of work due to redundancy or retirement, or changes in relationships
◆ Stress management

- Problems associated with the use of alcohol or drugs
- Interpersonal and relationship problems
- Sexual problems
- Family planning
- Infertility
- HIV/AIDS
- Psychological and less severe psychiatric problems
- Decision-making about the best course of treatment when the patient has alternatives to choose between.

Surveys suggest that the most common issues referred to counsellors are relationship problems, depression, anxiety and bereavement (Clark *et al.* 1997).

Many of these issues are discussed in more detail elsewhere in this book. It is not unusual for several issues to be closely related. For example, the diagnosis of a major illness will not only be the start of a process of personal adjustment but may also involve the patient in planning what to tell a partner, and perhaps reassessing personal relationships. There may also be a need to learn how to manage personal anxiety better. When someone presents with multiple issues, the counsellor's role is to help them prioritize the issues to be addressed. Typically the choice is made on the basis of what is most urgent, or causing greatest discomfort, or most likely to create the possibility of other successes if it improved. Depressed patients are an exception to this general rule for prioritizing the issues. Often it is better to start with the most manageable issue and work progressively towards the most demanding so that a sense of confidence and of regaining control can emerge. This approach counters the sense of helplessness and dispiritment associated with depression.

An important factor to take into consideration in deciding who could benefit from counselling is the aptitude of the counsellor. His or her training and experience may be decisive in who will be the most helped by counselling. However, counselling is possible only when the client becomes actively committed to the process. Therefore, the most important factor is the client's attitude to the offer of counselling. A positive attitude considerably increases the likelihood that the client will take advantage of the opportunities offered in counselling.

Who is unsuitable for counselling?

Not everyone is suitable for counselling. However, there appears to be no agreed classification of the situations unlikely to be helped by counselling. Probably the aptitude of individual counsellors is a more important factor than any general list. None the less, experience suggests that some situations may be less suitable for counselling. These include:

1 The person who does not want counselling. Counselling requires the active involvement of clients and, therefore, is essentially a voluntary activity.

2 The person who consistently externalizes problems on to other people or attributes his/her problems to his/her state of physical health. For example, a client who

attributes her emotional fluctuations exclusively to premenstrual tension and is unwilling to take any role in managing her situation other than to demand tablets from a doctor is unlikely to be suitable for counselling. In contrast, someone who wants to do what she can to improve her situation or is willing to explore whether there could be other factors contributing to her changes in mood is much more suitable for counselling. The counselling is most likely to complement any medical treatment.

3 Someone who has no insight into his/her condition due to a personality disorder or severe psychiatric disorder is unlikely to benefit from short-term counselling.

4 People with undiagnosed clinical conditions which would account for their problems. For example, counselling cannot help a tired, weepy patient who has untreated thyroid deficiency or pernicious anaemia because the appropriate tests have not been conducted. This situation is quite different from the patient who has done the rounds of all the possible medical specialities without any physiological explanation for the problems being discovered. In these circumstances, counselling may help a client to explore whether the problems could have psychological or social origins.

Some clients may be suitable for counselling but can be made unsuitable by being given unrealistic expectations of the counselling. It is important that the referrer conveys a realistic hope that counselling will be beneficial. Counselling can sometimes help people to solve problems. However, in many situations there is no immediate solution. Counselling cannot bring a loved relative back to life or remove the inevitable tensions of looking after an adolescent dependent, but it can help people manage their bereavement or difficult relationships better.

Effectiveness of counselling versus acceptable outcomes

It is important to consider the effectiveness of counselling and what are the outcomes. There are problems in answering these questions. Some of the problems relate to the nature of counselling itself. It is difficult to quantify the input of the counsellor in comparison to a medical or surgical procedure. Psychosocial factors are by nature often elusive and difficult to quantify. Many workers in primary care recognize the difficulty in assessing the contribution which verbal communications and the emotional climate of the relationship make to the well-being of the patient. There are also potential difficulties in identifying what changes can be ascribed to particular aspects of the counselling.

For example, I remember seeing someone after an attempted suicide who was experiencing social isolation, difficulties with her mother, and problems arising from an inability to say 'no' to people in need of her help. The counselling, at her direction, focused on these last two problems, but when I asked her what had been most useful, her response surprised me:

> It is the experience of being listened to. You remember when I started I talked about my loneliness and feeling I am the only one with these problems. I have taken you as a model and have started listening to other people and I have discovered many other people have similar problems.

The other topics addressed in counselling had been useful but for her this was the most useful.

It is also possible that beneficial changes are due not to the counselling but to events occurring in other aspects of the client's life.

The final methodological hurdle to be overcome is in deciding what constitutes a beneficial outcome in order for counselling to be considered effective. Is it sufficient that the client reports feeling better? Or is some more observable physiological or behavioural change required? In Chapter 5 of this book, these issues are examined from a researcher's perspective and are outlined in ways in which qualitative and quantitative methodologies have been applied to assess the effectiveness of counselling. Studies about the effectiveness of counselling are increasingly important for the medium- and long-term development of counselling, especially in a context where there is a strong expectation that practice can be justified by scientific evidence of effectiveness.

Primary health care teams require more readily available indicators of the results achieved by investing resources in counselling. In some cases these gains may be demonstrated better by secondary indicators. In the opinion of Dr Graham Curtis Jenkins, the Director of the Counselling in Primary Care Trust, acceptable outcomes might include:

◆ Reduction in GP consultations

◆ Patients in receipt of counselling making more appropriate use of consultations with health care staff

◆ Reduction in prescribed medicines

◆ Reduced referrals to psychiatric outpatient and psychiatric patient clinic admissions

◆ Reduced costs in managing some patients.

Eventually the monitoring of these secondary gains may accumulate to be used as benchmarks for the effectiveness of a particular counselling provision. Changes in the secondary gains may reflect changes in the quality of counselling being provided, if the kind of issues referred and the method of referral are constant.

Monitoring counselling

Regular and systematic monitoring of the counselling is important. There are different levels of complexity and sophistication in monitoring. At one time it was considered desirable to keep monitoring relatively simple. One of the reasons for doing this was to maximize the time available for delivering counselling. Generally there is only very limited time available for counsellors outside face to face contact with clients in primary care (Clark *et al.* 1997). The British Association for Counselling (1992) originally suggested restricting routine monitoring and auditing to: how many patients are seen, how often, from which partner, appointment failures and reasons for referral. This can be done at six-monthly intervals, and the results can appear in the annual report.

Even such basic auditing will expose important issues, such as whether referrals are evenly spaced across the practice or are mainly from a few sources. Changes in the pattern of appointment failures may be indicative of the underlying problem. It is reasonable to start with the rebuttable assumption that failure to attend first appointments may indicate problems with referral or reception. On the other hand, increases in failure to attend second or subsequent appointments may indicate dissatisfaction with the counselling facilities or with the counsellor, or the patient's deteriorating mental or physical health.

During my study of good practice in HIV counselling (Bond 1992), counsellors and their managers were invited to identify the criteria for monitoring the quality of counselling being provided. I have adapted their suggestions to primary care as possible ways of augmenting the simple audit already mentioned.

1 *Service delivery*
    (a) *Pre-counselling information*: is a leaflet or other means of explaining to patients what counselling entails readily available?
    (b) *Approachability*: are the counselling services attractive to intending clients? Are they provided by people who are acceptable to the clients in terms of gender, and ethnic, cultural and social background? Can clients choose a counsellor who is likely to satisfy their requirements?
    (c) *Accessibility*: has the location of the counselling sessions been considered in terms of its nearness to likely users of the service and its accessibility by public and private transport? Is access to the premises possible for people with difficulties with mobility or in wheelchairs? Are there arrangements for counsellors to visit clients in hospital, at home or at other venues if these are more appropriate?
    (d) *Availability*: does the availability of the service correspond to clients' needs, for instance during weekdays, evenings or at weekends?
    (e) *Continuity*: are the services provided with sufficient continuity to gain the confidence of potential client groups? Is counselling staff turnover taking place at an acceptable rate?
    (f) *Confidentiality*: are the established practice and procedures about confidentiality understood and implemented by staff? Are any limitations on confidentiality communicated to clients?
    (g) *Statement of standards and ethics*: is there a readily available statement or code of practice which sets out the standards and ethics of the counselling? Is the code available to clients?

2 *Client participation in monitoring*
    (a) *Client feedback*: is client feedback sought regularly about the service provided to them?
    (b) *Complaints procedure*: is there a procedure to deal with complaints from clients? How does the agency respond to the complainant? How does the agency learn from complaints and revise its practice?

3 *Staffing*
    (a) *Selection*: what are the selection criteria for counsellors? What are the selection procedures?

(b) *Training*: what provision has been made to ensure counsellors receive appropriate basic training for their role? What provision has been made for the continuing training of counsellors?

(c) *Supervision and support*: what are the arrangements for supervising counsellors by management, and for independent supervisors for counselling supervision/consultative support?

4 *Co-operation with others*

(a) *Liaison with other staff and agencies*: how effectively do counsellors and their managers liaise with other service providers within the same agency and between agencies?

(b) *Reputation of the counselling service*: what is the reputation of the counselling service amongst other agencies? How are these views collected and responded to?

5 *Counsellors can contribute to the monitoring by the following methods*

(a) *Client's manner*: changes in the client's manner towards becoming more competent and assertive in counselling sessions are generally thought to be positive indicators.

(b) *Changes attributed to counselling by clients*: constructive changes that are attributed to the counselling by the client are considered to be positive indications of the usefulness of the counselling. However, the counsellor also needs to consider the possibility that the changes were exclusively due to other factors or a combination of counselling and other factors.

(c) *Clients keeping prearranged appointments*: attendance at prearranged second and subsequent counselling sessions may be an indication that the client is getting something of value from the sessions.

(d) *Returning for further sessions*: clients who return for further sessions after an interval without counselling may be demonstrating with their feet a belief that counselling has helped them previously.

(e) *New clients recommended to seek counselling by former clients*: the recommendation of counselling by former clients is generally considered to be a very positive indicator.

(f) *Informal feedback from clients*: some counsellors ask for informal feedback at the end of sessions about what has/has not been useful to the client. This can be extremely informative.

6 *Other members of the primary care team or the practice manager may wish to participate in the use of any of the following*

(a) *Monitoring attendance for appointments*: significant changes in the frequency of non-attendance for appointments usually indicates changes in the client group's perception of the counselling service. Generally, a reduction in missed appointments is considered to be a positive indication unless there is evidence of excessive dependence on counsellors.

(b) *Distributing questionnaires to current and former clients*: questionnaires can be a useful means of obtaining information from clients who are able to read and write and who are confident enough to express their views in writing.

An alternative approach is to use structured/semistructured interviews by a skilled interviewer, although problems over confidentiality often make this approach impossible.

(c) *Using an independent consultant*: the independence of the consultant adds to the credibility of the monitoring.

(d) *Monitoring complaints and unsolicited positive feedback*: reviewing complaints and unsolicited feedback can be very informative.

This list is the accumulation of methods adopted by a variety of agencies. It is not envisaged that any single practice would attempt to undertake all the activities suggested in any single review. The list is intended to stimulate consideration of alternative methods and issues to be taken into account during monitoring. One way of using the list would be to select one topic from the list for specific attention during routine monitoring and to change the topic periodically so that over an extended period there has been a wide-ranging consideration of the quality of the counselling available.

An increasingly popular and well-respected approach routine to the monitoring of counselling services has been developed by the CORE systems group in the Psychological Therapies Research Centre at the University of Leeds. This has the advantage of a professionally developed and progressively refined system that would ordinarily be outside the areas of expertise of even reasonably well-informed counsellors. It is also proving to be a valuable method of accumulating anonymized data on a significantly large scale to make meaningful contributions to assessing the effectiveness of counselling generally and in specific settings (Mellor-Clark & Barkham 2000).

Formal monitoring is no substitute for regular meetings between the counsellor and other members of the primary health care team. If a new counsellor has been appointed, these meetings are necessary in order to establish how the counsellor works and to provide opportunities for team members to express their hopes and misgivings and to plan the detailed integration of the service into the work of the practice (McLeod 1992). Extra meetings are a burden on professionals who have many other demands on their time. However, it has been shown that regular meetings are beneficial both to the primary health care staff and to counsellors (Marsh & Barr 1975). They are the best means of ensuring that referrals are appropriate and that expectations are realistic. Of benefit to the counsellor is the breaking down of isolation. These meetings do not need to be all of the same kind. June McLeod (1992) suggests different ways of meeting members of the primary health care team:

1 Discussing particular patients with particular doctors or other staff.

2 Reporting back in general terms, particularly the discussion of practical problems.

3 Opportunities for more detailed discussions of referrals and outcomes, and opinions about the counsellor's role.

4 Using the counsellor to offer support and training in basic counselling skills for other team members.

A variety in the kinds of meetings between the counsellor and other staff reduces the burden on any individual member of staff and helps to disseminate knowledge about the service throughout the practice.

Conclusions

Counselling is a relatively new activity in primary health care, not withstanding its rapid adoption by large numbers of practices. The need to establish sound professional standards is paramount. A great deal of progress has been made by the British Association for Counselling and Psychotherapy, the Counselling in Primary Care Trust and the Royal College of General Practitioners. Work about clarifying the nature of counselling, the implications of its particular values and methodology will be continued within national bodies such as these. However, the justification for the provision of counselling must be the outcomes for individual patients and their level of satisfaction with the service in the first instance, and the secondary benefits this additional service brings to the work of other members of the primary health care team. The rapid growth of counselling provision in primary care has been generated by the high level of demand by patients for help with relationship and emotional problems. Many general practitioners have found counselling a useful resource for responding to these needs. However, the future scale of counselling provision seems uncertain unless those committed to the provision of counselling services can establish evidence-based justifications for these services and can sustain an argument for services that extend beyond the usual scope of mental health. These challenges are considerable and the outcome is uncertain. The evidence of demand-counselling services and the way counselling has adapted in the past to the demands of providing a professional service within the primary care team give grounds for optimism about its future, but more is needed to secure that future.

References

Argyle, M. (ed.) (1981) *Social Skills and Health*. Methuen, London.

Bond, T. (1989) Towards defining the role of counselling skills. *Counselling*, **69**, 3–9.

Bond, T. (1992) *HIV Counselling: Report of National Survey and Consultation*. British Association for Counselling, Rugby and Daniels Publishing, Cambridge.

British Association for Couselling (1984) *Code of Ethics and Practice for Counsellors*. British Association for Couselling, Rugby.

British Association for Counselling (1985) *Counselling: Definition of Terms in Use with Explanation and Rationale*. British Association for Counselling, Rugby.

British Association for Counselling (1992) *So You Want to Start a Counselling Service: Advice to Doctors*. British Association for Counselling, Rugby.

British Association for Counselling (1997) *Code of Ethics and Practice for Counsellors*. British Association for Counselling, Rugby.

Burnard, P. (1999) *Counselling Skills for Health Professionals*. Chapman & Hall, London.

Clark, A., Hook, J. and Stein, K. (1997) Counsellors in primary care in Southampton: a questionnaire survey of their qualifications, working arrangements, and casemix. *British Journal of General Practice*, **47**, 613–617.

Corney, R.N. (1986) Marriage guidance counselling in general practice. *Journal of the Royal College of General Practitioners*, **36**, 424–426.

Counselling in Primary Care Trust (1992) *Work Specification for Counsellors Working in GP Practices*. Counselling in Primary Care Trust, Staines.

Culley, S. (1990) *Integrative Counselling Skills in Action*. Sage, London.

Dryden, W. (1996). A rose by any other name: A personal view on the differences among professional titles. In I. James & S. Palmer (Eds.), *Professional therapeutic titles: Myths and realities*. Leicester: British Psychological Society, pp. 29–30.

Feltham, C. (1995) *What is Counselling? The Promise and Problem of the Talking Therapies*. Sage, London.

Herlihy, B. and Corey, G. (1992) *Dual Relationships*. American Counseling Association, Alexandria, VA.

Heron, J. (1990) *Helping the Client—Creative Practical Guide*. Sage, London.

Inskipp, F. and Proctor, B. (1989) *Skills for Supervising and Being Supervised*. Alexia Publications, St Leonards on Sea, UK.

Jacobs, M. (1999) *Psychodynamic Counselling in Action*. Sage, London.

James, I. and Palmer, S. (eds) (1996) *Professional Therapeutic Titles: Myths and Realities*. British Psychological Society, Leicester.

Marsh, G.N. and Barr, J. (1975) Marriage guidance counselling in group practice. *Journal of the Royal College of General Practitioners*, **25**, 73–75.

McLeod, J. (1992) The general practitioner's role. In *Counselling in General Practice* (Sheldon, M., ed.). Royal College of General Practitioners, London, pp. 8–14.

Mearns, D. and Thorne, B. (1999) *Person-Centred Counselling in Action*. Sage, London.

Medical Defence Union (1998) Membership news. *Journal of the Medical Defence Union*, **14**, 4.

Mellor-Clark, J. and Barkham, M. (2000) Quality evaluation: methods, measures and meaning. In *Handbook of Counselling and Psychotherapy* (Feltham, C. and Horton, I., eds). Sage, London, pp. 255–270.

Mellor-Clark, J., Simms-Ellis, R. and Burton, M. (2001) *National survey of counsellors working in primary care: evidence for growing professionalism?* (Occasional paper 79) Royal College of General Practitioners, London.

Murgatroyd, S. (1985) *Counselling and Helping*. British Psychological Society, Leicester and Methuen, London.

Pearsall, J. (1998) *The New Oxford Dictionary of English*. Clarendon Press, Oxford.

Rowland, N. (1992) Counselling and counselling skills. In *Counselling in General Practice* (Sheldon, M., ed.). Royal College of General Practitioners, London, pp. 1–7.

Sheldon, M. (1992) Preface. In *Counselling in General Practice* (Sheldon, M., ed.). Royal College of General Practitioners, London.

Silverman, D. (1996) *Discourses in HIV Counselling*. Sage, London.

Smith, S. and Norton, K. (1999) *Counselling Skills for Doctors*. Open University Press, Buckingham, UK.

Thorne, B. (1990) Person-centred therapy. In *Individual Therapy in Britain* (Dryden, W., ed.). Harper & Row, London, p. 106.

Trower, P., Casey, A. and Dryden, W. (1988) *Cognitive-Behavioural Counselling in Action*. Sage, London.

Truax, C.B. and Carkhuff, R.R. (1967) *Towards Effective Counselling and Psychotherapy Training and Practice*. Aldine, Chicago.

Chapter 2

Developing a role for counselling in the primary health care team

Jane Dammers and Jan Wiener

Introduction

This chapter describes our view of past, present and possible future directions for counselling and its relationship to general practice. We have worked together as GP and psychotherapist for two decades, exploring how to build bridges across our two professions to bring medical and psychological models of work together to help patients with mental health problems. Our thinking, writing and the conferences and workshops we have helped to convene have emerged from a common starting point—a belief in the value of a psychodynamic approach to work in a general practice setting. GPs and psychodynamic counsellors share a longitudinal approach to acquiring information and understanding about their patients relatively slowly over time. Patients' presenting problems are seen in the context of past medical, social and personal histories. A psychodynamic approach appreciates the role of unconscious forces in shaping attitudes and behaviour. These forces are likely to affect not only the relationships between patient and GP, patient and counsellor, and indeed between GP and counsellor, but also the larger institutional and organizational dynamics within a practice. Multidisciplinary work is not easy as projections based on a lack of understanding of one another's work and expertise can lead to stereotyping and rivalry between professional disciplines. Defences against differences, such as the extremes of idealization and its opposite, denigration, may arise. As you may imagine, our work together has therefore not always been easy.

Our approach emphasizes relationships; relationships between mind and body, between individuals and between disciplines, as well as a space for thinking about 'what things mean'. The present culture of 'action', rapid change and short-term solutions presents dangers of 'malignant understanding' (Britton 1998), where the essential values integrated into our work, such as the uniqueness of the individual and the value of clinical integrity, are misunderstood in such a fundamental way as to produce chaos. Making time together to think about patients, what we do and how we work becomes ever more necessary.

In this chapter we explore the history of how ideas and practice derived from psychotherapy and counselling have been assimilated into primary care. We describe the attractions of the work and the potential role of generic practice counsellors. We discuss what is likely to help and what might get in the way of their proper integration into practices, including important issues surrounding confidentiality and sharing information in a primary care team. We look forward to developments in community-based mental health services and the role of counselling in the future.

Evolution of ideas and practice over the last 50 years

By tracing ways in which psychodynamic thinking and models of counselling have evolved and been put to good use in primary care, we hope to shed light on the dramatic proliferation of attachments and schemes to employ counsellors in general practice, from the first reference by Marsh and Barr (1975) to the present day when there are an estimated 3500 part-time counsellors covering approximately 50% of all practices in England and Wales (Counselling in Primary Care Trust 2000, personal communication). Many GPs have felt increasingly dissatisfied with the limitations of biomedical models—models of treatment and cure, models which separate mind and body, models which are grossly inadequate to deal with the emotional and psychological distress brought by their patients every day. The application of pharmacological interventions to what are fundamentally psychosocial problems, for example the widespread prescribing of antidepressants, is disturbing. This has left GPs receptive to offers of other kinds of help for their patients. It appears that the growth of counselling has been highly valued by both GPs and patients, despite the difficulties of proving that counselling is effective (Hemmings 2000). A MORI poll of the general public found that 85% of respondents considered counselling to be the treatment of choice for depression (MORI 1992).

The metaphor of an adopted child getting to know a new parent, rather than a blood relation, may be helpful in trying to illustrate the birth and development of these liaisons which have involved the coming together of people from different origins, disciplines and allegiances. These are people who speak different languages and have to struggle to create a common language, while at the same time seeming to need one another, holding many values in common and sharing many similarities in their commitments to help others.

In the 1950s, Carl Rogers' humanistic ideas led to a client-centred approach to counselling. He emphasized the qualities of empathy, warmth and genuineness on the part of the listener who could help the client to explore, understand and reframe his or her experiences (Rogers 1951). Rogers believed that patients were the best, and probably the only, people able to find appropriate solutions to their problems and offers of gratuitous advice were likely to be unhelpful. Around the same time Michael Balint, a psychiatrist and psychoanalyst, with his wife Enid Balint, also a psychoanalyst, pioneered research work exploring the doctor–patient relationship and the potential for introducing psychoanalytic ideas into general practice (Balint 1957). Balint saw the personality of the doctor as the most powerful 'drug' available to treat emotional problems and wanted to find out how this 'drug' could be most effectively used, when it might be harmful and what its side effects might be. In his group work with GPs, attention was given to thoughts, feelings, flashes of insight and fantasies generated by the doctor's encounter with the patient. He encouraged GPs to make use of transference and countertransference, central tools of psychoanalysis. Balint also wrote about the difficulties of developing a common language between psychiatrists and GPs, contrasting highly developed medical terminology with the less precise diagnoses in psychiatry. We see a continuation of these struggles today with the difficulties of establishing proper dialogue between counsellors and GPs, of truly integrating counsellors into primary health care teams and in trying to develop models of joint work.

Balint and Rogers both stimulated interest in 'the doctor–patient relationship'. The advent of vocational training for doctors in general practice in the late 1960s, becoming mandatory in the 1970s, saw half-day release study groups begin to adopt a Balint-style approach to case discussion, offering trainees valuable opportunities to explore difficult issues and develop reflective practice. Balint groups co-led by psychoanalytic psychotherapists and Balint-trained doctors sprang up and the Balint Society flourished. More recently 'developing reflective practice' has become an explicit component of undergraduate medical curricula as well.

The late 1960s and 1970s saw rapid progress in building large health centres, associated with the development of group practices. This enabled health visitors, district nurses and midwives to work alongside groups of GPs. The primary health care team was born with opportunities for others to work alongside and within it. Generic social workers were created in 1968 and some were placed in health centres to address the needs of the local population. Their work addressed the patients' emotional and psychological needs as well as offering practical help with benefits, housing and so on (Graham & Sher 1976). Many of the pioneering models of counselling in primary care came from this work, including Brook (1967) who worked in surgeries with a psychiatrist and later with a psychotherapist (Brook & Temperley 1976). In response to the White Paper *Better Services for the Mentally Ill* (Department of Health and Social Security 1975), that emphasized the need to develop community care services, some hospital departments began to place clinical psychologists in general practice. Beck's cognitive therapy work on anxiety and phobias (Beck 1979) and on depression (Beck *et al.* 1979) came into the arena with GPs starting to use rating scales for depression. Family systems theory (Bateson 1972) was helpful in developing thinking about GPs' work with families and we began to see child guidance clinics and child specialists liaising more intimately with primary care, establishing clinics in some of the large health centres.

However, by the early 1980s, increasing awareness of child abuse led most social workers into statutory work, forcing them to abandon their placements and counselling roles in general practice. Their contribution was sadly missed at a time when GPs were becoming increasingly aware of the emotional and social components of their work and wanting to develop their own counselling skills. At the same time many women doctors were coming into general practice; there was a struggle to develop a holistic approach to problems of the mind and body. The pressure of demand from patients encouraged doctors to look around for more help and, significantly, many did not turn to secondary mental health services for that support. Some sought help from complementary therapists, employing or referring patients to acupuncturists, homeopaths, osteopaths and others. Many turned to something called 'counselling', which was rather ill-defined, but was becoming more desirable and fashionable in popular culture.

What was it that GPs were looking for? From our own work with counsellors and doctors we understood that they were looking for somebody with whom to share the burden, not 'out there' but within the practice; somebody who would both understand the difficulties and complexities of the work and also help with the sheer volume of the workload. Motivation came not only from a desire to provide a better service to patients, but also from a need for support and understanding for doctors and their work and a wish to have another member of the team who could help to think about some of the patients whom the practice found hard to manage.

In the early days of practice-employed counsellors, a minority were members of co-ordinated schemes, such as those with whom we were involved in London—the Paddington Centre, now the Parkside Clinic within Brent, Kensington, Chelsea and Westminster Mental Health Trust and a scheme in the Department of General Practice and Primary Care, Kings College Medical School. Many were employed through personal contacts and most were women with extremely varied training and experience. They included psychotherapists, ex-social workers, community psychiatric nurses, counsellors in other fields, general nurses and those with no formal training at all. They were employed under all sorts of guises, for example as 'receptionists' to qualify for the staff reimbursement scheme, or on a voluntary basis. In a curious way this lack of definition of counselling was attractive to general practice which was looking to mould something into what it needed rather than importing another discipline with a strong identity of its own, such as clinical psychology. Counselling was seen to be allied to lay practice rather than to a medical model and was, therefore, presumed to be more acceptable and accessible to patients, carrying less stigma than most activities in the field of mental health within the NHS. Given the shortage of clinical psychologists, long waiting lists and limited access to mental health services, later confirmed in the government review of strategic policy (Department of Health 1996), this choice was also realistic. There is no doubt that financial constraints and expediency were also important. Counsellors were, and still are in many cases, poorly paid but highly motivated to do the work.

By the early 1990s, a rather fragmented situation had developed, surveyed by Sibbald et al. (1993) who found that many practices knew nothing about their counsellor's training and had little idea of how to appraise new recruits. Slowly attempts were made to bring some kind of order. Relate, or as it was then, the National Marriage Guidance Council, the first service to place a considerable number of counsellors in general practice in the 1980s, issued very helpful guidelines on good practice, recognizing the complexity of work in primary care and the need for highly trained, flexible counsellors with good supervision (National Marriage Guidance Council 1985). Accreditation standards of the British Association of Counselling (BAC) were helpful, although way beyond the qualifications of many counsellors employed at that time, and were adopted as a 'gold standard' qualification. The needs for specific training and models of work to suit the particular circumstances of general practice were recognized and began to be developed and the Counselling in Medical Settings (CMS) division of the BAC drew up the first published guidelines for the employment of counsellors in general practice (Counselling in Medical Settings 1993).

Since then we have seen a proliferation of schemes throughout the UK. Primary care counselling is now struggling to establish a professional identity, set standards of accreditation, registration and training prerequisites, and codes of practice and regulation against a background of major structural changes within the NHS. It is not surprising that this has been an uphill struggle, as we observed that many of those who came into counselling were leaving other core professions to work freelance and part-time, probably with the hope of escaping bureaucracy, regulation and professionalism. The development of Primary Care Groups and Trusts have posed threats, as well as opportunities, for the continuation of counselling schemes and have forced urgent political issues onto the agenda for those who have been threatened with the loss of their jobs. Some counsellors may take some small comfort from the observation that there are many GPs who chose general practice because of the relative autonomy and clinical freedom it offered, and who now find themselves beset with issues of clinical governance, evidence-based medicine and re-accreditation.

The need for a strong political voice to fight for counselling as a core profession has led to the establishment of the Counselling and Psychotherapy Forum in Primary Care* aimed at bringing together nine interested organizations: British Association for Counselling (BAC), Association of Counsellors and Psychotherapists in Primary Care, Counselling in Medical Settings Division of the BAC, Counselling in Primary Care Trust, Relate, Research Council for Complementary Medicine, SMG Smithson Mason Group, United Kingdom Association for Therapeutic Counselling, and United Kingdom Council for Psychotherapy. Other interested organizations with relevant expertise include the Royal College of General Practitioners, the British Confederation of Psychotherapists, the Society of Analytical Psychotherapy and, most recently, the new Primary Care Section of the Association of Psychoanalytic Psychotherapy in the NHS.

The move now is towards managed services in many regions and an intensified struggle to prove the value and effectiveness of counselling. Unsettling rivalries between disciplines in the mental health field have surfaced in the market place of commissioning and purchasing. Much of the rest of this book is devoted to these issues, in the context of how counselling can best be employed in many different areas of primary care.

Attractions of the work

There is no doubt that many trained professionals want to do this work; it has an in-built attractiveness. This is supported by the fact that in recent years, for each job advertised, the number of applications received can sometimes reach three figures. The attractions of the work may be described under six main headings (Wiener & Sher 1998).

A bridge between psyche and soma

The old Cartesian split between mind and body has had an undermining effect on the entire field of mental health. Doctors can overvalue the 'objective' body, neglecting

---

* The Counselling and Psychotherapy Forum in Primary Care can be contacted c/o Mole Conferences, 26 Church Road, Portslade, Brighton BN41 1LA, UK. E-mail: enquiries@mole-conferences.com

patients' subjective experience of their bodies; counsellors and psychotherapists are often tempted to ignore or interpret away patients' actual medical symptoms (Wiener 1996). Counsellors who come to work in a surgery have a unique opportunity to learn more about general medicine and a range of medical conditions which may have psychological sequellae, or take the form of psychological symptoms. They can learn about appropriate medication for depression, psychosis and anxiety and when such treatments are likely to be most helpful. They can come to know the work of the practice nurse, the health visitor and other specialists such as clinical psychologists who may have attachments to the practice and use different, complementary skills to counsellors.

Work at the coalface

For counsellors and psychotherapists, the rewards of involvement in a process at its inception are compelling. For most patients, the GP is the first port of call when they are in difficulty, permitting counsellors the opportunity to see patients when some problems are fresh and before they become chronic. Primary care is the 'real world' of mental health problems, where counsellors are likely to be called upon to adapt and develop flexibly all the training skills they possess. It is also an opportunity to experience personally, on site, the nature of the professional expertise of GPs and other members of the primary care team. While the pace and pressures here are undoubtedly faster and greater than in the more rarefied atmosphere of private practice, the range of patients will help counsellors learn whom to take on for treatment themselves in the surgery, whom to refer to other suitable specialists and whom to return to the GP.

A wide variety of patients

For counsellors who wish to broaden their skills and clinical experience, in particular their ability to make comprehensive mental health assessments, this is an ideal work environment. Working in an organization with colleagues helps counsellors to feel more secure and contained. This is especially important if they take on disturbed, borderline patients. They are likely to encounter a more diverse range of problems than in private practice, such as patients from different ethnic groups, elderly patients and patients with entrenched psychosomatic symptoms. This kind of setting, where many families are registered with the practice for some years, also means that counsellors will have opportunities to work with young people and adolescents, couples and families as well as doing individual therapy.

Teamwork

Counsellors who are drawn to working in GP surgeries, rather than the more introverted atmosphere of private practice, will find a multidisciplinary team of people struggling to work together to provide good quality patient care. Unlike the tightly boundaried dyadic model of one-to-one work in private practice, working as part of a team brings exciting opportunities for the shared care of patients who are best helped when GP and counsellor can collaborate to manage and treat problems. Clinical and philosophical discussions between individuals from different backgrounds can be enlightening ways to inform thinking and practice and keep counsellors in touch with contemporary issues, new research data and treatments, as well as political trends in primary care.

A flexible style of work

The character of a GP surgery means that counsellors will inevitably have to find a more flexible *modus vivendi* than the models advocated by their supervisors and teachers from their own training institutions. While the central attitude to the work, in our case a psychoanalytic perspective, may remain constant, counsellors will most probably have to find creative ways to manage their work when faced with a large numbers of referrals and insufficient time to treat everyone adequately. While training-led dogmas such as 'six sessions for all patients' make for more easily audited patient information and may protect the counsellor from difficult decisions about equity in terms of numbers of sessions offered to patients, they are not always in the patient's best interests. Many patients are well served by less regular sessions, or even shorter sessions.

Missionary work

Working in primary care permits counsellors to make their approach to helping patients in difficulty more accessible to other professionals. GPs, practice nurses and health visitors are offered alternative perspectives about patients, families or situations of concern to the practice as a whole. The rewards of such liaisons, where different aspects of patients' communications may be integrated, are truly gratifying and keep the motivation to continue the work buoyant.

Potential roles of a counsellor in a primary health care team

Many opportunities present themselves to a counsellor who comes to work in primary care. Clearly the prime task is to provide a service to patients and deal with referrals. Sometimes these tasks progress smoothly, but at other times, despite the best efforts of GP and counsellor alike, unconscious factors can undermine this triangular relationship. We hope to illustrate how this can happen while we explore some of the roles a counsellor can adopt in a practice.

Assessment

The initial task is assessment of the referral, made on the basis of the information provided by the referrer and an interview with the client. Assessment is an important and challenging part of counsellors' work and some will initially feel ill-prepared for the wide range of patients and problems encountered in primary care. A good supervisor who is familiar with the primary care setting is invaluable. It is helpful to keep in mind a distinction between assessment and treatment as it is important to make an assessment of the patient's difficulties, defences and probable ability to use counselling productively before treatment begins. One of the functions of assessment is to decide which patients not to treat. It is essential, therefore, that counsellors should be able to tell the referrer if they feel that a patient is unsuitable. We know that this can be difficult if counsellors do not have a good standing within the practice, or if there seems to be nowhere else for the patient to go because of under-resourcing in secondary care. However, counsellors then risk seeing patients who are inappropriate to their level of training.

Edwards (1983) outlines five categories of patient for whom individual counselling or psychotherapy seems to be contraindicated:

1 Many cases of psychosis, borderline and latent psychosis where dangers exist of the development of persisting psychotic transferences and the release of primitive aggression.

2 People with dependent personalities who form attachments that cannot be resolved and for whom separation, or its threat, leads to disintegration.

3 People with personality disorders or psychoneuroses with rigid defences of an obsessional, paranoid or schizoid type.

4 People with histrionic personalities who have shown intense acting out, self-destructive, attention-seeking or manipulative behaviour including eating disorders.

5 People with severe addictions to alcohol, cannabis or opiates.

It is also inappropriate to take on severely depressed patients who are at risk of suicide, as the risk of self-harm may be exacerbated by counselling, particularly in the initial stages. Others who are severely depressed may be too incapacitated to be able to use therapy and may benefit from a course of antidepressant medication before they are taken on.

Referrals

When counsellors work as integrated members of the practice team, they will also be interested in the practice and why a particular doctor is referring a particular client at a particular time. Some referrals are straightforward, but many are complicated. Most counsellors will be familiar with the fact that they are often asked to see some of the patients whom the practice finds most difficult to manage: somatizers, clients with eating disorders, complex family problems and so on. Tom Main (1957) explains that some patients can be difficult because they convey great suffering, but at the same time have an insatiability so that 'every attention is ultimately unsatisfying'. Behind this suffering he believes that there is an in-built attack which demands that the helper takes what can be a masochistic responsibility: 'you must go on helping me as so far nothing you have done is making me better'. These patients may be subject to many different referrals and very probably will come to the counsellor at some stage.

Counsellors may notice patterns in referrals and that individual doctors have difficulties with particular sorts of patients reflecting some of their personal experiences. The patients and their problems sometimes mirror problems in the practice as a whole. The following example illustrates how a doctor experienced a particular group of patients who mirrored a difficult issue in her own life and how this group also came to be a symptom of the practice dynamics.

Case history

One of the female partners who had been in the practice for about six months began to refer to the counsellor a number of middle-aged, depressed women who were struggling to make a life for themselves after their children had left home. Their husbands were emotionally unavailable. The counsellor realized that some of these women did not really want to see her, but had been 'sent' by the doctor. She had a good relationship with this GP and was able to explore with her what was going on. It emerged that the doctor had been left with a large number of older, middle-class women when another woman partner left the practice. The new doctor came to see that she was experiencing difficulty with these women because they reminded her of her own mother, who had recently been widowed. The referrals reflected some of the difficulties experienced by the practice in adjusting to changes in the partnership, as well as something of the doctor's personal internal struggles.

Isabel Menzies Lyth (1988) believes that primitive anxieties are always present in any organization or social structure. Influenced by the writings of Klein and Bion, she explored how the very structure of an institution can be seen as a form of defence, designed to avoid or minimize personal experiences of doubt, guilt, anxiety and uncertainty. However, these structures may at times be antisupportive to staff. 'Busyness' in general practice is surely a good example of a defence against uncertainty and anxiety. The six- or even 10-minute consultation could be seen as a defence against really getting to know the patients and some referrals are undoubtedly defensive, having more to do with the referrer getting rid of a problem rather than being in the best interests of the patient. It is helpful to review referrals at regular meetings and reflect on the feelings, motivations and expectations of both the person making the referral and the patient. This may help to minimize those, often unconscious, actions that are actually unhelpful to patients. Patients who present a 'muddle' and generate some of the most intense feelings and divergent opinions among the professionals are often those from whom most can be learned.

Effect of patients on the doctor–counsellor relationship

Patients are powerful and can consciously and unconsciously undermine even the best efforts to work collaboratively. A psychodynamic approach can be very helpful in permitting counsellors to think sensitively about the unconscious processes at work. These include transference and countertransference phenomena which both affect and inform what is happening in the relationships between GPs and patients, counsellors and patients, and so on.

In our own work we found that the following groups of patients can be difficult for both doctors and counsellors:

1 Psychosomatic patients can generate anxiety about the possibility of missing real physical disease.

2 Some patients present problems of such enormity and urgency as to be overwhelming and create intense pressure to 'do something immediately'.

3 Seriously depressed patients can project their depression, paralysing professionals and engendering feelings of hopelessness.

4 Self-destructive patients, including those with addictions, can induce feelings of anger in their helpers.

5 While professionals may enjoy a certain amount of dependency because it makes them feel needed, highly dependent and vulnerable patients can foster high levels of anxiety.

6 The patient's problem may be too close to home. For example, a recent bereavement may make it hard for a professional to work with loss for a while.

7 Patients who are out of touch with their feelings can leave professionals feeling remote and out of touch too.

8 Professionals may 'act out' inappropriately in response to a patient they like very much.

9 There are those patients who, for one reason or another, doctors or counsellors do not like and want to 'get rid of'. These patients are likely to be neglected.

10 Finally, patients who could benefit from psychological help to manage a physical illness are often not referred to the counsellor. GPs can be possessive about physical symptoms, forgetting that counsellors could have a vital role to play.

The professionals' difficulties in working with some of these patients can be manifest by their feeling undermined in the consultation, making unnecessary referrals, behaving uncharacteristically, experiencing splits with colleagues, and maintaining unhelpful divisions between body and mind.

Joint management of difficult patients

Counsellors can work alongside the doctor with patients who are hard to bear. We have found that sometimes doctors make referrals because they need someone else to know how hard it is to be with or work with a patient. This may not be explicit in the referral, but counsellors will discover that while these patients are often not suitable for counselling, it can be helpful to see them a couple of times themselves, or together with the doctor in a joint consultation. Armed with these insights, counsellors may be able to help the doctor to continue to work with the patient and/or make a different referral. Over time and when there is trust between doctor and counsellor this supportive role may become an important part of a counsellor's work, conducted through discussions without the counsellor seeing the patient. These discussions may not be formalized on a regular basis, but we recognize them as a form of consultation/ supervision and appropriate to experienced and highly trained counsellors. This role may be extended to helping the whole practice deal with difficult and distressing situations, such as cases involving child protection, serious complaints, the death of a child and so on. Counsellors are also often approached 'for a chat' by individual team members with personal problems. Many would consider getting too involved here to be outside their remit, particularly if they are practice employees, but might suggest other avenues for help.

Treatment

Having made an assessment, various treatment pathways are open to counsellors. For some patients the referral and initial assessment alone may have had considerable therapeutic impact and may be as much as they want or can bear at that time. They may decide that counselling is not for them. If counselling continues, many counsellors adopt a strategy of short-term work; indeed many contracts impose strict limits on the number of sessions available and a time period which must elapse before a client can be seen again, for the sake of equity and managing waiting lists. A more flexible approach has been allowed to develop in some practices where counsellors take on a minority of clients for longer term work, not necessarily on a weekly or even on a regular basis. This 'revolving door' approach, whereby clients can make contact again if necessary, is much closer to models of work adopted by other members of the primary health care team and we think it encourages proper integration of counsellors into the team. Approaches to treatment vary according to patients' problems and counsellors' training and skills. We have noticed that as counsellors become more experienced in general practice they tend to draw on a wider range of skills, techniques and therapies and often embark on further training to broaden their areas of expertise.

Counsellors may also make referrals for treatment to a member of the mental health team, to a specialist organization such as an alcohol counselling service, or to a community group. Patients may prefer to be referred to the private sector depending on their own and local resources. Counsellors can develop a useful role in facilitating links with specialist services and providing good up-to-date information to the practice about local resources, particularly in the voluntary sector. In JD's practice, the counsellors co-ordinated a book recording all referrals made to agencies outside the practice, with comments on usefulness, waiting times, special interests and so on. We suggest that this role is best developed if counsellors are able to make direct contact and referrals, rather than going back to the GP or through a central agency. It is essential, however, that information about such referrals is fed back to the appropriate people. In this way counsellors are more likely to develop insight into the management of mental health problems in the practice as a whole and the full potential of their own roles in particular. They can become involved in discussions about the appropriateness of referrals to different professionals in primary, secondary and voluntary agency care. In our own practices this has been facilitated by holding regular meetings among all the mental health workers and doctors in the practice.

An extended role for counsellors

We suggest that counsellors have potential for work in many different areas in the practice. Indirectly they bring skills, models of work and ways of thinking that can permeate into the practice and encourage a more psychologically minded approach among those who are receptive. The counselling model values space and time to think. It provides clear guidelines about setting boundaries and limits and is very careful about confidentiality. Counselling, like social work before it, also introduces the important concept of supervision, a notion previously rather alien to medicine. It recognizes the inherent difficulties of the work, the emotional burdens to be carried by all who work in general practice, the need to distinguish the professional's difficulties from those of the patient, and the value of having a regular supervisor with whom to discuss cases and central issues. The values which counsellors bring can help to strengthen and develop similarly held values and beliefs throughout the whole practice from receptionists to doctors. We can see that counsellors have a much greater contribution to make to a practice than just 'seeing patients'.

It usually takes time, at least a year or two, for an extended role to evolve within a practice as this is dependent on insight, good management, good humour and a willingness on all sides to engage in dialogue and regular meetings. Recognition of each other's competencies and potential is essential. Without these commitments, counsellors may remain satellites to the practice, or commonly a satellite to a number of practices, working only a few hours a week in each. Here, information about patients at the time of referral is usually minimal and counsellors do not discuss the case except to inform the doctor when counselling is starting and finishing, unless there are serious concerns about harm to self or others. We know of counsellors working in this way who have become a dumping ground for many of the practice's most difficult patients. Counsellors can become very isolated, struggling with these patients with no established structure for thinking with the practice about what is going on. This can lead to feelings of demoralization and lack of self-esteem.

Models of confidentiality

When counsellors are truly integrated into the primary care team, have a flexible approach to their work, are interested in and value the work of the doctors and others and share information and ideas with them, anxieties may surface surrounding issues of confidentiality. Indeed, if issues of confidentiality cannot be explored, discussed and thought about, then it is unlikely that counsellors will move from a position of satellite to one of proper integration into the practice team. At times 'confidentiality' may be used as a defence against confronting the anxieties involved in moving from the first to the second position.

We have a responsibility to provide high standards of service to our patients, in particular to respect our patients' rights to confidentiality. Issues concerning confidentiality come under the general rubric of ethics and, as Higgs (1999) points out, 'ethics are concerned particularly with issues of conduct or character, with values and veracity, with rights and respect'. The Hippocratic oath states that 'all that may come to my knowledge in the exercise of my profession … which ought not to be spread abroad I will keep secret and never reveal'. The question arises when working alongside GPs as to why knowledge 'ought not to be spread abroad'; whether abroad means 'to the GP' or 'outside the practice' and whether counsellors are doing the patients any favours if they do not pass on some information on a 'need to know' basis.

A conceptual distinction between privacy, secrecy and confidentiality is helpful at this point. Privacy is a universal professional principle, 'a fundamental right that allows individuals to decide the manner and extent to which information about themselves is shared with others. Self-determination in this respect is also central to preservation of safety and dignity and the integrity of the individual' (Wiener & Sher 1998). Secrecy frequently imbues what patients tell us about themselves, their lives and their inner worlds. We may distinguish between 'ordinary' secrets, part of the fabric and texture of everyday therapeutic work, and 'extraordinary' secrets, when the boundaries between what is fantasy and what is reality become blurred and counsellors should ask themselves whether they should be doing anything about it or should be telling someone else. Most commonly this occurs when a patient is becoming psychotic, threatening to commit suicide, or telling us they may harm someone.

Confidentiality is about a commitment to maintain boundaries to secure an atmosphere of trust, without which patients may not agree to be treated. It implies a policy of 'no action'. For counsellors the temptation to take action is dependent on their personal and moral principles, codes of ethics, clinical judgement, the role of the law and the setting in which they are working. They break these boundaries with the knowledge that if patients do not implicitly or explicitly believe that the thoughts, fantasies and feelings they bring to therapy will be confidential, they will not come (Wiener 2001).

Confidentiality presents us with a central paradox. On the one hand, sharing of certain critical information may be seen as in the public interest, to protect adults or children; it is good multidisciplinary working together; and sometimes is compliant with reporting laws. On the other hand, it can be a betrayal of patients' and clinicians' rights to privacy and the violation of our rights to practice our profession within established boundaries. Our codes of ethics provide us with etiquettes and structures to guide our practice and behaviour—moral principles if you like. However, these are often insufficient when we are struggling with our ethical principles, which can be described as 'an attitude achieved through judgement, discernment and conscious struggle, often between conflicting rights or duties' (Solomon 2000).

Most practices, with teamwork in mind, use a model of confidentiality not of a patient–counsellor couple, but one operating within the bounds of the practice team. They see a broad cohort of patients including many with physical or psychosomatic problems who require physical and psychological help. A GP might well ask what the point is of having a therapist in the practice who does not talk to him or her. In primary care we are not usually practising formal and long-term counselling or psychotherapy. In the case of psychodynamic counsellors, we use a psychodynamic attitude to the work to understand the conscious and unconscious matrix of relationships within the surgery and the effect patients have on us. Coltart's (1993) phrase 'adventures of the spirit', conveys something of the atmosphere of the work; trying out new things with the possibility of using fresh approaches. Where exchanges between patients and counsellors are absolutely confidential as a matter of course, without considering the nature of the patient's situation, counsellors are in danger of rigidly adhering to a private practice model which leaves them isolated and marginalized in the surgery in which they work. Patients' expectations when seeing a counsellor in the surgery may be different from a presentation in private practice. Patients may see the surgery as a building housing a number of professionals to whom they seek access at different times. It can be containing to have two figures/parents, counsellor and GP, who talk together. Elder delivers words of wisdom to counsellors, 'if you live in a very exposed spot (GP) it is hard not to look for shelter, but if you live in a rather sheltered spot (counsellor) you may begin to forget that outside the shelter lies the wilderness. As mental health professionals move closer to the world of general practice, interesting things begin to happen in response to the new setting, and some of the boundaries and apparent distinctiveness of different approaches begin to melt away, and then re-form as a response to new challenges (Elder 1996, p. 61).

Elder's quote is good evidence to support a model of confidentiality which advocates the appropriateness of regular dialogue about patients between counsellors, GPs and other members of the practice team. In this way, the surgery's patients who are seen by counsellors will be getting a more integrated and comprehensive mental health service.

The future

In the future, it is likely that the commissioning of mental health services will be increasingly primary care led and attempts will be made to involve service users and carers much more actively in deciding what is needed and how resources should be allocated. There are still many unanswered questions among interested professional groups—psychiatrists, psychotherapists, clinical psychologists, community psychiatric nurses, counsellors, voluntary agencies and GPs. Who should do what and for whom? What particular skills, attitudes and training are required to fulfil identified needs? How are specialist skills best used: at a secondary care level or disseminated more widely in primary care? Is there a need for 'secondary' care at all? Should a model be embraced in which care is based entirely in the community, except for a few in-patient beds? Suggestions have been made to train generic, community-based mental health workers, each with some specialist skills, who together would form a team to work in primary care.

There are fears that specialisms will be denigrated and that important professional skills and ideas will be lost. A trend towards dismantling the core professions and creating generalists can be understood as a defensive manoeuvre during a time of stress. Obholzer (in Obholzer & Roberts 1994) describe three layers of anxiety in organizations, which must be understood if they are to be addressed. These are, firstly, primitive anxieties for which we expect the institution to have a containing function; secondly, anxieties arising out of the nature of the work when primary tasks tend to be avoided as a defence; and thirdly, personal anxieties which are unique to the individual. Institutions are supposed to protect us from these three layers of anxiety. However, when the organizations themselves (government strategies, general practice, counselling structures) are all in flux, we are in danger of psychotic thinking. As Obholzer says, 'the failure to recognise the anxiety-containing function of institutions means that even the best intentioned organisational changes often create more problems than they solve, since they lead to the dismantling of structures which were erected in the first instance to defend against anxiety' (Obholzer & Roberts 1994, pp. 206–207).

All this leaves many mental health workers, especially practice counsellors, with major anxieties about their future roles and employment and fosters the tendency towards rivalry and competition between different disciplines. It is likely that the number of managed schemes for counsellors will increase. While we know of some excellent schemes of this kind, they present great challenges in truly integrating counsellors into primary care, particularly if the management is at a secondary care level. We know that there are still vast gulfs of misunderstanding between primary and secondary care in mental health. Schemes tend to become beset by rules such as 'six sessions only per patient', 'patients not to be seen again for six months', 'clients not to be over 65 years old', 'every practice must have a counsellor', 'counsellors must use their non-attendance time in lieu of administrative work and meetings', and so on. Many of these rules are formulated in the name of 'equity', a seemingly admirable objective. However, we would argue that if a service is spread so thinly and so inflexibly as to make the development of relationships almost impossible and if the main tool of evaluation is the number of patients seen and the 'did not attend' rate, without taking into account the quality of the work and the much wider role a counsellor might play, then the managed counselling service is only achieving a fraction of its potential.

There are also moves to train more 'specialist' counsellors: for patients who are bereaved, or have diabetes, or have had a heart attack etc. This seems to be a defensive move against dealing with the real difficulties of integrating mind and body and dealing with the relatively undifferentiated problems encountered in general practice. Everyone in the UK has a doctor to whom they can bring their symptoms, concerns and problems in an unformulated state, creating opportunities to develop holistic approaches to care. Our outline of the history of counselling demonstrates the desire for more generic counselling help at the general practice level.

What is certain is the need for continuing professional development and the imperatives of deciding on primary tasks and finding new skills and tools to tackle complex issues together. We face the challenge of tackling the question of social inclusion outlined in the National Service Framework for Mental Health (Department of Health 1999), which highlights the need to address high levels of mental health problems among the unemployed, children in the poorest households, those abused in childhood, victims of domestic violence, the homeless, black and ethnic minority groups, refugees, people with alcohol and drug-dependency problems and those with physical illness. These are the real challenges in which counsellors are being asked to participate.

We will need to work together to promote teamwork and an integrated approach to patient care (Pritchard 1995). We need a space in which to think and to reflect together; to be open and to learn from our mistakes; to develop interprofessional understanding, trust and respect; and to share explicit goals and tolerate differences. This can only happen if we establish a dialogue and a common language; if we agree to meet and talk both formally and informally; and if we strive for consciousness, innovation and excellence in our work. In the end, it is only if counsellors foster good personal relationships with GPs and other practice staff that the counselling profession in primary care will flourish.

References

Balint, M. (1957) *The Doctor, His Patient and the Illness*. Pitman, London.

Bateson, G. (1972). *Steps to an Ecology of Mind*. Ballantyne, New York.

Beck, A.T. (1979). *Cognitive Therapy of Anxiety and Phobic Disorders*. Centre for Cognitive Therapy, Philadelphia.

Beck, A.T., Rush, A.J., Shaw, B.T. and Emery, G. (1979) *Cognitive Therapy of Depression.* Guildford Press, New York.

Britton, R. (1998) Subjectivity, objectivity and triangular space. In *Belief and Imagination: Explorations in Psychoanalysis.* Routledge, London, p. 54.

Brook, A. (1967) An experiment in general practitioner–psychiatrist collaboration. *Journal of the Royal College of General Practitioners,* 13, 126–131.

Brook, A. and Temperley, J. (1976) The contribution of a psychotherapist to general practice. *Journal of the Royal College of General Practitioners,* 26, 86–94.

Coltart, N. (1993) *How to Survive as a Psychotherapist.* Free Association Books, London.

Counselling in Medical Settings (1993) *Guidelines for the Employment of Counsellors in General Practice.* Counselling in Medical Settings, Rugby, UK.

Department of Health (1996) *NHS Psychotherapy Services in England: a Review of Strategic Policy.* Department of Health, London.

Department of Health (1999) *National Service Framework for Mental Health: Modern Standards and Service Models.* London: DOH.

Department of Health and Social Security (1975) *Better Services for the Mentally Ill.* CMND 6233. HMSO, London.

Edwards, A. (1983) Research studies in the problems of assessment. *Journal of Analytical Psychology,* 28, 299–311.

Elder, A. (1996) Primary care and psychotherapy. In *Conference Proceedings: Future Direction of Psychotherapy in the NHS: Adaptation or Extinction. Psychoanalytic Psychotherapy,* Suppl. 10, 58–63.

Graham, H. and Sher, M. (1976) Social work in general practice. *Journal of the Royal College of General Practitioners,* 26, 95–105.

Hemmings, A. (2000) *A Systematic Review of the Brief Psychological Therapies in Primary Health Care.* Counselling in Primary Care Trust and the Association of Counsellors and Psychotherapists in Primary Care, Staines, Middlesex.

Higgs, R. (1999) Depression in general practice. In *General Practice and Ethics: Uncertainty and Responsibility* (Dowrick, C. and Frith, L., eds). Routledge, London, pp. 134–150.

Main, T. (1957) The ailment. *British Journal of Medical Psychology,* 30, 129–145.

Marsh, G.N. and Barr, J. (1975) Marriage guidance counselling in a group practice. *Journal of the Royal College of General Practitioners,* 25, 73–75.

Menzies Lyth, I. (1988) *Containing Anxiety in Institutions: Selected Essays.* Free Association Books, London.

MORI (1992) *Attitudes Towards Depression.* Research study conducted for the Defeat Depression Campaign, MORI, London.

National Marriage Guidance Council (1985) Surgery counselling: guidelines for marriage guidance work in health centres or medical group practice. *Practice Outlook,* 1, 7–13.

Obholzer, A. and Roberts, V. (eds) (1994) *The Unconscious at Work: Individual and Organizational Stress in the Human Services.* Routledge, London.

Pritchard, P. (1995) Learning to work effectively in teams. In *Inter-Professional Issues in Community and Primary Health Care* (Owens, P., Carrier, J. and Horder, J., eds). Macmillan Press, London, pp. 205–232.

Rogers, C.R. (1951) *Client Centred Therapy.* Constable, London.

Sibbald, B., Addington-Hall, J., Brenneman, D. and Freeling, P. (1993) Counsellors in English and Welsh general practices: their nature and distribution. *British Medical Journal,* 306, 29–33.

Solomon, H.M. (2000) The ethical self. In *Jungian Thought in the Modern World* (Christopher, E. and Solomon, H.M., eds). Free Association Books, London, p. 191.

Wiener, J. (1996) Looking out and looking in: some reflections on 'body talk' in the consulting room. *Journal of Analytical Psychology*, **39**, 3.

Weiner, J. (2001) The sanctum, the citadel and the souk? Confidentiality and paradox. In *Values and Ethics in the Practice of Psychotherapy and Counselling* (Murdin, L. and Palmer Barnes, F., eds). Open University Press, Buckingham, pp. 144–163.

Wiener, J. and Sher, M. (1998) *Counselling and Psychotherapy in Primary Health Care: a Psychodynamic Approach*. Macmillan Press, London.

Chapter 3

General practitioners and counselling in primary care

Simon Cocksedge

Introduction

The GP has a unique place in society in the UK. He or she has traditionally been the 'gate keeper' to the British NHS and, as such, the first port of call for anyone needing non-emergency access to medical care of any description. GPs form a (generally) valued part of all communities in the UK. The strength of this system of primary care lies in the immediate local accessibility and availability of health care professionals who will often have a long-term relationship with, and knowledge of, the individual and their social and family context.

The role of the GP in relation to counselling in primary care must be seen in the light of the overall role of the GP which has been defined by the Royal College of General Practitioners (1972) as:

> A doctor who provides personal, primary and continuing medical care to individuals and families… He [sic] accepts responsibility for making an initial decision on every problem a patient may present to him, consulting with specialists when he thinks it appropriate to do so… His diagnoses will be composed in physical, psychological and social terms. He will intervene educationally, preventively and therapeutically to promote his patient's health.

Despite the many organizational changes in primary care since this definition was written, it remains valid and important.

For a GP to compose a diagnosis and begin a therapeutic intervention for a patient who may require counselling, a variety of skills are required. The GP must first hear the cues offered by the patient and then make a decision on the most appropriate course of action. This might involve no further intervention, further consultations with the GP, or referral to another health care professional. Such a professional might be within the primary health care team (PHCT), such as the practice counsellor or attached community psychiatric nurse (CPN). Alternatively, referral might be elsewhere, such as to the community mental health team (CMHT) or the psychiatrist.

This chapter explores, firstly, the role and the skills of the GP, as a clinician, in identifying people needing listening or counselling and initiating their management. It goes on, secondly, to consider the managerial role of the GP as employer and provider of counselling services.

The GP as clinician

Recognizing that listening is needed—hearing the cues

Recognizing that someone needs attention, in the form of time to talk, or to be listened to, during the consultation in the middle of a busy surgery, is part of the day-to-day work of the GP (see the example given in Table 3.1). This recognition of need will vary for each GP, each patient and each context.

Cues may arise as a natural consequence of a consultation about a physical problem. A presentation with dyspepsia which has worsened since relationship difficulties started may lead to consideration of those difficulties in the consultation. Often the physical problem is being used as a 'ticket' to consult about other issues — attendance with a respiratory infection followed by 'could this be related to stress doctor?' and a discussion about, for example, pressures at work. The person who makes an aside just as they are leaving ('Oh, by the way doctor...'), which gives away the real reason for the consultation, is well recognized in general practice. Cues do not have to be spoken out loud — body language, dress and manner must all be assessed. Similarly, the person who attends the surgery several times in quick succession, having avoided GPs for several years, may be sending a covert message. Patients who somatize will generally not realize that their physical symptom is a manifestation of a different problem.

The potential variety and multiplicity of cues means that the GP has constantly to be aware of the possibilities. The ability to recognize the cue, verbal or otherwise, during the consultation is a core skill for the GP. There is no doubt that many cues given by patients to their doctors go unrecognized, even by the most highly skilled GPs.

Once the initial identification of a cue has taken place, a decision must be made by the GP that may or may not involve the patient. This choice involves the options of:

- Hearing the cue and choosing either to listen now or to listen on another occasion
- Hearing the cue and referring the patient on for listening elsewhere
- Ignoring the cue.

Table 3.1 Example 1

During a consultation about vague join pains ...

  'I've nothing else physical wrong with me doctor'

Response 1 might be:

  'Good, well I suggest we try this medication...'

Response 2 might be:

  'Nothing physical ...?'

  'Well the main problem is my son ...'

The cue was the word *physical*, which could be completely ignored or missed, or picked up and explored.

Hearing the cue and choosing to listen

The GP who hears the cues given by the patient must decide whether to attend to them now, in this consultation, or to ask the patient to return on another occasion, perhaps for a longer appointment (see below). Either way, some preliminary exploration must go on in this consultation to identify the need and the issues behind the cues. Then, a variety of factors must be taken into account in deciding whether to spend time listening and exploring these issues further.

Sometimes it will be inappropriate to explore a particular cue in the consultation. For example, a person presenting with chest pain needs the physical problem (i.e. the chest pain) managing before an exploration of the other factors involved (e.g. threatened redundancy, family problems). These can be revisited at a later date.

Structural factors within the practice must be considered. It may be possible to give patients extra time in normal surgery, perhaps accepting that the surgery will over-run. Alternatives include asking the patient to attend again for an ordinary appointment, a double appointment, the last appointment of the surgery, an extra appointment away from normal surgery times, or a visit at home by the GP.

The most fundamental personal factor is the valuing of listening as a therapeutic tool. Some GPs find listening easier than others and a natural inclination in this direction is likely to influence personal priorities in attending to the needs of the patient. It may take the novice GP some years to realize that time spent listening, perhaps only for a short time and without any other intervention, is often highly therapeutic for the patient. It is also likely to lead to a deepening of the doctor–patient relationship in both the short, and the long, term.

Another factor is the skill level of the GP, which will depend on previous training and experience. In addition to finding time for the patient in a busy working day, the GP who chooses to listen requires skills in communication which have only found their way onto the curriculum of most medical schools in the last few years. At a basic level, these include such tools as using open questions, reflecting, pausing, using silence and summarizing. Some GPs undertake further training in either listening skills or counselling, and a few in psychotherapy. Such training, combining counselling and/or psychotherapeutic skills with everyday general practice, will undoubtedly add much to a GP's level of understanding and job satisfaction. However, it is hard to combine counselling or psychotherapy with day-to-day general practice without allocating specific time to these activities. Further consideration of these issues can be found in the writings of Sue Culley (1991), John Holland (1995), John Salinsky (1993) and Kenneth Sanders (1986).

Hearing the cue and referring the patient

Once a GP has heard the cues given by the patient and identified the issues behind the cues, a decision may be made to involve another health care professional. Who this is and when and how they are involved will depend on local availability. A working knowledge of the therapeutic options and the services available in the locality is another of the core skills of the GP. Interprofessional referral may be to members of the immediate PHCT, including the practice counsellor, the midwife for antenatal and postnatal issues, the health visitor and the surgery-based CPN. Referral outside the PHCT may involve the psychiatrist and hospital mental health team, the psychologist, the psychotherapist and the CMHT, who are likely to be reserved for more complicated problems such as overt mental health issues and personality disorders. Other agencies who might be accessed include Relate, alcohol advice services, drug addiction services, eating disorder clinics, local bereavement services, social services, the Citizens Advice Bureau and the Member of Parliament (the latter three being for practical issues such as housing and finance).

The Derbyshire Counselling Scheme has published guidelines for GPs making referrals to counselling and mental health services (Table 3.2). The guidelines, which are not intended to restrict individual freedom of referral but rather to offer some assistance, suggest that counselling services should be used for the mild to moderate range of the psychological/mental health problem continuum, and that mental health services should be used for the moderate to severe range. Some GPs may be unclear about the precise role of different members of the mental health team and particularly about the distinction between the role of the counsellor, the psychologist and the psychotherapist. A locally agreed referral policy, which takes into account the strengths of the different professionals involved, will help to clarify the situation and facilitate liaison between members of PHCTs and CMHTs.

Ignoring the cues

All GPs put boundaries on their willingness to spend time listening, consciously or unconsciously, for a variety of reasons. The most common reason for choosing to ignore the cues is pressure of time. It can be very hard, even when the GP knows that listening is needed, to sit back and be non-directive while still having one eye on the clock and the thought of other patients in the waiting room. Time pressures may be created by constraints within the practice. There may be several doctors away, or urgent visits and extra consultations needing attention. There may be pressures from patients with multiple problems or particularly demanding situations. There may also be pressures within the GP—some GPs strive to stick accurately to their appointment times whereas others are more relaxed in this respect. Some GPs may feel guilty at their inability to fully listen, they may feel unfulfilled by listening, they may just be tired and having a bad day, or they may feel pressured by external personal circumstances such as family or financial issues.

Ideally, the GP's decision not to listen will be made consciously and the cue noted for a future consultation with that patient. Having boundaries, and sometimes choosing not to listen, is an inevitable part of current general practice in the UK. Such choices may put pressure on the GP who may need to acknowledge the inevitability of such decision-making and perhaps to share the difficulties involved.

The GP as manager and employer

The other role of the GP, in relation to counselling in primary care, is as a manager in providing counselling services within the practice. Increasingly, this role is likely to be carried out in collaboration with other practices in the primary care organisation (PCO).

Table 3.2 Making referrals to counselling services and mental health services (Derbyshire Counselling Scheme 1997)

These guidelines are designed to help PHCTs make appropriate referrals to counselling and mental health services.Psychological or mental health problems are often seen as ranging along a continuum from mild to moderate to severe. These guidelines suggest that counselling services should be used for problems in the mild to moderate range and that mental health services be used for those in the moderate to severe range. Counselling and mental health services are available across the adult age range, including elderly people.

Counselling services
The Derbyshire Counselling Scheme in general practice offers at the first point of contact a professional counselling service, specifically for those patients with emotional or psychological problems. There is a substantial psychosocial element within general practice consultations because people generally seek help initially from their doctor. Practices that employ a counsellor offer their patients a treatment choice and ease of access to a professional counselling service within a primary care setting.

A counsellor can enable the process of change by helping people to express their feelings, clarify thoughts, reframe their problems and consider potential solutions so that they can understand themselves better and be able to manage their lives more effectively.

Problems appropriate for counselling services
(Mild to moderate problems)
Depression
Relationship difficulties
Anxiety
Bereavement
Emotional and psychological difficulties
Response to physical illness
Life cycle development issues
Response to trauma
Sexual difficulties

Mental health services
Mental health services, through the care programme approach, offer a comprehensive and multidisciplinary range of options for people with significant mental health problems and their carers and families. Specialized therapies, support, practical help, hospital admission and rehabilitation are all available. Caselink, the Supervision Register and the Section 117 Register are used as indicated.

Although many clients will be people who are seeking help and are aware of their difficulties, mental health services also work with people who are less willing or able to engage in relationships with others. Referrers should use mental health services when they are seeking a mental health assessment or diagnostic advice.

Problems appropriate for mental health services
(Moderate to severe problems)
Schizophrenia and related disorders
Mania and hypomania
Depressive disorders
Cognitive impairment or dementia
Risk of suicide, violence or self-neglect
Hypochondriasis
Obsessive compulsive disorder
Post-traumatic stress disorder
Eating disorders
Substance abuse
Personality and behavioural disorders
Severe anxiety

The first steps in providing such services are establishing the level of need and considering the pros and cons of practice-based counselling. These questions are discussed elsewhere in this book in more detail (see Chapters 1, 2 and 4), but there is no doubt that such a local and easily accessible service, requiring no additional travel and carrying minimal stigma for the patient, is very well received. It may be useful for the

PHCT as a whole, and is likely to reduce referrals elsewhere, hence reducing costs and waiting times.

Having decided to provide a practice based counselling service, there are several hurdles for the GP or PCT. These include devising a job description, finding a suitable person and appointing them, employing them (with a contract), providing systems and space within the practice for the service, and then making appropriate referrals. The Association of Counselling and Psychotherapy in Primary Care (CPC) (2000) *'Guidelines and protocols: defining psychological therapy in primary care'* and the Derbyshire Counselling Scheme (1997) *'Guidelines and Protocols for the Employment of Counsellors in General Practice'* provide further information in some detail, as do the Counselling in Primary Care Trust and the British Association for Counselling and Psychotherapy (see *Useful contacts* below). Some points that must be taken into consideration are discussed in the following sections.

Employing a counsellor

A job description and a contract need to be devised. These should outline the role of the counsellor and include the time allocated for counselling 'face-to-face', supervision, administration (e.g. writing notes and letters), professional development, meetings (including liaison within the practice), and training. It should also include terms and conditions of service and to whom the counsellor is accountable within the practice. Whether the counsellor is self-employed or an employee of the practice or PCG/PCO will depend on local funding arrangements.

Part of the job description needs to be clear about the type of work that the practice expects from the counsellor. The Derbyshire Counselling Scheme, for example, aims to provide short-term focal counselling for adults aged 18–70 years registered with the employing practice, with an initial assessment session and a total of six to 12 sessions of counselling. There are other models of providing counselling in primary care with a different balance of assessment, short-term and long-term work. While the ideal has yet to be found, there is an emphasis on short-term work in many practices, and it is essential that a practice counsellor is capable of undertaking brief focal work.

The approach to counselling taken by different counsellors may puzzle their would-be GP employer. There are a variety of types of counselling (from transactional analysis to Gestalt to psychodynamic and more) and the specific method used is probably secondary to the overall relationship between the counsellor and the patient/client. It is almost certainly more important to find the person who fits the practice and the PHCT than to worry about their specific approach to counselling.

Appointing a counsellor

Where to start in finding the right person? The training available to counsellors in primary care has changed a great deal in the last decade. In order to ensure that the person appointed has adequate skills, the GP should require at least BACP accreditation as a minimum qualification (see Derbyshire Counselling Scheme (1997) for a description of the accreditation process, or contact BACP), preferably with additional specific training for counselling in primary care. The ideal candidate would have a background in mental health care, nursing or social work.

Help with the process of appointing can be sought from the local Health Authority (who may have an adviser for counselling services), other practices who employ a counsellor, or possibly local training courses for counsellors. Additional advice may be given by BACP or the Counselling in Primary Care Trust. Advertising could be via the Health Authority, in the BACP Faculty of Healthcare for Counsellors and Psychotherapists journal or via the local press. It may be particularly helpful to ask a trusted third party (for example, the Health Authority counselling adviser) to be involved with the process of short listing and interviewing.

A counsellor in the surgery—practical issues

For the employing practice, there are a number of practical issues which will need to be considered in taking on a counsellor. These are mentioned only briefly here as they are covered more fully elsewhere (British Association for Counselling 1996; Derbyshire Counselling Scheme 1997).

A *quiet room*, with adequate privacy and no interruptions (by people or telephones), is a prerequisite for counselling. Counselling will work best in the same room each week, preferably with clinical equipment (such as sphygmomanometers and bare couches) removed or covered up. Two comfortable chairs are needed with an adequate distance between them—whatever the pressure on space, counselling cannot really be done in a cupboard! Like other staff, the counsellor needs to be able to summon aid quickly should the situation arise, perhaps by using a panic button.

A suitable *referral system*, with agreed protocols on who to refer, must be set up along with an appointment system which suits the patients, the office staff, the GPs and the counsellor. In some practices, the doctor refers to the counsellor, who then gets in touch with the patient by letter or by telephone. In others, after talking to the doctor, the patient is asked to fill in a short form giving their personal details and a brief outline of why they would like to see a counsellor. Asking patients to take this initiative may eliminate those who do not really want counselling. Some practices also have an appointment book at reception, so that patients can refer, or re-refer, themselves.

Record-keeping and levels of confidentiality must be considered. Most practices include the counsellor within the boundary of confidentiality of the whole practice, with access to the patient's medical record. It is helpful if the counsellor makes an entry in the records when the counselling starts, each time the patient is seen and when the counselling finishes. It is also extremely useful to know if the patient does not attend, as they often come to see the doctor instead, who may then discuss why they have not taken up the offer of counselling. A few patients may not want any record of their visits to the counsellor to be in the notes. The amount of written information passing between doctor and counsellor seems to vary enormously. The initial referral may be a detailed typed letter, or just a name in an appointment book. Some counsellors copy their initial assessment to the doctor and/or write a summary when the counselling is finished. Others communicate nothing at all in writing.

All counsellors should keep proper *records* of their work for their own benefit and for medicolegal reasons. It would be extremely unusual for these to be kept in the patient's notes, and suitable locked storage is needed for the counsellor's private use. Under the Data Protection Act, patients have the right to see their medical records. It is unclear whether this would include the notes of a counsellor employed by the practice, but it is probably safest to assume that it might.

The *boundaries of confidentiality* for doctor–counsellor–PHCT communication vary considerably between practices. They need to be agreed by the doctors and the counsellor and explained to the patient at the beginning of any counselling. Broadly, confidentiality can be approached in two ways. Either the counsellor does not discuss or pass on anything, without specifically asking for the patient's consent in each instance, or confidentiality is shared with the doctor and/or within the PHCT. In the latter case, which is the normal medical model in primary care teams, the patient can expect the counsellor to discuss whatever is appropriate, although the patient can stipulate if there are specific matters which are to remain entirely confidential to the counsellor. Should counsellors also tell patients about their own supervision, and perhaps about case discussions outside the practice if they attend groups or seminars? When would confidentiality be broken because of concern about risks to the patient or to a third party? These issues need to be considered and the boundaries clearly shared with counselling clients.

Liaison with the doctors and the practice team (for example, by attending PHCT meetings) must be an allocated part of the counsellor's role, along with regular audit and feedback. It is important to remember that all members of the PHCT, not just the GPs, spend time listening to and supporting their patients, and will benefit from liaison, either informal or formal. Counsellors should be encouraged to meet and liaise closely with other mental health professionals in the locality such as the CPN, the CMHT, the psychology team and the local hospital mental health team. They should also be aware of the care programme approach to the management and risk assessment of mental illness and be able to link appropriately with CMHTs to institute this if needed.

Knowledge of local resources and agencies is also needed. The counsellor may, for example, need to occasionally refer patients on to other counsellors locally, operating outside the National Health Service, or to specialist services (e.g. alcohol or drugs teams).

Support for the counsellor is required, both within the practice (meeting with a specific doctor or another member of the team) and elsewhere (there are often regular meetings of counsellors in primary care locally or nationally). Paid time for supervision and adequate secretarial backup are also essential.

Other practical issues are around what to do with patients who 'DNA' ('do not attend'), where to refer for longer term counselling or psychotherapy (if this is not provided in the practice), and how often patients can attend for a 'repeat episode' of counselling or for an occasional 'top up' session.

The wider scene

This chapter has outlined briefly the role of the GP in counselling in primary care, both as clinician and initial point of access for health services in the UK, and as employer and manager. GPs must also note that they have a wider role as part of the changing structures of general practice. They may need to argue the case for continuing, establishing or expanding counselling in primary care services in their locality, or within their PCO. This may involve assessing priorities and critically reviewing established patterns of mental health care provision in the community.

References

Association of Counsellors and Psychotherapists in Primary Care (2000) *Professional Counselling and Psychotherapy guidelines and protocols: defining psychological therapy in primary care.* CPC, Bognar Regis, Sussex.

Culley, S. (1991) *Integrative Counselling Skills in Action.* Sage, London.

Derbyshire Counselling Scheme (1997) *Guidelines and Protocols for the Employment of Counsellors in General Practice.* North Derbyshire Health and Southern Derbyshire Health.

Holland, J. (1995) *A Doctor's Dilemma—Stress and the Role of the Carer.* Free Association Books, London.

Royal College of General Practitioners (1972) *The Future General Practitioner.* Royal College of General Practitioners, London.

Salinsky, J. (1993) *The Last Appointment—Psychotherapy in General Practice.* Book Guild, Lewes, Sussex.

Sanders, K. (1986) *A Matter of Interest—Clinical Notes of a Psycho-Analyst in General Practice.* Clunie Press, London.

Useful contacts

Association of Counsellors and Psychotherapists in Primary Care. Telephone: 01243 870701; website: www.cpc-online.co.uk
British Association for Counselling and Psychotherapy. Telephone: 0870 443 5252; website: www.bacp.co.uk
Counselling in Primary Care Trust. Telephone: 01784 264300; website: www.cpct.co.uk

Chapter 4

Managed counselling in primary care

Joan Foster

Introduction

The key word in the title of this chapter is 'managed': a concept which has not been part of the culture of counselling in the past. This chapter will look at the growth of counselling in the NHS and the changes that have taken place with the introduction of 'the new NHS' since April 1999. The particular areas of equity of provision and clinical governance will be discussed. These have had major implications for primary care counsellors in many areas. One of the results will be more a widespread introduction of managed counselling services. What this means in concrete terms will be explored, from both a management and counselling perspective. The consequences in terms of both gains and losses will also be addressed.

'The new NHS'

Twenty years ago there was hardly a counsellor in a general practice surgery in the country. By 1998 there were counsellors in 51% of the surgeries in the UK (Mellor-Clark *et al.*, 2001). By any reckoning this is a dramatic growth. In the mid-1990s, primary care counselling had been particularly strong in fund-holding practices, where the GPs had more autonomy over their budget, could see the benefits of primary care counselling, and particularly wished to provide services in primary care rather than refer their patients to secondary services. However, its growth was patchy and often dependent on an entrepreneurial counsellor and a psychologically minded GP who knew each other and decided to introduce counselling into primary care. As a cultural phenomenon of growth of a non-statutory service within a statutory service, primary care counselling deserves exploration and reflection.

The Labour government's changes to the NHS following their White Paper 'The New NHS' (Department of Health 1997) have included a restructuring of primary care. In England, all general practices were required to form themselves into primary care groups (PCGs) with a target patient list of 100 000. However, geography and politics resulted in PCGs with patient populations of anything between 47 000 and 257 000 (NHS Confederation 1999). In 1999, there were 481 PCGs in England. In Wales all general practices were required to join local health groups, which were similar to PCGs. Twenty-two local health groups were set up in Wales with a similar spread of patient population. The structure is different in Scotland where they have set up local health co-operatives. There were initially 70 of these with a patient population spread of 25 000 to 150 000 (NHS Confederation 1999). It was not mandatory for general practices in Scotland to join a local health co-operative but as of May 1999 it was estimated that 95% had done so (Health Service Journal, May 1999). In England each PCG had to appoint a board made up of:

+ A minimum of four to a maximum of seven GPs

+ One to two nurses

+ A local social services department representative

+ A lay member

+ A Health Authority non-executive representative

+ The PCG chief executive/manager (as a full *ex officio* member) (Department of Health 1997).

The PCG had to appoint a chief executive or general manager, who created an administrative structure. The PCG also had to appoint a 'mental health lead'. This person was responsible for mental health, was normally a GP and usually sits on the PCG board. The result of these wholesale changes was the establishment of PCGs in varying stages of readiness to perform the tasks with which they were charged. The national tracker survey of PCGs and primary care trusts (PCTs) reported that 81% provided practice-based counselling (it is not stated whether this provision was for some or all of the practices in each primary care organisation or PCO) (Wilkin *et al.* 1999).

Equity of provision

One critical point for counsellors is that a key aim of the government, as stated in the NHS circular *Primary Care Groups: Delivering the Agenda* (Department of Health 1998b), is 'equity of provision'. This meant that if one practice provided a service, all practices in a PCG should. With the laudable intent of resolving the two-tier service caused by fund-holding, the government set the task of providing an equal service across a PCG. It is, of course, likely that inequity of provision will also be evident on a larger scale, between PCOs instead of between individual practices. Many PCGs are moving to PCT status, which may involve responsibility for the provision of a wide range of community-based health services currently seen as part of secondary care. At the time of writing, 19 of the 481 PCGs have submitted applications to be considered for PCT status from 1 April 2000 (Health Service Journal 1999).

Readers may well be wondering why all this information is relevant to a counsellor working in primary care. The answer is that the era of the individual self-employed counsellor, which seems to have been the most common model up to now, reported as 60% in a national survey of primary care counsellors (Mellor-Clark *et al.*, 2001), is almost certainly over. The primary care counsellor will have to belong to some structure in the future. In addition they will have to think both in terms of their PCO as well as their individual GP surgery or practice. More decisions are being made at PCO level and not at individual practice level. This, of course, also impacts upon the current providers of counselling: NHS Trusts and in some cases private providers. For primary care counsellors to survive, they need to understand the changes and their consequences. This is a well-nigh impossible task for any individual, part-time counsellor, perhaps working five or six hours a week in a GP surgery. A number of organizations have been set up to inform and support counsellors through this time of change and details of these are given at the end of the chapter.

Many primary care counsellors have had a very uncertain time through 1998 and 1999, and this is likely to continue into the twenty-first century. They have not known if they would still have a job, how they would be employed, how much they would be paid and whether they would have to work under different conditions of service. The principle of 'equity of provision' could have the profoundest impact on primary care counsellors. The intent is that if one surgery has access to counselling, all surgeries in the PCO should have access to counselling on a pro rata basis. From the figure of 51% of practices employing a counsellor, it is evident that counselling resources risk being stretched very thinly over an entire PCO. Of course, the situation on the ground is very varied. While some PCOs had only one or two practices with counsellors, the proportion was up to 75% in others. Whatever the number of counsellors, three options for the future have emerged:

1 Spread the existing counselling resources across all the practices—this would cost no more money but could result in doubling the waiting lists and the risk of a totally inadequate provision of clinical hours for the patient population.

2 End the provision of primary-care-based counsellors completely.

3 Increase the counselling provision to at least match the existing provision in practices which had a counsellor. This would mean more money would have to be allocated.

As of December 1999, all three options are being pursued by PCOs, with the majority taking the first option, a very small number taking the second and some taking the third.

Models of provision

Primary care organisations are taking decisions on commissioning services on a group-wide basis. An almost inevitable result of this will be managed counselling services in primary care. It is unlikely that a chief executive of a PCO with, say, 25 practices, some single-handed, spread over both rural and urban areas, would wish to employ 25 individual counsellors. Neither would he or she want to decide their number of clinical hours, to appoint them to surgeries and be responsible for the audit and evaluation of their service. It is much more likely that managers will wish to allocate a sum for the primary care counselling provision to a provider of counselling services who would be responsible for managing the service.

There are a number of different models of provision emerging (Counsellors in Primary Care 1999c). These are for primary care counselling to be provided by:

1 NHS Mental Health Trusts.

2 Private providers of counselling, such as Relate.

3 Associations or consortia of existing primary care counsellors.

4 Other NHS Trusts.

All these models will offer some form of a 'managed counselling service'. The tightness of the structure may vary, but there will be features common to all. Management of a service means structure, organization and accountability. It means standardizing provision, audit and evaluation. It means cross-fertilization of ideas and approaches. It gives the opportunity to work with specialists, to offer male or female counsellors, and to set up groups. It can benefit from economies of scale.

A possible structure is given in the Cousellors in Primary Care (CPC) (1999a) guidance document *Outline Proposal for a Managed Counselling Service* (Fig. 4.1).

A private counselling service provider would also require access to a consultant psychiatrist for case consultation.

This structure can be employed within the NHS or by private providers. However it raises important issues for a profession that has traditionally been one of private practice. Christopher Butler (1999) states: 'I feel that the realities of the organisational context have not really been addressed in the counselling world'. He observes that situating counselling within an organizational structure is often referred to negatively and there is little counterbalance looking at the benefits of organizational involvement. In the context of the NHS, an additional variable is that private health care has an established relationship with the NHS. Referrals may be made both privately and on the NHS. The primary care counsellor has often received both and run the two modes of provision in parallel. Hence there is a culture of both free and paid-for health care within the same system. In future the primary care counsellor will need to ensure there are clear and distinct boundaries between private and NHS work.

A managed service approach is a major shift for counsellors who have come from a counselling world that does not yet seem to have come to terms with counselling within an organization and whose training organizations on the whole prepare counsellors for individual private practice. Indeed it could be argued that this very individuality, autonomy and independence were the qualities that attracted many people into counselling in the first place. For many counsellors who were the first to work in their GP surgery there has been an element of being 'counter NHS culture'. They offered an individual service, took pride in not keeping clients waiting and worked from a position of unconditional positive regard. It is generally understood that the introduction of a holistic approach into a GP surgery usually working within a medical model has often been a struggle, but when achieved has had very positive effects. So from this

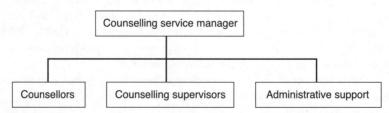

Fig. 4.1 A possible structure is given in the CPC guidance document 'An Outline Proposal for a Managed Counselling Service' (Counsellors in Primary Care 1999a).

background, moves towards structure and management may well not be viewed with enthusiasm! Indeed for many counsellors the benefits of working within a managed structure are not easily perceived and may not be recognized at all.

An additional issue is that the vast majority of primary care counsellors work part-time. They are often involved in a range of other counselling activities. However, the costs of running a PCO-wide service would be reduced by employing as few counsellors as possible working in more than one surgery. A consequence of the introduction of a managed counselling service could be that even though the number of counselling hours provided is not reduced nationally, the number of posts may be significantly lower.

A managed counselling service

In such a managed service, the counselling services manager would be required to have relevant training and experience and demonstrate good clinical practice, and administrative and management skills. The manager would be expected to interview and appoint staff, co-ordinate and represent the service, and be responsible for continuing professional development and audit and evaluation. It would be desirable for the manager to continue in counselling practice to ensure an understanding of current clinical issues. Further information can be obtained in a guidance sheet *Criteria for a Counselling Services Manager* (Counsellors in Primary Care 1999b). Decisions would have to be taken as to the number of clinical contact hours to be delivered, ensuring that the number of counselling hours was no less than 1.5 hours per 1000 of the adult population (Counsellors in Primary Care 1999a).

To run an effective service, counsellors need to be paid for both administration and clinical contact time. Counselling has almost totally been a part-time profession, traditionally paid on an hourly self-employed rate for clinical contact hours only. Once counsellors are employed they should expect to be paid to attend meetings (including those of the PCTO), and for supervision, as well as for note taking and audit/evaluation. The Counselling in Medical Settings division of the British Association for Counselling (1995) recommended a minimum of 70% clinical contact time and 30% administration time. To counsellors, it may appear that they are being paid at a lower rate, but the hourly rate reduction would be compensated for by payment for additional administrative hours. The reality is that the NHS pays less than the private sector, but that there are benefits such as holiday and sick pay as well as pension and employment rights. In addition all the existing work that had been done by the counsellor in his/her spare time should now be covered by their paid work.

The manager of a counselling service would expect detailed returns to be made. These returns could comprise:

- Number of clients
- Age/sex of clients
- Presenting problems
- Number of sessions
- Cancellations

- 'Did not attends' (DNA)
- Re-referrals to referrer
- Referrals to other services.

In addition, to measure outcomes it would be expected that a service provider would wish to use a credible audit and evaluation tool, such as the clinical outcomes research evaluation (CORE) system (CORE System Group 1998).

It would be expected that a managed counselling service would set agreed referral guidelines as to suitable presenting problems for primary care counsellors. CPC, in their referral guidelines (Cousellors in Primary Care 1999d), list the following presenting problems that may be suitable:

- Pathological bereavement
- Coping with injury or illness
- Depression—reactive, circumstantial
- Developmental or life crises
- Emotional, physical or sexual abuse issues
- Family relationship issues
- General anxieties and phobias
- Lack of direction, alienation or existential problems
- Loss, for example relationship, employment, health, etc
- Self-image and identity issues
- Stress and trauma—pre and post event
- Issues of sexuality.

The following may not be suitable for primary care counselling, unless the counsellor has specific, relevant skills:

- Sexual dysfunction
- Poor communication ability
- Self-destructive behaviour which, over time, has shown very little change, i.e. prolonged substance misuse, eating disorders
- Severe mental disorders
- Severe challenging behaviours, i.e. aggression, violence, severe learning disabilities.

It would be expected that there would be standardization of paperwork within a managed service, which would include letters to clients, the information provided about counselling and appointment sheets. Procedures would have to be agreed on note taking and keeping and confidentiality, both within the service and with relation to the primary health care team.

I perceive a managed counselling service to have a number of strengths. The service is openly accountable, both to the employer, the referrer and the client. The management can set standards of training and experience and be aware of the issues at national level concerning the movements to self-regulate the profession of counsellors in primary care. In addition, management has the opportunity to learn from other providers, in particular through the National Network of Counselling in Primary Care Service Providers (see 'Useful contacts' below). There is always a great danger that operating in isolation means that perfectly good wheels are continually being reinvented. Becoming part of a service will also enable the individual counsellor to learn and to teach good practice. It is also realistic to say that there may be more protection available to an individual counsellor, in this increasingly litigious world, if the counsellor is part of a counselling team.

With a service approach, there is the possibility for extending the service provision. For example, crisis counselling could be offered and long-term counselling. In addition, a wider choice of specialisms might be made available to clients. These could include: couples counselling, psychosexual counselling, family therapy and group work. Boundary issues that clients may have with a particular counsellor could be resolved with a wider team to refer to. In particular, the service could offer both male and female counsellors.

Clinical governance

This is defined as follows:

> ... a framework through which NHS organisations are accountable for continuously improving the quality of their services and safeguarding high standards of care by creating an environment in which excellence in clinical care will flourish (Department of Health 1998a).

Satisfying the requirements of clinical governance represents a substantial challenge for all counsellors in primary care. It is almost certainly easier to meet this challenge by collaborating as groups of counsellors by utilizing the organizational potential of managed services rather than by individual counsellors working in isolation from other counsellors. In either case, clinical governance requires the development of agreed national standards. An essential prerequisite is that counselling has to be recognized as part of statutory NHS provision in primary care. However, a great deal of very good work has been done already at both individual and organizational levels. The CORE system is being used by over 100 services as of December 1999, with an additional 50 services having their data analysed and 'benchmarked' by Psychological Therapies Research Centre (PTRC) researchers (Mellor-Clark 1999).

A requirement of clinical governance will be to demonstrate continuing professional development. Counselling in primary care is relatively new and at the time of writing it seems that the majority of counselling training courses do not adequately prepare counsellors for primary care work. There are two issues here. The first is to ensure that practitioners are appropriately trained for primary care work. A national forum of organizations concerned about this area worked together through 1999, culminating in a conference on 'Quality, Standards and Excellence' held on 14 November 1999 (further information can be obtained from the CPC). The second issue is to provide existing primary care counsellors with the opportunity to formalize the learning many have done 'on the job'. Again, the strength of a managed service is the opportunity for training to be provided for practitioners.

Supervision

Whilst many of the issues for practitioners of counselling in primary care are being addressed urgently, it seems to me that supervision too often is not adequately considered. It is of note that there is no separate chapter in this book concerning supervision of primary care counsellors. There are questions concerning who should supervise primary care counsellors, what training they should have and what accountability they should have to the service provider. Concerns are expressed about the isolation of primary care counsellors, which can only be compounded if the supervisor has no experience of primary care and the issues that will confront the primary care counsellor.

The establishment of a managed counselling service is an opportunity to ensure that supervision is provided by appropriately trained counselling supervisors with congruent theoretical approaches. As the decisions are made as to who provides the counselling service, it is essential that counsellors believe they are being appropriately managed and supervised. Further discussion of this issue can be found in Supplement 3 of *Supervision* (CPCT, Aug 1997) and Foster (2000).

Gains and losses

At the time of writing, it seems likely that the only way forward is for counsellors to work in some form of a managed counselling service. In discussions with counsellors at workshops round the country, concerns were raised as to the hierarchical nature of a managed counselling service structure. This is an inevitable reality when becoming part of an organization but it may be difficult for many current practitioners who have created their own role in their surgery. Being told what to do and having to fit into a structure that is bound to be imperfect will not be easy, especially when the counsellor may have created his/her own structure in the first place.

It is to be hoped that there will be increased understanding of primary care counselling as it is being practised at the turn of the century. It is an integrative approach, delivered by counsellors, psychotherapists and counselling psychologists with a scattering of clinical psychologists and behaviour therapists for good measure! It is usually time-limited, offering between six and 12 sessions. Some practitioners have never worked to a time limit, but offer open-ended counselling. They often find that this averages out to approximately five to eight sessions per client. It is to be hoped that as the profession matures, employers will have the confidence in the professional competence of the practitioner to let go of the need for rigid control of time boundaries. However, *realpolitik* means that at present, in many primary care settings, it is a huge enough task just to establish counselling itself, before the decision about the length/number of sessions can be left to the service manager or the practitioner. At present, it is largely short-term counselling that is offered in primary care, with some services offering the flexibility for a longer term option (Pietroni & Vaspe 2000). Psychotherapy is sometimes available in secondary care. However, there is a large group of clients for whom short-term counselling is not enough, but they are either not ill enough for secondary mental health services or are considered inappropriate for psychotherapy. A managed service could expand to offer open-ended counselling.

That said, I do believe that it is essential for practitioners to believe in the effectiveness of short-term counselling, to view it in the context of a life crisis and recognize that it may be needed again. It may also act as a bridge to further work. In addition it should be emphasized that short-term work can produce long-term change and for many clients is the treatment of choice.

Conclusions

In conclusion, it might be helpful, not too seriously, to look at a managed counselling service approach using two different languages. The first could be described as 'management speak', the second as 'counselling speak'.

'Management speak'

A managed service will be structured hierarchically, employing the existing counsellors in the PCO. The counsellors will be allocated to cover all surgeries in the PCO. A manager will be appointed who will assess the counsellors and identify areas for improvement. A group supervision structure will be established. The supervisors will also be part of the service and accountable to the management. All members of the service will have professional responsibilities and be expected to contribute on a clinical and administrative level as required. Team members will be required to undertake a specified number of hours (say 25) of continuing professional development per year.

'Counselling speak'

A managed service is an opportunity for isolated counsellors to come together as a group and work for the benefit of their clients. They may have the opportunity to work in more surgeries. The group will recognize that they need a spokesperson to represent them at meetings and to co-ordinate the information they will collect. This person will also be responsible for the appointment of staff. They will be able to identify their individual strengths and weaknesses and support each other. They will be encouraged to improve their skills and knowledge. They will come together in supervision groups and can ensure important issues are debated and understood. The supervisors will also be able to work together as a team for the good of both clients and counsellors. All involved will ensure they have the opportunity to be part of the decision-making process but be alive to the realities of operating in a difficult and changing environment.

Whilst this is a light-hearted attempt to translate what is happening to counsellors into some more acceptable wording, it does reflect the process that has taken place over the last 20 years. Counselling language has been introduced into primary care and there is much more awareness of a holistic rather than medical model. The establishment of a managed counselling service, whilst it will result in loss, will also result in major gains. The battle that all counsellors have fought for so long, to be respected and recognized, may well continue in the public arena, but it is to be hoped that as we embark on the twenty-first century, there will be gains and opportunities within the NHS.

Primary care counsellors are, therefore, facing major changes. Change can be both an opportunity and a threat. The opportunity is that there will be an increase in counselling provision, pay and conditions will be improved, and standardized and primary care counselling will be recognized by the Department of Health as a distinct discipline. One would not like to say 'wishful thinking'! The threat is that the primary care counsellor will disappear. All those representing primary care counsellors are working very hard to ensure that primary care counselling survives. What I hope is clearer from this chapter is that the structure of the NHS has changed and the aims of equity of provision and improved clinical governance have resulted in unavoidable changes for primary care counsellors. These changes will mean a new structure for many counsellors in a managed counselling service. I expect this to result in improvements in quality and equity of provision. It is to be hoped that the information in this chapter may be of use to those counsellors who have been, are or may be, involved in discussions as to the implications of a managed counselling service, as well as to those GPs and others who are making decisions about whether and how to commission such a service for primary care.

References

British Association of Counsellors/Counselling in Medical Settings (1995) *Guidelines for the Employment of Counsellors in General Practice (Revised)*.

Butler, C. (1999) Organisational counselling: the profession's shadow side. *Counselling,* 10 (3), 227–231.

CORE System Group (1998) *CORE System (Information Management) Handbook*. CORE System Group, Leeds.

Counsellors in Primary Care (1999a) *Outline Proposal for a Managed Counselling Service*. Association of Counsellors and Psychotherapists in Primary Care, Bognor Regis, UK.

Counsellors in Primary Care (1999b) *Criteria for a Counselling Services Manager, Guidance for Commissioners*. Association of Counsellors and Psychotherapists in Primary Care, Bognor Regis, UK.

Counsellors in Primary Care (1999c) *Information Sheet: Possible Models of Counselling Provision*. Association of Counsellors and Psychotherapists in Primary Care, Bognor Regis, UK.

Counsellors in Primary Care (1999d) *Information Sheet: Referral Guidelines*. Association of Counsellors and Psychotherapists in Primary Care, Bognor Regis, UK.

Department of Health (1997) *The New NHS. Modern, Dependable*. CM3807. HMSO, London.

Department of Health (1998a) *A First Class Service—Quality in the new NHS*. HMSO, London.

Department of Health (1998b) *Primary Care Groups: Delivering the Agenda*. Health Service Circular 1998/228. HMSO, London.

Foster, J. (2000) Counselling and the new NHS. *British Journal of Guidance and Counselling,* 28 (2).

Gould, M. (1999) Nowhere plans for nobody? *Health Service Journal,* 109, 12–13.

Mellor-Clark, J. (1999) *CORE System Manager*. Psychological Therapies Research Centre, University of Leeds, Leeds.

Mellor-Clark, J., Simms-Ellis, R. and Burton, M. (2001) *National Survey of Counsellors Working in Primary Care: Evidence for Growing Professionalisation?* (Occasional Paper No 79). Royal College of General Practitioners, London.

Millar, B. (1999) Skye's the limit. *Health Service Journal*, **109**, 14.

NHS Confederation (1999) *The Pocket Guide to the NHS.*

Pietroni, M. and Vaspe, A. (2000) *Understanding Counselling in Primary Care—Voices from the Inner City.* Harcourt Publishers, London.

Wilkin, D., Gillam, S. and Leese, B. (eds) (1999) *The National Tracker Survey of Primary Care Groups and Trusts. Progress and Challenges 1999/2000.* University of Manchester, Manchester.

Useful contacts

The National Network of Counselling in Primary Care Service Providers is an informal organization of providers of counselling. Contact: The Counselling in Primary Care Trust, First Floor, Majestic House, High Street, Staines TW18 4DG, UK. Telephone: 01784 441782.

The Association of Counsellors and Psychotherapists in Primary Care (CPC) was launched in November 1998 with the following aims: to represent counsellors and psychotherapists working in primary care and to lead the way in establishing national standards and guidelines for further development of professional and effective counselling throughout NHS primary health care.

It has been working, as have the Counselling in Primary Care Trust (CPCT) and the Faculty for Healthcare Counsellors and Psychotherapists (FHCP) in the British Association for Counselling and Psychotherapy (BACP) to inform and support counsellors through this time of change.

Contact: CPC, Queensway House, Queensway, Bognor Regis PO21 IQT, UK.

email: cpc@cpc-online.co.uk

website: www.cpc-online.co.uk

Part 2

Debates about counselling

Chapter 5

Counselling research and evaluation

Nancy Rowland and Stephen Goss

Introduction

As an emerging professional group, counsellors, especially those who work in primary or secondary care, are taxed with questions about the utility of the work they do. Does counselling work? What interventions work best for which patients? Are counsellors providing a safe and effective service? Further questions focus on the cost of counselling. How much does it cost? Is counselling cost-effective? Is it good value for money? How does it compare in terms of cost and effectiveness with other interventions designed to alleviate mental health problems in primary care? These questions about effectiveness and cost-effectiveness are framed in the context of current health service policy, with its emphasis on quality of care, evidence-based practice and cost-effective services.

The notion of quality of care is central to counselling and informs the Codes of Practice and Ethics (e.g. British Association for Counselling 1997) which guide counsellors in their work. The added value of counselling is quality—it is perhaps the main justification for the provision of counselling services in primary care. Issues about quality of care are discussed throughout this chapter. The drive towards evidence-based health care, and the government's commitment to effective and cost-effective services present a challenge for counsellors, who are increasingly called upon to provide evidence to justify their practice. This chapter begins with a brief overview of the government's current policy for a knowledge-based NHS, the Department of Health's research and development (R & D) strategy which underpins it, and the supporting organizations which generate evidence and produce guidelines.

This leads us to reflect on the knowledge base for counselling. What do we know about counselling? What sort of evidence do we have? What is the nature of the evidence and which methods are used to generate it? Counsellors and researchers will be the first to admit that counselling is not easy to evaluate, partly because the process is so difficult to define and to standardize. Counselling is offered by a range of practitioners with different professional backgrounds and different levels of training, skills and experience. There are a range of theoretical models of counselling and counsellors in primary care, who tend to be generalists and pragmatists, will often draw on several methods in treating patients. Again, counselling is provided for a range of patients with different characteristics and problems. Given the different practitioners, methodologies, patients and aims, it is not surprising that the evaluation of counselling has proved difficult. The challenges involved in the evaluation of counselling, including problems of definition, measurement and outcome, will be discussed here, along with a brief critique of the research methods that have been used. An awareness of the nature of the problems that beset counselling research enhances a critical appreciation of reports of efficacy or effectiveness. Finally, the chapter concludes with a discussion of how individual practitioners can evaluate their own practice. Supervision is a fundamental part of counselling; the notion of reflective practice informs both the individual practitioner and the evaluative culture of counselling. Counsellors can also engage in audit, practice research networks and research into counselling—from single case studies to controlled trials. Both individual practitioners and their representative organizations need to influence and extend the evaluation of counselling and to contribute to the evidence base for counselling in primary care.

The drive towards evidence-based health care

The drive towards evidence-based health care started with the medical profession. Sackett *et al.* (1996), defined evidence-based medicine as the conscientious, explicit and judicious use of current best evidence in making decisions about the care of individual patients. The practice of evidence-based medicine means integrating individual clinical expertise with the best available clinical evidence from systematic research. Evidence-based health care can thus be narrowly defined as the conscientious, explicit and judicious use of current best evidence in making decisions about any aspects of health care (Li Wan Po 1998). It is an umbrella term which includes, for example, evidence-based medicine, evidence-based nursing, evidence-based patient choice— the list of terms is almost endless. Evidence-based counselling is not, as yet, a widely used term. It is, however, beginning to be debated.

The present government is explicitly committed to improving quality in the NHS, including support for the drive towards an evidence-based health service. In 1990, the government introduced a formal structure for R & D in the NHS, spawning the movement for evidence-based health care in the UK. The purpose of the NHS R & D strategy (Department of Health 1991, 1993) is to build a knowledge base to inform all decisions made by NHS managers and clinicians. The strategy consists of an information strategy, a research commissioning strategy and an implementation strategy. The underlying aim of the strategy is to assist in effecting a culture change within the health service—towards a knowledge-based service (Baker & Kleijnen 2000). The rationale for the strategy is straightforward: it recognizes that it is impossible for health care professionals to keep abreast of the vast amount of research into new health technologies or service developments. The information strategy aims to provide and disseminate up-to-date critical reviews of research, and clinical practice guidelines informed by existing knowledge. The research commissioning strategy aims to extend the evidence base, and the implementation strategy, perhaps the least developed of the three arms, exists to get evidence into practice.

The NHS R & D initiative has supported the founding of some flagship infrastructures that have become of international importance. The Cochrane Collaboration is an international collaboration which aims to prepare, maintain and disseminate systematic reviews of health care. It has published systematic reviews of over 150 000 controlled trials concerned with mental health (Department of Health 1999). (The synthesis of evidence, in systematic reviews and guidelines, is described later in this chapter.) The NHS Centre for Reviews and Dissemination at York (CRD) also undertakes systematic reviews of certain topics—for example, the treatment of depression or schizophrenia—and publishes the results with guidance for practitioners and commissioners in a series of Effective Health Care bulletins. Other organizations support the NHS drive towards evidence-based health care. There is a Centre for Evidence Based Nursing at York and a Centre for Evidence Based Medicine at Oxford—as yet there is no centre for evidence-based counselling. These centres aim to amass, review and critically assess existing research and to undertake further research to fill the gaps in the evidence base—gaps that are often enormous.

The National Institute for Clinical Excellence (NICE) has been established to provide clinical guidance to the NHS in England and Wales, including guidance on the clinical and cost-effectiveness of new and existing clinical conditions. NICE thus has an overarching role to play in the commissioning and dissemination of guidance on a range of issues identified by ministers at the Department of Health. It will also, in consultation with appropriate organizations, produce guidance for patients and carers on the implications for them resulting from its recommendations.

There are two further national initiatives of particular interest to counsellors and those who work with them: the clinical practice guidelines on treatment choice in psychological therapies and counselling (Department of Health 2001) and the government's focus on mental health policy as documented in the National Service Framework (NSF) for mental health. We will briefly describe these initiatives here, as they are likely to directly impact upon service provision.

The Department of Health commissioned an umbrella group representing six organizations—the British Association for Counselling and Psychotherapy, the British Psychological Society, the Royal College of Psychiatrists, the Royal College of General Practitioners, the UK Council for Psychotherapy and the British Confederation for Psychotherapists—to produce clinical practice guidelines to aid decisions about which forms of psychological therapy are most appropriate for which patients. The chair of the committee, Glennys Parry, writes in the Preface to the guidelines (Department of Health 2001) that the recommendations, based on generalizations from a systematic review of the research evidence and expert clinical professional consensus, are an aid to informed decision-making but cannot and should not replace professional judgement in assessing the individual case. None the less, the guidelines on psychological therapies in primary care form the basis for an approach to talking therapies which could benefit patients by clarifying how much (and how little) we currently know from research, or can agree between experts. The result may be better research and more systematic practice. The report concluded that there is strong evidence to suggest that psychological therapy should be routinely considered as a treatment option when assessing mental heath problems. None the less, the guidelines indicate that the evidence base for counselling and other psychological therapies, while improving, suffers from methodological shortcomings.

Mental health policy

In *A First Class Service* (Department of Health 1998), the government explains how NHS standards will be set by NICE, delivered by clinical governance (a framework for assuring quality within the NHS), underpinned by professional self-regulation and informed by lifelong learning, monitored by the Commission for Health Improvement, the National Performance Assessment Framework and the National Survey of Patients. The importance placed upon mental health is demonstrated by the fact that it is identified as one of the most significant causes of all health and disability in England and is covered by one of the first NSFs. The NSF for mental health focuses on the mental health needs of working age adults up to 65 years, most of whom are cared for by their GP and primary care team. The standards and service models in the NSF are based on the evidence of effectiveness, including cost-effectiveness, currently available. Standards two and three focus on primary care and access to services. Counselling in primary care receives barely a mention, and the only reference to counselling is negative. Thus the NSF concludes that non-directive counselling is less effective than structured therapies such as cognitive behavioural therapy, brief focal psychoanalytic therapy and interpersonal therapy (Department of Health 1999). This brief reference to counselling reflects the fact that the evidence base is limited. None the less, even since the publication of the NSF, three controlled trials of counselling in primary care evidence have been published, thus expanding the evidence base (King *et al.* 2000; Simpson *et al.* 2000; Chilrers *et al.* 2001) and a systematic review of the effectiveness and cost-effectiveness of counselling has been completed (Rowland *et al.* 2001) and updated (Bower *et al.* in press). There is a pressing need for the expansion of the knowledge base. Until it is able to demonstrate efficacy, counselling risks losing funding and being side-lined as an ineffective intervention.

The dangers of evidence-based health care

Parry (2000) notes that one of the dangers of evidence-based health care is that funding decisions will be driven by research reviews and clinical practice guidelines. Systematic reviews of research can only reflect findings for types of therapy which have been extensively researched, and generally speaking, these have been briefer, more structured and focal therapies, particularly, but not exclusively, cognitive behavioural therapy. Where research evidence is lacking for other approaches, such as counselling, it is easy to jump to the conclusion, as the NSF suggests, that such approaches are ineffective, when in fact they are merely not proven. The lack of an evidence base can lead to cuts in funding, with the consequence that potentially valuable and effective therapies are lost to the NHS.

The implications of this brief overview of current NHS policy are clear: therapeutic interventions must be based on good evidence of effectiveness; where there is no evidence, research must be done; if an intervention is found not to be substantiated by robust evaluation, it should be dropped in favour of those interventions which can demonstrate effectiveness. The implications for counselling in primary care are very clear: evaluate or be damned. We shall now review the evidence base for counselling.

What do we know about evidence for counselling?

Uncontrolled trials

The first case reports of counselling in primary care (Rutledge 1972; Harray 1975; Marsh & Barr 1975; Anderson & Hasler 1979; Waydenfeld & Waydenfeld 1980) describe the employment of a counsellor in general practice and the benefits that appeared to accrue. Benefits included patient preference for an on-site counselling service rather than the stigma associated with referral to the psychiatric services; a reduction in doctors' consultation and prescription rates; and high levels of patient and professional satisfaction. The reduction in prescriptions, referrals and consultations led advocates of counselling to infer that counselling was not only effective, but cost-effective. Later studies (e.g. Coe *et al.* 1996; Booth *et al.* 1997; Baker *et al.* 1998) added to the weight of anecdotal evidence that counselling works; counsellors and GPs believe it to be a valuable therapeutic tool and a substantial proportion of patients report that they have been helped (Keithley & Marsh 1995). However, these studies reflect an enthusiasm for counselling which appears to be unsubstantiated by the evidence base. The studies were limited by small sample size, short timescales and follow up, scant information on patient selection criteria or description of treatment offered, and lack of control groups. Such methodological problems led Craig and Boardman (1997) to comment that the efficacy of generic counselling is far from certain. It has been suggested (King *et al.* 1994) that counselling needs to be rigorously evaluated and that the best way to do this is by randomized controlled trials.

Previous reviews

Previous reviews of psychological therapies report mixed results. In a meta-analysis of 475 psychotherapy trials, Smith *et al.* (1980) reported that psychotherapy is effective; they estimated an average effect of 0.85 for all types of therapy, clients and outcomes. (This means that there was a large positive change in favour of therapy.) However, most of the trials took place in educational (56%) and hospital (12%) settings, rather than in general practice.

A meta-analysis of 11 UK studies (Balestrieri *et al.* 1988), comparing specialist mental health treatment with usual GP care, found that specialist mental health professionals had a 10% greater success rate than usual GP treatment. However, Freidli and King (1996) comment that some of the studies did not use randomized control groups, and only two studies compared counsellors with usual GP care.

A recent review of the efficacy and effectiveness of the psychotherapies (Roth & Fonagy 1996) included a chapter on counselling and primary care interventions. The section on counselling in primary care consisted of a narrative review, which suggested that the efficacy of counselling is difficult to assess because of the lack of specificity and control in studies, the diversity of patient groups studied, the variation in treatments administered and the heterogeneity of contrast treatments. Roth and Fonagy conclude that if counselling services are to be extended within primary care settings, urgent research is required to examine the efficacy of counselling interventions across a wide range of psychological disorders.

A systematic review of the effectiveness and cost-effectiveness of counselling in primary care (Rowland *et al.*, 2001) reported results from four randomized controlled trials of non-directive counselling by BACP accredited (or equivalent) counsellors. The authors concluded that patients who receive counselling are more likely to have improved psychological symptom levels than those who receive usual GP care, and that levels of satisfaction with counselling are high. There is limited information about the cost-effectiveness of counselling; one study reported no clear cost advantage with either counselling or usual care. Data from the trials were statistically significant when pooled, but the clinical significance of the findings is unclear. The review has recently been updated (Bower *et al.* in press). The authors now conclude that counselling for psychological problems is better than usual GP care in the short term and that patients who receive counselling are more satisfied. However, in the long term, counselling is not any better than usual GP care.

In a recent review of the efficacy and effectiveness literature, Hemmings (2000) concluded that systematic reviews of research using randomized controlled trial methodology produce equivocal results because the research methods themselves are narrow and flawed and inadequately evaluate counselling. In contrast, effectiveness research, which evaluates an intervention in clinical settings, has relevance and meaning but lacks rigour. We will return to this issue in the discussion of research methods below.

Finally, a recent review of the efficacy and the effectiveness of counselling in primary care (Friedli & King 1996) concluded that despite the popularity of counselling with GPs and their patients, there is still no good evidence that counselling is clinically or cost-effective. The authors write that it is paradoxical that in an era when evidence-based health care is assuming ever greater importance, challenging us to provide evidence for the effectiveness of medical and social interventions, counselling services are expanding rapidly without such evidence. There is an urgent need to establish which type of counselling intervention is effective for which patient, and direct resources accordingly.

Generating the evidence

How can we assess the results of previous research so as to draw conclusions from the findings? A brief overview of the methods for evaluating counselling, their strengths and weaknesses, will help critically assess the evidence to date. There are various methods to generate evidence about counselling. The methods can be broadly divided into quantitative and qualitative methods. As their names suggest, the two approaches utilize a range of methods to generate different sorts of data. Put simply, quantitative methodology includes questionnaires, surveys and trials; qualitative methods include interviews, observation and narrative. There is, of course, no reason why both approaches should not be used in the evaluation of a treatment—counselling might be assessed by a randomized controlled trial supplemented by a series of qualitative interviews to understand the clinical significance of any statistical findings. A recent book on evidence-based counselling and psychological therapies focuses on the types of methodology used to evaluate counselling (Rowland & Goss 2000). In this section, we will do no more than provide a brief overview.

Controlled trials

Cochrane (1972), writing 30 years ago, noted his concern about the increase of NHS counselling and psychotherapy services based on conviction rather than evidence of value, and advocated investigation by controlled trial. That this recommendation has been mostly ignored can be seen by the proliferation of largely unevaluated counselling services in the UK. Controlled trials are a widely accepted means of applying experimental methods to a clinical setting and have been advocated as the gold standard for comparing and evaluating different treatments. King (1997) suggests that only controlled trials will give clear evidence of efficacy.

In health care settings, clinical trials are usually undertaken in order to evaluate whether a treatment works or not. In these trials, the outcome of one group of patients receiving treatment is compared to the outcome of another group who receive no treatment or treatment of another kind. As Corney (1995) points out, the need for a control group is crucial as many patients with depression and anxiety (those patients most likely to be referred to a counsellor) will get better and resolve their problems with or without outside help. Moreover, patients will normally be referred to a counsellor at a point when their problems are likely to be at their worst. This means that many patients are likely to show some improvement at a follow-up interview, even without treatment. In order to demonstrate genuine treatment effects a control group, or comparison group, is necessary.

Randomized controlled trials

Control groups protect against bias with one all important proviso: all other things need to be equal. However, bias can creep into controlled trials and distort the results. One of the major distortions is that of selection bias. For example, if there are baseline differences between the patients allocated to counselling and those allocated to the control group, so that one group has more severe levels of depression than the other, or so that one group has higher levels of motivation for treatment, it is possible that outcomes may be determined not by the difference in interventions, but by the difference in patient characteristics. Such bias will threaten the validity of the results.

Randomization is the method used to minimize bias. An important feature of the randomized controlled trial is that patients who have provided informed consent to participate in a trial are randomly allocated to either one or more 'active' intervention groups (such as counselling or the prescription of antidepressants) or to a control group (the baseline or 'do nothing' option). The purpose of randomization is to reduce systematic bias in outcomes related to differences in the characteristics of individuals included in each group. The outcomes of interest from each option are measured over the trial period and the differences between them tested for statistical significance using a standard test such as Student's t-test or chi-square (Altman 1991). The principle is that if the difference in outcomes is statistically significant then a null (or baseline) hypothesis, that there is no difference in the effectiveness of the options, can be rejected. Or, as Cochrane (1972) wrote, a randomized controlled trial allows the researcher to test the hypothesis that one treatment is better than another and express the results in the form of the probability of the differences found being due to chance, or not. The randomized controlled trial is most frequently used in clinical research to establish the efficacy of health care interventions under controlled conditions; their strengths are manifest for comparing and evaluating different treatments.

However, various problems arise when attempting to conduct controlled trials in clinical settings. It is immediately apparent that it is impossible to compare counselling with no treatment, as it is considered unethical to offer 'no treatment' to patients who seek help from their GP for their condition. So instead of an experimental design, where counselling is tested against no treatment, a pragmatic approach is adopted—that is, a comparison between two treatments. Thus, for example, counselling in primary care might be compared with usual GP care or with the prescription of antidepressants. While reflecting the reality of clinical settings, it must be noted that a comparison of two treatments makes it more difficult to compare treatment differences, particularly when evaluating two generic interventions such as counselling and GP care. In addition, controlled trials require that those participating are 'blind' with respect to the treatment group to which they have been allocated, to try to ensure that prior expectations do not distort the results. This is hardly feasible in a trial that compares a counselling with a drug intervention.

There are other problems in conducting pragmatic trials of counselling in primary care. Trials aim to standardize the type of counselling offered (sometimes through manualization, i.e. a written specification of the content and process of the therapy according to its theoretical description), to standardize the training and experience of the counsellors (e.g. only counsellors accredited by the British Association for Counselling and Psychotherapy are involved in the trial), to standardize the type of problems that patients have (so that, for example, entry to a trial might include only patients with a certain level of depression) and to standardize the duration of the intervention (e.g. six to 12 sessions). This level of control enables the researchers to make recommendations about which therapeutic techniques appear to have efficacy. However, Parry (2000) points out that outside the clinical trial, such adherence to a pure form of therapy is rare—real therapists aim for a balance between uniform application of therapy and making adaptive choices in order to maintain the integrity both of the treatment and the therapeutic alliance. Patients are rarely 'just depressed'—they may be anxious and depressed and drinking too much alcohol—and co-morbidity is common among presenting patients. Again, length of treatment is rarely uniform, and patients may have a series of sessions, followed by a break, with 'top up' sessions later on. The standardized treatments to standard patients over a standard length of time may not represent the reality of a service in primary care; and may thus have little relevance as an evaluation of the 'real' work of counsellors. In the main, trials consist of a series of trade-offs between internal and external validity. A rule of thumb is that the higher the internal validity (i.e. the higher the level of control, or standardization, of patients, type of problems, intervention and so on), the lower the external validity (representativeness) and vice versa.

Controlled patient preference trials

Triallists report problems in conducting randomized controlled trials of counselling in primary care, suggesting that this is an area in which public awareness is high and genuine equipoise about counselling compared with usual GP care is rare

(Fairhurst & Dowrick 1996).With the widespread availability of counselling today, it is less acceptable to patients of GPs that a randomization procedure bars people from a counselling intervention (King 1995). True randomization may lead to patients being allocated to treatments that they would not normally accept, which is an unreasonable test of an intervention (Pringle & Churchill 1995). Furthermore, interventions such as counselling or medication need a high degree of involvement on the part of the patient and may succeed only if they are in line with the patient's expectations. Controlled patient preference trials, in which patients with a strong preference for a particular treatment are not randomized, but are allocated the treatment of their choice, are thus an innovative form of assessing counselling in primary care. Only those patients who do not express a preference for one treatment over another are randomized; the rest are allocated to the treatment of their choice. The increased acceptability of the trial to patients and participating clinicians may increase recruitment rates and the representativeness of the patient population, and the results from the randomized and preference cohorts can be used to investigate the influence of preference on outcome. There are problems in analysing data from patient preference trials—it may be, for example, that selection biases operate in variables other than their preferences—and for a full discussion of patient preference trials and randomized controlled trials the reader should refer to Bower and King (2000).

Qualitative research

The goal of qualitative research is the development of concepts that help us to understand social phenomena in natural, rather than experimental, settings, giving due emphasis to the meanings, experiences and views of all the participants. Qualitative studies are concerned with answering questions about the nature of counselling and how and why counselling varies in different circumstances. Quantitative methods cannot address question such as these, but a qualitative approach can (Mays & Pope 1996). Mays and Pope (1996) believe that the rigid demarcation of qualitative and quantitative research as opposing traditions is unhelpful; that the approaches can complement rather than exclude each other. They argue that qualitative research can be conducted as an essential preliminary to quantitative research, as for example in using qualitative techniques of focus groups, observation and in-depth interviews to provide a description and understanding of a situation or behaviour. Thus, for example, a researcher might want to understand a referral process to a primary care counsellor by observing the staff at the reception desk and by interviewing practice staff and patients, before designing and conducting a survey to assess whether or not the system is working efficiently.

Qualitative work can also supplement quantitative work as part of the validation process, as in 'triangulation', where three or more methods are used and the results compared for convergence (for example, a large-scale survey, focus groups and a period of observation). Combining methods can help to build a wider picture. Thirdly, qualitative research can explore complex phenomena or areas not amenable to quantitative research such as in studies of health service organisation and policy.

The methods used by qualitative researchers include individual interviews, focus groups, diaries and case notes, transcripts of therapy sessions, open-ended questionnaires or reports, narrative responses to projective techniques, ethnographic participant observation, biographies and novels (McLeod 2000). Rigour is ensured through the process of systematic and self-conscious research design, and data collection, interpretation and communication. Mays and Pope (1996) exhort qualitative researchers to create an account of method and data which can stand independently, so that another trained researcher could analyse the data the same way and come to the same conclusions; and to produce a plausible and coherent explanation of the phenomenon under scrutiny. The interested reader could do no better than read their excellent text on qualitative research methods to further understand the techniques used to ensure validity, reliability and generalizability.

Synthesizing the evidence

Systematic reviews

Previous reviews of the counselling literature—and indeed of any literature—were not systematic. Traditional reviews of health care research have tended to rely on the author's selection of papers and knowledge of the field, so that the results of the review have tended to reflect the views of the author, including his or her intellectual bias. It is no longer sufficient for an author to open the filing cabinet and pull out the papers which have gathered dust over the years, or to rely on summarizing the results of trials with interesting, usually positive results; this results in the production of a biased review. Traditional reviews undertaken by content experts are subjective and lack methodological rigour (Oxman 1995). In the face of growing dissatisfaction with the lack of transparency of methodology and lack of trust in the conclusions of traditional review articles, the systematic review emerged (Gilbody & Sowden 2000). Systematic reviews differ from other types of review in that they are explicit in their methodology and adhere to a strict scientific design in order to make them more comprehensive, to minimize the chance of bias, and so ensure their reliability. A systematic review aims to locate, appraise and synthesize evidence from scientific studies, ideally randomized controlled trials. In some cases, it is appropriate to produce a pooled summary statistic of the effectiveness of an intervention from several different studies. This is known as meta-analysis (NHS Centre for Reviews and Dissemination 1996). Systematic reviews of research evidence are invaluable scientific activities. They establish whether scientific findings are consistent and can be generalized across populations, settings and treatment variations, and they highlight areas of uncertainty. Both qualitative and quantitative systematic reviews, with their explicit methods, will limit bias and improve the accuracy and reliability of the conclusions and recommendations (Mulrow 1995). They are therefore valuable sources of information for decision-makers.

Clinical practice guidelines

Clinical practice guidelines are systematically developed statements to assist practitioner and patient decisions about appropriate health care for specific clinical circumstances (Field & Lohr 1990). They are being put forward in the UK as a means of promoting evidence-based practice and clinical effectiveness and reducing variation in standards and outcomes of clinical care (Cape 1998). When developed properly, they summarize current research evidence and clinical consensus on best practice in a given clinical situation, and can be a useful tool to help practitioners make clinical decisions. They can also be used to set audit standards, that is, as benchmarking tools.

Just as systematic reviews differ from traditional reviews, synthesizing research evidence in a rigorous way to minimize bias, clinical practice guidelines differ from standard guidelines in the manner of their construction. Clinical practice guidelines use a systematic and explicit development process, usually involving a representative guideline development group, and a systematic approach to identifying, evaluating and incorporating evidence in the guideline. Clinical guidelines may be developed by local groups of clinicians or by national bodies or agencies (Cape 1998). There is evidence that locally produced guidelines are more likely to be followed, although nationally produced guidelines are more likely to be valid (Grimshaw & Russell 1993). Best practice may result from local practitioners adapting national guidelines to local circumstances.

Their development in relation to psychological therapies is relatively recent, although, as noted above, the Department of Health (2001) has recently published systematically developed guidance on psychological therapies in primary care.

Cost-effectiveness

The *ad hoc* expansion of counselling services places increasing demands on an overstretched health care service. The government is explicit in its desire to provide cost-effective services. What evidence is there for the cost-effectiveness of counselling? Counsellors tend to believe that their employment in general practice can lead to improved patient outcomes and a reduction in NHS resource use, including fewer referrals to psychiatric services, fewer prescriptions and fewer GP consultations. These claims have been challenged (Sibbald *et al.* 1996; Cape & Parham 1998) and need further evaluation. The ideal basis for an economic evaluation is a randomized controlled trial carried out in a realistic situation (i.e. a pragmatic trial) to investigate effectiveness. The economic evaluation of counselling in the NHS involves utilizing information about the costs and effects of counselling and making decisions about the allocation of resources to finance counselling. In essence, economic evaluation entails drawing up a balance sheet of the advantages (benefits) and disadvantages (costs) associated with an intervention or service, so that choices between treatments can be made. Although the precise forms of economic evaluation may vary, the 'cost–benefit' framework is common to all of them and constitutes the distinctive feature of the economic approach (Robinson 1993).

Psychotherapists began to discuss the issue of the costs and benefits of long-term psychotherapy in the 1980s—over 20 years ago (McGrath & Lowson 1986)—but the cost-effectiveness of counselling largely remains unevaluated.

Types of economic evaluation

There are several types of economic evaluation, all of which can be applied to counselling in medical settings. The choice of technique depends upon the objectives of the evaluation and the time and money available for collecting data on effectiveness. The main types of economic evaluation are cost minimization, cost-effectiveness, cost–benefit and cost utility analysis. In each case the outcomes of different interventions are compared using a common unit such as life years gained. Cost minimization explores the total cost consequences of using, for example, different medicines to give identical outcomes in each case. Cost-effectiveness relates the cost of therapies to their different outcomes and produces measures such as cost per successfully treated patient or cost per life year gained. Cost–benefit analysis uses money as the common unit to compare the benefits of a given therapy with the associated costs to determine whether the benefits outweigh the costs or vice versa. Cost utility analysis is a special form of cost-effectiveness analysis that relates to the cost of different therapies to improvements in the quantity and quality of life. The QALY (quality-adjusted life year) measure has been developed to measure outcomes in cost utility analysis. In addition, descriptive information can be provided from a cost analysis which assesses the costs of a disease to the NHS, to patients (social burdens) and to the economy as a whole (Tolley & Rowland 1995).

The main purpose for undertaking an economic evaluation is to assess how efficiently resources are being used in the pursuit of an objective or a set of objectives. Efficiency is achieved if the resources used on one option have no other use which can be shown to be more worthwhile, that is, if it provides the greatest benefit at the least cost. The pursuit of efficiency only arises because of the existence of limited resources.

Economic factors in health care are becoming more important as demands on health care systems increase, often beyond the ability of these systems to satisfy them (Goodwin *et al.* 1990). When demands for resources exceed supply, decisions must be made regarding the allocation of resources. This in turn calls into view questions about treatment effectiveness and treatment cost. Economic analysis provides useful information on both costs and effects and is therefore an aid to decision-making. It is not prescriptive, but provides essential information to help decision-makers to make informed decisions.

Conducting an economic evaluation

There are a number of steps in conducting an economic evaluation. First, a clear definition of the objective of the evaluation is required. For example, the primary objective might be to discover the most cost-effective approach to treating depression in primary care. Second, a clear description of the options to meet this objective is needed. For example, viable options might be to employ a specialist counsellor, to train a GP or other practice staff to provide counselling, or to do nothing (which is in fact the active control—usual GP care). Third, an appropriate study design needs to be chosen for collecting data and measuring the effectiveness of each option. The fourth step is the identification of costs and the main outcomes or benefits of each option. In a cost-effectiveness analysis, an appropriate outcome measure needs to be chosen by which to compare options, for example, the reduction in the level of depression among patients visiting the GP. In a cost utility analysis, outcomes are usually measured using QALYs and in a cost–benefit analysis monetary values are used. Finally, a clear presentation of the cost-effectiveness results relating to each option should be provided. To go into detail about the methods of economic evaluation is beyond the scope of this chapter. Those practitioners interested in the practical application of cost-effectiveness analysis in health care settings are referred to Tolley and Rowland (1995).

Research into cost-effectiveness

Counsellors tend to believe that their employment in genral practice can lead to improved patient outcomes and a reduction in NHS resource use, including fewer referrals to psychiatric services, fewer prescriptions and fewer GP consultations. A systematic review (Bower and Sibbald 2000) suggests that this may occur for mental health professionals generally, but that the effects are limited in scope and consistency. In a recently updated review of counselling in primary care in the U.K. (Bower *et al.*, in press) four trials have reported economic analyses which aim to determine the relationship between clinical benefits and costs (Harvey *et al.* 1998; Friedli *et al.* 2000; Bower *et al.* 2000; Simpson *et al.* 2000). Two studies showed that the provision of counselling has been associated with increases in some costs in the short term (Friedli *et al.* 2000; Simpson *et al.* 2000). However, in the longer term, the overall costs to the NHS and society associated with counselling appeared to be broadly similar to those incurred when patients receive usual GP care. It may be that patients under the care of counsellors reduce their use of other NHS resources (such as consultations with the GP, anti-depressant medication and specialist mental health services). However, the relatively small numbers of patients in these trials suggests that the economic analyses are likely to be underpowered and should be treated with caution.

There is much rhetoric about the need to purchase cost effective therapies, but there is limited evidence on which to make decisions about the cost effectiveness of counselling.

Individual versus population health

There is a paradox in current health care practice. On the one hand, in the moral climate of the NHS, medical ethics dictate that individual practitioners try to maximize the health of individual patients. To this end, the practitioner will give as much time and treatment as necessary to assist in this goal. This ethic rests on the assumption that the over-riding principle governing a practitioner's actions towards a patient should be that the most is done for that patient; treatment should not rest on mathematical calculations about cost-effectiveness. And yet, at the same time, such an attempt ignores the opportunity cost to other patients—and, possibly, future patients. Williams (1992) argues that it cannot be ethical to ignore the adverse consequences on others of the decisions you make, which is what 'cost' represents. 'What will it cost?' means 'what will have to be sacrificed?' and this may be very different from the amount of money with which we have to part. Unlike medical ethics, economics embraces a concept of social as well as individual ethics. Thus, while economics in the field of health has as an objective the maximization of health in the community, subject to resource constraints, medical ethics pushes individual doctors to try to maximize the health of their individual patients (Maynard 2000). Commissioners are constantly making decisions about resource allocation—who to prioritize; how long to treat; who will benefit and so on. Mooney (1984) suggests that certain institutional alterations within the NHS, for example, new budgeting structures and the acceptance of efficiency as a social goal, are required in order to promote the type of behavioural change which will make doctors act in the interest of the common good to a greater extent than is now the case.

There are many sides to the ethics argument. In essence, the major standpoints are as follows. Medical ethics are fundamental in the health service and in doctor–patient relationships. Health care outcomes involve basic issues relating to the quality and quantity of life. Resources are scarce and decisions need to be made about their allocation. Should doctors act for individual patients or for the community as a whole, or should they leave such decision-making to health service managers (thus not compromising their relationship with patients)? If managers and politicians make decisions, how can this be done fairly and will doctors be happy to live with the consequences?

What does this mean for those who advocate the development of counselling in general practice? Proponents of counselling will need to consider the costs and benefits of counselling to general practice and to the health service as a whole, bearing in mind that the allocation of resources to counselling will necessarily mean that other treatments are foregone. The issue of ethics and economics is, as yet, unexplored for counsellors, but one that cannot be ignored. In a paper that questioned the place of psychoanalysis and psychotherapy in the health service, Wilkinson (1986) wrote that various aspects of choosing priorities in health care touch on medical ethics. He believes that it is not a question of a choice between ethics or economics. Without a wide use of economics in health care, inefficiencies will abound and decisions will be made less explicitly and hence less rationally (and ethically) than is desirable. Wilkinson argues that there are pressing clinical, research, economic and ethical reasons for an urgent review of the extent and impact of psychotherapeutic practices in the NHS. Such an understanding is needed to ensure the provision of efficient and effective mental health services within the context of general health services. The price of inefficiency, inexplicitness and irrationality in health care is paid for in death and sickness. Food for thought for counsellors.

How to get involved in research and evaluation

Supervision and case studies

The most common form of evaluation of counselling in Britain is through supervision of the counsellor's work. Supervision is considered essential to the ethical and competent practice of counselling. This form of reflective practice is the process by which adequate standards of counselling can be maintained through the continuous assessment of the counsellor's work. Not only does supervision monitor counselling by providing a setting in which individual counsellors or groups of counsellors have the opportunity to discuss their counselling regularly, but it operates at an organizational level. The cumulative effects of all individual experiences of supervision pervade the culture of counselling both at a national level, within its representative organization, the British Association for Counselling and Psychotherapy, and at a local level, in the practice setting.

While the peer review system of supervision is an essential part of the evaluation process, it takes place between individuals or groups of individuals—the insights gleaned remain confidential to those involved. A great deal of the material presented in supervision could be considered an informal type of case study (Tolley & Rowland 1995). It is a small step from supervision to documentation. Given that part of the aim of supervision is to establish good standards of practice, to develop the counsellor's knowledge and skills and to work with the counsellor's response to conducting the counselling, there is no reason why counsellors (with client permission) should not tape record their sessions, both as a learning tool and as a prelude to writing up the work as a case report. Case reports have a long history in clinical practice, but they are rarely reported in the counselling journals.

Preparation of case studies or case series studies (including a number of clients with clinically relevant characteristics in common) can be seen as part of on-going professional development (Parker 1995). As with other forms of qualitative research, what is lost in numerical precision is compensated for with accuracy of representation of the individuals concerned and their vivid direct insights.

Reflective practice should also demand that practitioners are informed of the findings of trials and systematic reviews as well as the content and status of current practice guidelines. Practice must be influenced by evidence even when not driven by it (Goss & Rowland 2000).

Audit

Audit is a useful tool for evaluating counselling. Audit is the process of critically reviewing clinical practices or services, and assessing the use of resources and outcomes for patients. As a result of the review, clinical standards, or standards of service provision, are defined and agreed. These must be capable of translation into explicit objective audit criteria, including expected outcomes. A period of implementation follows, after which the service is re-audited, to assess the extent to which standards are being met. The process of audit is on-going and cyclical.

Audit is a fairly simple evaluative process and many counsellors engage in it. Making use of routine audit and evaluation as part of everyday work ensures that standards and benchmarks for effectiveness are rigorously applied. Audit data can also provide evidence of a wider interest, especially if it can be collated with compatible forms of data from other agencies with large datasets, such as contributing to a practice research network.

Practice research networks

Practice research networks are valuable means to take clinical effectiveness audit and research forward. Parry (2000) describes the function of a practice network and gives examples of practice research networks in the UK. Typically, a practice research network consists of NHS departments whose members have agreed to gather and pool data relating to clinical outcomes, using the same set of measures, in order to enable analysis of aggregated and anonymized national datasets. These networks help practitioners to take a research-based approach to exploring outcomes in their own services, sharing the findings, and contributing to the development of national databases. With the advent of standardized packages for audit and evaluation, powerful indications of trends should be possible. Issues around equity of access, or different outcomes between different client groups or case types, may be more readily identified and addressed than at present. One example of such a network is the Society for Psychotherapy Research, which is a northern England collaboration of NHS psychotherapy services co-ordinated through the University of Leeds Psychological Therapies Research Centre. The British Psychological Society's Clinical Outcomes Research and Effectiveness Unit at University College, London, also co-ordinates a network in relation to patients with long-term, severe mental health problems.

Collaboration in trials

Whereas participation in audit and collaboration in a practice research network are feasible for most counsellors, other forms of research, such as conducting a controlled trial, or undertaking an economic analysis, may be more difficult to achieve. It is difficult, time-consuming and expensive to carry out large trials of counselling in primary care. Small trials will probably continue to be carried out, but they often do not have the power (number of patients) to detect differences in outcomes between groups. It is increasingly likely, and perhaps desirable, to undertake collaborative multicentre trials. The benefits of co-ordinating research include increased numbers and increased uniformity. Triallists and counsellors need to collaborate on the recruitment of patients, the intervention provided, the outcomes to be evaluated and the instruments utilized to measure them. Increased uniformity, enabling data to be pooled in a meta-analysis, can provide an estimate of the overall treatment effect across a large number of patients. This strengthens our understanding of the results of research (Rowland *et al.*, 2001).

Conclusions

Finally, it is important to return to the notion of quality. In his book, *Effectiveness and Efficiency*, Archie Cochrane (1972) wrote that we all recognize quality when we see it and particularly when we receive it. In cure, outcome plays an important part in determining quality, but it is certainly not the whole story. Other really important factors are kindliness and the ability to communicate well on the part of all members of the medical team. In care, these factors become very much more important. It is vital to remember that, as members of the primary care team, counsellors try to offer care as well as cure, and to consider both factors in evaluating counselling. There is a good deal of qualitative research to be done to understand the care and the cure, the treatment process and the outcomes that are desired by patients and GPs, and to incorporate this understanding into the measures we use to evaluate counselling. This is not to undermine any attempt to measure efficacy, but to emphasize the need for pragmatic, randomized controlled trials of counselling in primary care that have a greater emphasis on subjective symptoms, daily functioning and quality of life (King 1995) and on the qualities of the interventions which make patients feel better (Rowland *et al.*, 2001).

References

Altman, D. (1991) *Practical Statistics for Medical Research.* Chapman & Hall, London.

Anderson, S. and Hasler, J. (1979) Counselling in general practice. *Journal of the Royal College of General Practitioners*, **29**, 352–356.

Baker, M. and Kleijnen, J. (2000) The drive towards evidence-based health care. In *Evidence Based Counselling and Psychological Therapies* (Rowland, N. and Goss, S., eds). Routledge, London, pp. 13–29.

Baker, R., Allen, H., Gibson, S., Newth, J. and Baker, E. (1998) Evaluation of a primary care counselling service in Dorset. *British Journal of General P1ractice*, **48**, 1049–1053.

Balestrieri, M., Williams, P. and Wilkinson, G. (1988) Specialist mental health treatment in general practice: a meta-analysis. *Psychological Medicine*, **18**, 711–717.

Booth, H., Goodwin, I., Newnes, C. and Dawson, O. (1997) Process and outcome of counselling in general practice. *Clinical Psychology Forum 101*, **March**, 32–40.

Bower, P., Byford, S., Sibbald, B., Ward, E., King, M., Lloyd, M. and Gabbay, M. (2000) A randomised controlled trial of non-directive counselling, cognitive-behaviour therapy and usual general practitioner care for patients with depression. II Cost effectiveness. *British Medical Journal*, 321: 1389–1392.

Bower, P. and Sibbald, B. (2000) On-Site mental health in primary care: effects on professional practice. (Cochrane review) The Cochrane Library, Issue 3. Update Software, Oxford.

Bower, P., Rowland, N., Mellor-Clark, J., Heywood, P., Godrey, C. and Hardy, R. (in press) Effectiveness and cost effectiveness of counselling in primary care: updated. Cochrane Library.

Bower, P. and King, M. (2000) Randomised controlled trials in the evaluation of psychological therapies. In *Evidence Based Counselling and Psychological Therapies* (Rowland, N. and Goss, S., eds). Routledge, London, pp. 79–110.

British Association for Counselling (1997) *Codes of Ethics and Practice for Counsellors*. British Association for Counselling, Rugby.

Cape, J. (1998) Clinical practice guidelines for the psychotherapies. In *Rethinking Clinical Audit* (Davenhill, R. and Patrick, M., eds). Routledge, London, pp. 183–211.

Cape, J. and Parham, A. (1998) Relationship between practice counselling and referral to outpatient psychiatry and clinical psychology. *British Journal of General Practice*, **48**, 1477–1480.

Chilvers, C., Dewey, M., Fielding, K., Gretton, V., Miller, P., Palmer, B., Weller, D., Churchill, R., Williams, I., Bedi, N., Duggan, C., Lee, A. and Harrison, G. (2001) Antidepressant drugs and generic counselling for treatment of major depression in primary care: randomised trial with patient preference arms. *British Medical Journal*, **322**, 772–775.

Cochrane, A. (1972) *Effectiveness and Efficiency; Random Reflections on Health Services.* Nuffield Provincial Hospitals Trust and Cambridge University Press, Cambridge.

Coe, N., Ibbs, A. and O'Brien, J. (1996) *The Cost Effectiveness of Introducing Counselling into the Primary Care Setting in Somerset.* Somerset Health Authority.

Corney, R. (1995) The researcher's perspective. In *Counselling in Primary Health Care* (Keithley, J. and Marsh, G., eds). Oxford University Press, Oxford, pp. 286–295.

Craig, T. and Boardman, A. (1997) Common mental health problems in primary care. *British Medical Journal*, **307**, 576–577.

Department of Health (1991) *Research for Health.* Department of Health, London.

Department of Health (1993) *Research for Health.* Department of Health, London.

Department of Health (1998) *A First Class Service: Quality in the New NHS.* Department of Health, London.

Department of Health (1999) *National Service Framework for Mental Health.* NHS Executive, London.

Department of Health (2001) *Treatment Choice in Psychological Therapies and Counselling.* Department of Health, London.

Fairhurst, K. and Dowrick, C. (1996) Problems with recruitment in a randomised controlled trial of counselling in general practice: causes and implications. *Journal of Health Services Research,* 1, 77–80.

Field, M. and Lohr, K. (eds) (1990) *Clinical Practice Guidelines: Direction for a New Program.* National Academy Press, Washington, DC.

Friedli, K. and King, M. (1996) Counselling in general practice—a review. *Primary Care Psychiatry,* 2, 205–216.

Friedli, K., King, M., Lloyd, M. and Horder, J. (1997) Randomised controlled assessment of non directive psychotherapy versus routine general practitioner care. *Lancet,* 350, 1662–1665.

Friedli, K., King, M. and Lloyd, M. (2000) The economics of employing a counsellor in general practice: analysis of data from a randomised controled trial. *British Journal of General Practice,* 50, 276–283.

Gilbody, S. and Sowden, A. (2000) Systematic reviews in mental health. In *Evidence Based Counselling and Psychological Therapies* (Rowland, N. and Goss, S., eds). Routledge, London, pp. 147–170.

Goodwin, P., Feld, R., Warde, P. and Ginsberg, J. (1990) The costs of cancer therapy. *European Journal of Cancer,* 26, 223–225.

Grimshaw, J. and Russell, I. (1993) Achieving health gain through clinical guidelines l. Developing scientifically valid guidelines. *Quality in Health Care,* 2, 243–248.

Goss, S. and Rowland, N. (2000) Getting evidence into practice. In *Evidence Based Counselling and Psychological Therapies* (Rowland, N. and Goss, S., eds). Routledge, London, pp. 191–203.

Harray, A. (1975) The role of the counsellor in a medical centre. *New Zealand Medical Journal,* 82, 383–385.

Harvey, I., Nelson, S., Lyons, R., Unwin, C., Monaghan, S. and Peters, T. (1998) A randomised controlled trial and economic evaluation of counselling in primary care. *British Journal of General Practice,* 48, 1043–1048.

Hemmings, A. (1997) Counselling in primary care: a randomised controlled trial. *Patient Education and Counselling,* 32, 219–230.

Hemmings, A. (2000) Counselling in primary care: a review of the practice evidence. *British Journal of Guidance and Counselling,* 28, 233–252.

Keithley, J. and Marsh, G. (eds) (1995) *Counselling in Primary Health Care.* Oxford University Press, Oxford.

King, M. (1995) Evaluating the benefit of general practice based counselling services. In *Research Foundations for Psychotherapy Practice* (Aveline, M. and Shapiro, D., eds). John Wiley & Sons, Chichester, pp. 281–297.

King, M. (1997) Brief psychotherapy in general practice: how do we measure outcome? *British Journal of General Practice,* 46, 136–137.

King, M., Broster, G., Lloyd, M. and Horder, J. (1994) Controlled trials in the evaluation of counselling in general practice. *British Journal of General Practice,* 44, 29–32.

King, M., Sibbald, B., Ward, E., Bower, P., Lloyd, M., Gabbay, M. and Byford, S. (2000) Randomised controlled trial of non directive counselling, cognitive behavioural therapy and usual general practitioner care in the management of depression as well as mixed anxiety and depression in primary care. *Health Technology Assessment,* 4, 19.

Li Wan Po, A. (1998) *A Dictionary of Evidence Based Medicine.* Radcliffe Medical Press, Abingdon.

Marsh, G. and Barr, J. (1975) Marriage guidance counselling in a group practice. *Journal of the Royal College of General Practitioners,* 25, 73–75.

Maynard, A. (2000) Economics issues. In *Evidence Based Counselling and Psychological Therapies* (Rowland, N. and Goss, S., eds). Routledge, London, pp. 44–56.

Mays, N. and Pope, C. (1996) *Qualitative Research in Health Care.* BMJ Publishing Group, London.

McGrath, G. and Lowson, K. (1986) Assessing the benefits of psychotherapy: the economic approach. *British Journal of Psychiatry,* 150, 65–71.

McLeod, J. (2000) The contribution of qualitative research to evidence based counselling and psychotherapy. In *Evidence Based Counselling and Psychological Therapies* (Rowland, N. and Goss, S., eds). Routledge, London, pp. 111–126.

Mooney, G. (1984) Medical ethics: an excuse for inefficiency? *Journal of Medical Ethics,* 10, 183–185.

Mulrow, C. (1995) Rationale for systematic reviews. In *Systematic Rreviews* (Chalmers, I. and Altman, D., eds). BMJ Publishing Group, London, pp. 1–8.

NHS Centre for Reviews and Dissemination (1996) *Guidelines for Undertaking Systematic Reviews.* Report No. 4. University of York, York.

Oxman, A. (1995) Checklists for review articles. In *Systematic Reviews* (Chalmers, I. and Altman, D., eds). BMJ Publishing Group, London, pp. 75–88.

Parker, M. (1995) Practical approaches: case study writing. *Counselling,* 6 (1), 19–21.

Parry, G. (2000) Evidence based psychotherapy—an overview. In *Evidence Based Counselling and Psychological Therapies* (Rowland, N. and Goss, S., eds). Routledge, London, pp. 57–75.

Pringle, M. and Churchill, R. (1995) Randomised controlled trials in general practice. *British Medical Journal,* 311, 1382–1383.

Robinson, R. (1993) Cost effectiveness analysis. *British Medical Journal,* 307, 703–705.

Roth, A. and Fonagy, P. (1996) *What Works for Whom? A Critical Review of Psychotherapy Research.* Guilford Press, London.

Rowland, N., Bower, P., Mellor Clark, J., Heywood, P., Hardy, R. and Godfrey, C. (2001) Effectiveness and cost effectiveness of counselling in primary care. (Cochrane review). *The Cochrane Library,* Issue 3. Update Software, Oxford.

Rowland, N. and Goss, S. (eds) (2000) *Evidence-based Counselling and Psychological Therapies.* Routledge, London.

Rutledge, M. (1972) Counselling in general practice. *Australian Family Physician,* 1, 461–464.

Sackett, D., Richardson, W., Rosenberg, W. and Haynes, R. (1996) *Evidence Based Medicine.* Churchill Livingstone, London.

Sibbald, B., Addington Hall, J., Brenneman, D. and Freeling, P. (1996) Investigation of whether on site general practice counsellors have an impact on psychotropic drug prescribing rates and costs. *British Journal of General Practice,* 46, 63–67.

Simpson, S., Corney, R., Fitzgerald, P., and Beecham, J. (2000) A randomised controlled trial to evaluate the effectiveness and cost-effectiveness of counselling patients with chronic depression. *Health Technology Assessment,* 4, 36.

Smith, M., Glass, G. and Miller, T. (1980) *The Benefits of Psychotherapy.* John Hopkins University Press, Baltimore.

Tolley, K. and Rowland, N. (1995) *Evaluating the Cost Effectiveness of Counselling in Health Care*. Routledge, London.

Waydenfeld, D. and Waydenfeld, S. (1980) Counselling in general practice. *Journal of the Royal College of General Practitioners*, 30, 671–677.

Wilkinson, G. (1986) Psychoanalysis and analytic psychotherapy in the NHS—a problem for medical ethics. *Journal of Medical Ethics*, 12, 87–90.

Williams, A. (1992) Cost-effectiveness analysis: is it ethical? *Journal of Medical Ethics*, 18, 7–11.

Chapter 6

Counselling—the sceptical view

Myles Harris

No earthly good?

In rather leaden prose, the *Concise Oxford Dictionary* (1990) defines counselling as 'The process of assisting and giving guidance to clients especially by a trained person on a professional basis to resolve (esp.) personal, social, psychological problems and difficulties.' This tight, bureaucratic language does scant justice to one of the great phenomena of the twentieth century. There are said to be more counsellors in Britain today than GPs, and in the NHS the number of surgeries having direct access to a counsellor (usually in-house) has risen from around 5% in the early 1980s, to close to 40% today. An editorial in 1993 described 'an explosion of counselling' taking place in the UK (Laverty 1993).

Not surprisingly counsellors, given this increasingly pivotal role, often find themselves portrayed by society as priests. While in the past major accidents would be reported with photographs of chaplains kneeling by the side of the dead or dying, today the TV almost always announces that 'counsellors are present'. While this may not be true, viewers are often shown clips of a counsellor, usually a sympathetic, middle-aged woman talking perhaps of 'holding a patient in his/her distress'. This type of quasi religious language appeals to the public.

Counselling, however, is not a religious activity. It is a talking treatment aimed at getting patients to reveal their emotions. Counsellors believe that when patients are aware of their feelings they can act on them. What is considered important in a patient's conversation varies with a counsellor's training. There are many types of counsellor: non-directive therapists, dynamic therapists, interpersonal therapists, group therapists, cognitive behavioural therapists, Freudian, Jungian, Adlerian and Rogerian counsellors. Some counsellors are trained, some are not. Problems of definition abound.

Only one type of counselling, loosely termed cognitive therapy—psychological reconditioning and desensitization—is purely directive. Including such techniques as behaviour therapy and cognitive behaviour therapy, it offers symptom control rather than interpretation of the sufferer's anxieties. Most other forms of counselling are interpretations of human behaviour. Nearly all of them involve clients confessing their feelings and emotions to a therapist, often at great length. It is this latter type I will call 'confessional' counselling. In this chapter, unless cognitive or psychological methods (as opposed to purely psychotherapeutic methods) are specifically referred to, the word counselling means confessional counselling.

Confessional counselling is not just talking. It involves choice. Counsellors discuss choices of relationships, feelings, anxieties and fears entirely divorced from any over-arching code of right or wrong. Indeed both words tend to be excluded from their vocabulary. This is because counsellors say they are 'non-judgemental'. Actions are, for the counsellor, only 'appropriate' or 'inappropriate'. Confessional counselling seems to be a 'physiology' as it were, of social behaviour and the emotions, in which social gains or losses are like changes in metabolism or heart rate. They are either of net benefit to a patient or they are not. Because choice is ultimately dictated by how we feel, this represents man's first attempt to marry his physiology to his feelings.

Modern doctors frequently use the language of confessional counselling on their patients. Its vocabulary has invaded the consulting room in the past decade. A great deal of teaching in general practice employs counselling terms and ideas. Younger doctors talk about listening skills, mirroring, closure, empowerment, grief work and non-judgemental interviewing. The carefully non-discriminatory combination 'she/he' or 's/he' appears frequently in their writing and speech. These are all new words in the language of medicine, each with a specific moral and political meaning. What is interesting about counselling is that it has managed to pass itself off as quite the opposite—a neutral language. I believe this view is at best naive, at worst disingenuous. Counselling may well be a form of patient control. 'Words' as the astronomer Sir Fred Hoyle (1994) once said, 'are like harpoons, once you thrust them home they cannot be pulled out.'

History and sociology

It is important for doctors to be aware of the social, scientific and economic history of any treatments they use. This is especially true if the treatment is a language. Counselling dilemmas are regularly examined and discussed in magazines, the radio and on TV. Its theories have permeated into family and social life. So just as patients in the past expected antibiotics for a sore throat, today an increasing number expect to be referred to a counsellor. Moreover, as counselling skills become a compulsory part of a doctor's training, they will tend to be used more and more. If such treatment is ineffective or harmful a knowledge of its origins and development is a powerful tool in helping the doctor to decide not to prescribe it, or to explain to patients why they might not want to accept it.

Psychoanalysis and counselling share many similarities. Both are derived from the great confessional movements that swept Europe in the late nineteenth and early twentieth centuries. Although there is very little if any empirical evidence to support Freud's theory of the unconscious mind (Eysenk 1991), his belief in the therapeutic benefit of confessing one's hidden sexual desires to an analyst, was enthusiastically received by European intellectuals. Here was a secular explanation of our behaviour that dispensed with the superstition of religion, but retained the therapeutic benefits of confession.

Talking therapy, however, remained the province of the rich until the 1950s. Often taking months, years or even a lifetime, it was a pastime of those who did not have to go to a factory each day, stand waiting at a table or spend their days in the fields. It took the great American industrial boom in the early 1950s and in the 1960s to stimulate a demand for a form of relatively quick, affordable mass psychotherapy to a population that had more leisure to enjoy it. Along with fast food, cheap cars, mass air travel and widely available high fashion clothes, came an understandable desire for a new explanation of what constituted happiness. But it had, like the ever-growing piles of goods in the shops, to be cheap, easily available and simple to understand. Early counselling, which did not require years of training, and could be undertaken by almost anybody who could read (and some who could not) was born. Much of it was amateurish and silly, but gradually more serious, thoughtful philosophers such as Carl Rogers (1961) began to ponder how the self might be best developed in an increasingly material world.

Many models of counselling were developed. They have varied in popularity over the years. Rogerian counselling, problem-solving therapy, social work intervention, interpersonal therapy, psychodynamic counselling and Freudian analysis all have had their enthusiasts and their day. Of late, cognitive therapy has gained in popularity. Although many counsellors declare they are quite happy to use any treatment that works, it is hard to believe they do not have their 'first loves'; Jungians remain, in the heart if not in the head, Jungians for life.

Most lay people, however, are unaware there are many different types of counselling. When they talk about counselling they usually mean confessional counselling that relies heavily on the interpretation of questions such as 'Why am I nasty to my wife?', 'Why do I fear travelling on aircraft?' or 'Is fear of my mother the reason I cannot get an erection?'

From the 1950s to the 1980s, confessional counselling meant the teaching of the American therapist Carl Rogers (1902–1987). Rogers began life as a student minister at the Union Theological Seminary College in Wisconsin. He developed a theory of unconscious repression similar to Freud's, but one that did not dwell particularly on sexuality. Breaking with religious belief, Carl Rogers reasoned that people were only unhappy or neurotic because they were unaware of what was going on in their minds. People are essentially good and seek good. Blocks and prejudices cause us all to act irrationally. Rogers developed 'person-centred therapy' (which, unable to obtain certification as a psychotherapist, he later called counselling (Totton 1999)), in which the patient, helped by non-directive counsellors, uncovered the true nature of their psyche in a process called 'self-actualization'. Since only you can know the blocks in your mind, nobody else can judge your actions. Indeed to censure or criticize a person only made matters worse, thus the rigorous insistence of counsellors that they are 'non-judgemental'.

Rogers' ideas, a version of Rousseau's myth of inner nobility (Chambers 1984, pp. 1154–1155), particularly appealed to a deeply Christian nation that due to science had lost its belief in God. Some of this frustration was reflected in the beliefs of the hippie movement, which was much influenced by Rogers' ideas. 'Letting it all hang out' and 'doing your own thing' became warped interpretations of the master's suggestion that true freedom could only be obtained by self-knowledge. The hippie movement was hugely influential in America, especially among the middle classes, and even when it collapsed in squalor and drugs, its central beliefs of unfettered choice in sexuality, emotions and loyalties, left a lasting mark on American life.

Helped by the expanding sciences of marketing and business management, with which it shares a common vocabulary, counselling spread through churches, industry and government. Although the first university course in counselling began in the 1960s in Britain it was not until the 1980s, when counsellors achieved widespread television coverage at spectacular disasters such as the Kings Cross fire and the Zeebrugge ferry disaster, that counselling became popular. In these horrific accidents counsellors were rarely if ever seen on TV, but it was widely believed they were present. What exactly they were supposed to do for people with their legs trapped under fallen masonry, trembling with deathly cold after being fished from the North Sea, or deprived by death of children, husbands or wives was never explained. In the public eye counsellors began to take on almost magical powers as secular 'interpreters' of random catastrophes.

A similar myth, reflecting the helplessness and shock people felt in Britain at early defeats to the German Army in the Great War, was that of the angels of Mons (Terraine 1980). It was widely believed at the time that angels with flaming swords had been seen in the sky covering the British retreat from Mons in 1914. If help is not there, people invent it.

By 1990, like the angels of Mons, the counsellor entered global mythology. It was then that the writers of the cult science fiction TV series, *Star Trek*, the longest running series ever shown on worldwide TV, introduced a character called Counsellor Troi. Troi, a beautiful but rather forbidding woman, was an 'empath', a superior being from a distant planet whose inhabitants possessed an extraordinary sixth sense, an ability to read other people's feelings to perfection, or in a phrase so often used by therapists, 'to feel their pain'. In an episode in which Troi is deprived of this sense, and becomes just another human being, her grief and disorientation almost brings her to suicide. This is a parable of the twentieth century. The modern fall from grace is a loss of one's ability to feel another's pain. It is easy to sympathize with this in a world of brutalizing technology and mass production techniques applied to medicine. It is little wonder counselling has such a deep appeal.

Does it work?

Evidence for and against counselling is uneven. Those studies that show an advantage are often criticized on the grounds of methodology. Indeed, much of the evidence is flawed either by a lack of numbers, poor follow up or difficulties with definitions. In many studies it is difficult to discover what sort of therapy has been employed. As a result the results are very difficult for a doctor without statistical expertise to interpret, and there are some surprising disparities between theory and practice.

The first difficulty in any test of the effects of counselling is that the general public thinks it works. There is a built-in subjective bias in its favour. Churchill *et al.* (1999) in a review of the literature on randomized controlled studies of counselling report that the Defeat Depression Survey 'found that 86% of responders believed "counselling" to be an effective intervention for depression, and 90% agreed that people with depression should be offered it'. Therefore, in any trial of counselling, a large proportion of patients must be biased in its favour. You cannot blind a trial so people do not know if they are seeing a GP or a counsellor. Nor is this bias confined to patients. As Freidli *et al.* (1997) report: 'although most GPs were aware that no proof of efficacy for brief psychotherapy existed, general practitioners were never the less hesitant to refer patients in a randomised control trial in which there was only a 50% chance of seeing a therapist'. Balint and many others have pointed out how important the attitude of the doctor is in the success of a treatment. Such an attitude must transmit itself to patients.

This may be one of the reasons why, even in the absence of objective evidence, patients state they feel so much better after being counselled. In 1983, Ashurst *et al.* studied 726 neurotic patients aged between 16 and 65 years, randomly assigned to counselling or routine GP treatment. They had in the past received large numbers of sedatives and other mood-altering drugs. It was hoped that counselling would decrease their need for such medication. No significant differences were found, but the patients themselves were impressed with the help they got. This pattern—no other clear effect but satisfied patients—is common. In 1978, McCord traced 250 people who had received Rogerian counselling plus social skills training 30 years earlier and recorded that 80% said they benefited from treatment; however, 'they had a worse health, criminal and employment record than a matched 250 strong control group'. This is a finding which would be repeated in various forms over the years.

In 1997, Friedli *et al.* compared the efficacy of psychotherapists with GPs in family practice. 'Between one and 12 sessions of (Rogerian) psychotherapy were given over 12 weeks in 14 different general practices in North London. Of 136 patients with emotional difficulties, mainly depression, 70 were randomly assigned to the therapist (in the practice) and 66 to the general practitioner.' The trial was robust. Counselling sessions lasted 50 minutes; GP sessions were 'as usual'. While there were no significant differences in outcome between the two groups, those patients who received psychotherapy reported greater satisfaction than those treated by their GPs. Hemmings (1997), in a similarly well-structured trial, reported similar findings. There were no differences between those patients who received brief psychotherapy and those who saw their GP, but patients preferred counselling. Hemmings, however, thought that the lack of difference could have been affected by the fact that a GP representative and three counsellors met to discuss working practices.

In contrast, in 1994, Boot *et al.* in a randomized trial of counselling versus GP care found that a statistically significant number of counselled patients felt better compared with those who attended their GPs and used fewer psychotropic drugs. However, although the findings were statistically sound the authors report the level of drug prescribing in both those patients seen by their GPs and those seen by a counsellor was low to begin with. Follow up after six weeks was difficult to evaluate due to patient attrition. The authors felt the trial would have been more useful if the patients could have been assessed at one year. This did not prove possible.

Certain types of (non-confessional) counselling have a good record and are becoming increasingly popular. In *What Works for Whom*, Fonagy (1998) argues that highly structured psychological treatments seem to work better in a far larger number of disorders than psychodynamic therapies. Behaviour modification and cognitive behaviour therapy are highly effective in post-traumatic stress disorder, eating disorders, male impotence, social skills training phobias and school refusal and many workers regard cognitive behaviour therapy as the treatment of choice in obsessive compulsive disorder and agoraphobia. Churchill *et al.* (1999), comparing the effect of counselling with antidepressants in severe depression, found a benefit from social work counselling and problem-solving therapy, but complained that no studies had been published evaluating the effectiveness of generic counselling for depression. They suggested that GPs should be cautious in sending patients with major depressive illness to counsellors unless they knew exactly what sort of therapy would be used.

Is there then any role for confessional counselling? Even if counselling did not 'work' in the way that a hernia operation works, it may have a useful social role. Mental disorders account for 9% of all GP consultations (OPCS 1980). People like counselling and many GPs find counsellors a useful place to send their 'heartsink' patients, those on whom every other form of treatment has been tried without effect. Such patients are time-consuming and many present problems that have no solution. Counsellors not only free doctors to spend more time on less intractable problems, but they are less inclined to make pointless referrals to specialists. This keeps costs down. But whether counsellors are cheaper than GPs is arguable. P. Bower (personal communication) feels they are likely to be no more costly than GPs, but Rowland and Goss (see Chapter 5) write, 'It is dispiriting to note the lack of evidence of cost-effectiveness of counselling in primary care'. And Harvey *et al.* (1998) in a randomized controlled trial and economic evaluation of counselling in primary care found there was 'no clear difference in the cost-effectiveness of the two interventions. Purchasers should take account of these findings in allocating resources within primary care'. They should do. A GP (using the example of a locum and thereby discounting the various built-in allowances of full-time GPs) earns at current rates around £37–40 an hour, but sees one patient every eight minutes. Counsellors on the other hand expect to set aside at least an hour for each client.

In summary, the statistical, evidential and financial case is not proved for many types of counselling, and probably never will be. The difficulties of mounting large-scale trials, not least in attracting sufficient funds to carry them out, are great and the philosophical issues associated with counselling are too entangled with social and political bias to make for cool judgement. As we have seen, confessional counselling is not just a pure treatment, but a social and historical movement as well. This does not mean that talking to your patients is useless. Human beings are social animals and talking is as essential as food, but what sort of talk, to whom and for how long remains open to serious question. Some talk can be very dangerous indeed.

All true except the facts?

Counselling, like all professions, assumes certain ideas to be self evidently true. Physicists believe because the universe is continuously expanding at a vast speed it began as a single mathematical point, a singularity. Big bang is logical, but it is not necessarily true.

Counselling's 'big bang' is the sudden and widespread belief that talking about your troubles to a trained therapist is helpful, and the more helpful and unobtrusive the listener, and the more skilled, the more likely it is that patients will arrive at a true insight into their difficulties. However, what is obvious and what is true may not be the same thing at all. We have only to recall the belief that six weeks' strict bed rest following a myocardial infarct to 'rest' the heart seemed, 30 years ago, so obvious that only the perverse would question it.

Counselling's axioms

Assumption 1: talking to a properly trained counsellor rather than just a friend or relative is essential; only properly qualified and registered counsellors should practice in the primary care team; standards are important

While this may seem self-evident, Christensen and Jacobsen (1994), in an exhaustive review of 42 papers in the US literature, found only one study in which a trained therapist produced better results than an untrained one. This was not confirmed when the experiment was repeated. In 12 of the studies, paraprofessionals (untrained lay therapists) did better than trained ones. In the remainder of the studies there was no difference between trained and untrained therapists. Nor does experience seem important. Strupp and Hadley (1997) reported on two groups of disturbed college students sent for therapy. One group was assigned to either analytically or experientially orientated therapists with an average of 23 years of therapeutic experience. The other group was referred to a matched group of liberal arts college professors with no clinical experience or training. There were no differences in outcome. Stein and Lambert (1984) further compared the results of treating 'real clinical problems using such treatment approaches as psychodynamic client centred therapy and behavioural methods'. They found no difference in outcome between trained and untrained therapists. All these findings, because of their importance, were exhaustively re-analysed and meta-analysed, but the same result was always found.

Assumption 2: patients feel better if they are able to talk about a problem; 'getting it off your chest' makes for a swifter recovery

In 1996 a randomized controlled trial of psychological debriefing for victims of road traffic accidents, found that those who received debriefing had a worse result in respect of persisting symptoms and emotional distress than controls who were not debriefed. Despite the small numbers, the finding, reported the authors (Hobbs *et al.* 1996), 'was clinically convincing'. Bisson *et al.* (1997) carried out a randomized controlled trial of debriefing of victims of acute burns. Those debriefed did significantly worse than those left untreated.

Following a review of the Cochrane database (1999), which suggested that rapid or single-session debriefing significantly increased the risk of post-traumatic stress disorder, Wessely *et al.* (1999) advised, 'compulsory debriefing of victims of accidents should cease'.

Counsellors will say that this was because such debriefings were either too short or not of the 'right' type. That may be. The fact remains that in a highly specific, closely controlled set of circumstances, talking about a trauma or 'getting it off your chest' might worsen symptoms. Moreover in a separate study, the use of technique of 'a seven stage semi-structured approach covering an introduction, the facts, thoughts and impressions, emotional reactions and normalisation and planning for the future and finally disengagement' (Bisson *et al.* 1997) exactly mimics long-term counselling.

Assumption 3: having time to talk through problems with a patient is beneficial; it gives the patient time to clarify the issues in his or her own mind

This statement is difficult to reconcile with the quite small differences, if any, measured between 'as usual' treatment by GPs and treatment given by counsellors (Wessely *et al.* 1999). An 'as usual' GP consultation lasts about seven minutes. A counsellor often spends 50 minutes with a patient on several occasions. Even if we accept that counsellors are better at treating emotional difficulties, why are their results so disproportionately small?

This finding is further confirmed by a literature review by Churchill *et al.* (1999) who found no evidence that the length of time a patient is counselled made a difference to the outcome. A 'dose–response' relationship was not found. Do patients get better just by the act of being counselled, just as some patients recover from tonsillitis by the act of being given antibiotics?

Assumption 4: patients can suffer the effects of hidden traumas that can affect them psychologically; only when a skilled analyst or therapist helps them to remember, do they start on the road to recovery

In the 1980s in the United States a widespread belief gained ground that a large number of Americans had been sexually abused as children and the trauma was so severe they had repressed all memory of it. So-called 'recovered memory' is of particular interest because it incorporates all the essential beliefs of confessional counselling— repression, denial, unconscious memories, an inability to see one's emotions clearly, and disordered behaviour. (An account of this extraordinary mass delusion can be read in *Victims of Memory* by Mark Pendergrast 1997.)

Advocates of the recovered memory syndrome were convinced that hundreds of thousands of US adults, possibly even millions, had been sexually abused as children but had completely suppressed all memory of it. The result, they claimed, was a huge incidence of depression, neurosis, antisocial behaviour, marital breakdown, suicide and anxiety among Americans. Worse, the child molesters themselves, so the theory went, would, when confronted with the evidence, often themselves go into denial. Some zealots even believed that for someone to deny that the syndrome existed was strongly suggestive they too had been assaulted.

However in 'Creating false memories' in *Scientific American*, Elizabeth Loftus (1997) examined the ways in which patients could be induced to reconstruct their past. An experiment adding a false event, a trivial incident about spilling a bowl of punch at a party, to an anecdotal account of childhood, had no effect when it was offered to interviewees at the first interview, but was recalled by 18% at the second interview and 25% at the third interview. It seems a therapist can create a memory that he or she may later go on to treat.

Commenting on the phenomenon of repressed memory, in 1988 the *Lancet* (Lipian 1988) reminded its readers that evidence for unconscious repression of painful memories to protect the organism had 'never been empirically validated'. And 'contrary to theory and prediction', repressed memories of abuse 'often get worse rather than better as therapy proceeds and hidden traumatic memories surge forth' (Boakes 1995). Boakes reminds us that 'despite 60 years of attempts, efforts to study repression in the laboratory have failed to produce evidence in support'. Similar conclusions were reached by Pope and Hudson (1995).

The repressed memory phenomenon demonstrates how easy it is for a therapist, however unwittingly, to implant ideas and recollections into a patient's mind, only to have them retold as actual historical events. Moreover does this phenomenon only relate to the implanting of memories of distinct events? The possibility, merely by unconscious gesture and expression, of a counsellor 'microediting' a patient's account of their symptoms surely must be given serious consideration? Such 'microediting' need not have anything to do with child abuse. Pedestrian, but clinically significant, recollections could be suggested to patients with neither counsellor nor patient being aware they were false.

Conclusions and suggestions

Doctors and therapists are only too human and therefore constantly on the look out for a Holy Grail, whether it be the perfect antidepressant or an antibiotic to which bacteria will never develop resistance. Nearly all new treatments enjoy a vogue. Barbiturates, tranquillizers, tonsillectomies and antibiotics were all overprescribed when they first become available.

This is because there is a natural history of medical expectation. When an advance in treatment occurs there is initial scepticism, followed by cautious dabbling, and when it is found to work, overcompensatory enthusiasm. After some time doubts—usually voiced outside the profession—are raised, scandals about side effects exhumed, and opinions revised. In the end the treatment settles down to a compromise.

In addition, understanding of the true nature of a disease can be difficult. For example, stomach ulcers were said for many years to be caused by the non-specific but readily understood term 'stress'. But doctors were vague as to the reason for this, or what they meant by stress. Some psychoanalysts thought that a gastric ulcer was a symptom of a deeper desire to return to the mother's breast, a breast hunger! Surgeons on the other hand took a practical view of the problem. The stomach produces acid. Some stomachs produce more acid than others. In the latter, therefore, there is a higher risk of direct damage to the gastric mucosa. Had somebody suggested that ulcers might be caused by infection he would have been thought mad. Yet, as LeFanu (1999) points out, all the evidence was there to implicate bacteria in this disorder. Pathologists could see them in gastric washings. The obvious in science is often invisible until somebody points it out.

We smile and nod our heads at such blindness, but can we be sure we are not making similar mistakes? Is counselling one of these mistakes? And if it is an important mistake how might we protect our patients from its consequences?

It is for these reasons we should be cautious about allowing any further development of counselling in its present form in general practice. Not only does it not pass the sort of criteria we expect of new drugs or operations, it may also have extremely damaging social side effects.

Mental hygienism: a clean mind in a clean body

Counselling is not only a treatment, but a political, symbolic and religious language. It tries to explain why we are distressed or ill in terms of our feelings. Feelings demand explanations. But as with all religious or political explanations it is often the language that shapes reality, not the reality which shapes the language. This poses a danger of mental hygienism.

By the skilful use of language, counsellors hope to alter human behaviour. It is why counselling conversations are hedged around with ritually avoided words. The principle of 'unconditional regard' means that often accurate and useful descriptions of behaviour such as 'greedy' 'nasty' 'wrong' and 'wicked' are abhorred by counsellors.

'Judgementalism' they find worrying, although making judgements on other people is the very stuff of society. A non-judgemental society would collapse into anarchy and chaos. So would one based on symbolism—upon which much counselling language relies. A counsellor objecting to having to fill missed appointment slots with fresh patients to cut costs writes that 'the symbolic importance of the counsellor waiting, reflecting on the emptiness and receiving the (missing) patient's unconscious communication was outside the finance officer's repertoire of ideas' (Bravesmith 1999). But how long would it be before cardiac surgeons sat in empty operating theatres contemplating the resemblance of the room to an empty heart? Or entire medical out-patients sessions were kept deliberately empty as a symbol of man's flight from the prospect of death? All the staff, of course, would be on full pay.

And language used in this manner can rapidly become a straitjacket. In clinical discussions with a counsellor it is only too often necessary to put a guard on one's tongue for fear of giving offence. Only one type of language can be used, the correct, non-judgemental language. All other forms are banned. It is why outsiders so frequently comment on the rigid, conformist language of counsellors, their stereotyped gestures, their fear of certain types of words or phrases.

This conformism can rapidly translate to patients, who begin to talk in the same way as their counsellors. And because this language is often sterile and artificial it can, like religious language, be a substitute for real relationships, real conversation and real action. This is of particular danger in families where communications have broken down almost completely. Under intensive (and often addictive) therapy, patients can often retreat into a world of therapy and psychobabble, from which they refuse to emerge.

'Jane' (a composite) who is grossly overweight and very fond of chocolate has had back pain for years. No other treatment having worked, her GP, in desperation, suggests counselling. Some weeks later accompanied, as usual, by her silent, rather terrified-looking husband, she returns to the surgery announcing she is transformed. Her back pain continues undiminished but she tells the doctor she is now beginning to see what has been wrong with her life all along. As a second child, she was not given enough attention by her parents. Her multiplicity of symptoms, two failed marriages, her alienation from her family are all due to this. She is beginning to 'work through' her conflicts and with further 'exploration of her inner space' is confident she will be able to resolve her pain. She hints at the possibility of being abused as a child. When the GP tries to point out that she still weighs over 17 stone and has a large bag of sweets poking out of her handbag, and that her weight, rather than any childhood conflict, might be the cause of her back pain, she flounces out of the room. The GP listens to her bullying her husband down the corridor. Nobody, he thinks to himself, has ever had the courage to tell her she is fat, cruel, greedy and selfish.

Even more dangerous is the counsellor armed with powers of certification.

'Fred' and 'Mary' (composites), married for 20 years with a good home, apply to adopt a child and are sent to a confessional counsellor to assess their suitability. Although enormously fond of children, and very good with them, Fred refers to women as 'girls', calls all immigrants 'blacks' and the disabled 'crippled'. It transpires that Fred is a life-long devotee of fox hunting, believes that most illegal immigrants should be deported on the decision of an immigration officer, and is keen to see the death penalty restored for murder. He is uneasy at the idea of women working. He feels it undermines the cohesion of the family. He makes no secret of his beliefs to the adoption counsellor who in any event, alerted by his language, would have ferreted them out.

Is he likely to be recommended by the counsellor as a fit person to adopt? The answer to that is simply no. These views, interpreted by counsellors, and initially diagnosed by Fred's language, would suggest that the applicant has a rigid, unbending personality, harbours deep hostility toward certain disadvantaged groups in the community, feels threatened by an equal partnership with women and has a large streak of cruelty in his nature. He obviously needs extensive therapy. Yet he is only expressing legitimate political views, all allowed by law, which 40 years ago were the mainstream of respectable thought. And 20 years from now, such are the vagaries of fashion and politics, they may be respectable again. Nor is it unreasonable to suppose that had 'Fred' been the mirror opposite, politically correct in his language, a man devoted to womens' issues, sensitive to the plight of immigrants, abhorring all forms of violence, he would have gained a much more sympathetic hearing.

Yet both descriptions are 'only' language. In Fred's case it is his failure to conform to a particular language that proves his undoing. Counselling is just as much a belief system as Christianity, Hinduism, Socialism or Liberalism. Counsellors deny this vehemently, claiming they are apolitical and non-judgemental.

This assertion, however, fails in the face of what I call the state executioner conundrum. A theoretical case is put to a counsellor; a state executioner approaches her complaining of his unease while beheading people for crimes such as drug dealing, 'witchcraft' and sodomy. He is convinced these crimes merit the death penalty, but he finds the sentences increasingly difficult to carry out. He has developed a phobia of the large crowds that gather to watch him at work. As he wants to keep his job, which he considers an honourable and moral occupation, he would like a course of therapy to strengthen his resolve. Would the counsellor, being non-judgemental, offer him therapy on these terms? I have been unable to find a counsellor who would accept this commission! Doctors on the other hand asked the same question, say they are obliged to treat anyone, however repugnant their views or occupation. Medicine is politically neutral, counselling cannot be.

With these problems in mind we might look at a way that counselling could be of useful service to patients while avoiding the dangers of concealed judgementalism, dependence and politicization.

Friends and family rediscovered: the end of counselling as a state licensed friendship service

There seems an overwhelming case that counselling should be deprofessionalized. Patients need people to listen to them, not necessarily their doctors, but not a pair of ears paid for by the state (or private industry) that only listen for a set of psychological reflexes in tune with the latest politically correct nostrums.

Nor do we need a counselling service bent on unpicking family ties. A recent UK government proposal (Sunday Times 2000) suggests appointing a trained counsellor, or 'mentor' to every teenager aged between 13 and 19 in the country. In effect this is appointing state counsellors to interpose themselves between children, their parents, friends, schools and family. What is so terrifying about this is a mindset that has no concept of the important ties that bind society.

This idea, and similar proposals, stem from claims that in modern society people are lonely, isolated and have nobody to talk to. Few studies have been done to verify the claim that people are lonelier today than they were 50 years ago. But if these claims are true then further alienation stoked by professionals cannot be the answer. Given the serious objections raised to the intellectual and scientific basis of counselling it would surely be better to replace counsellors throughout the NHS (and the state in general) with a corps of unpaid, voluntary 'listeners'. They would be chosen perhaps by the same process we choose another cornerstone of our liberties, our lay magistrates, ordinary people prepared to sit and listen to the troubled, the grieving and the unhinged, but this time not to judge or punish, but to help. The advantage of 'listeners' over counsellors is that they would be drawn from a huge cross-section of society, of all views and opinions, and would more closely reflect reality for the patient, offering him the opportunity to talk not in the artificial and sterile context of 'therapy', but to a person as ordinary as themselves. One realizes that immediately there would be attempts to bureaucratize such volunteers with 'introductory' courses that quickly developed into 'management' courses, as there has been in the last few years with lay magistrates.

Lay magistrates used to be true amateurs. Here the law would be of help. Like the traditional lay magistrate, the listener's status as a true amateur would be defined in law, and protected from the attentions of the state or counselling.

It is likely they would do a good job, and would cost little. Prison visitors do an excellent job, as do lay pastors. To be a 'listener' would soon be a job of considerable status. Patients with various diseases such as diabetes, AIDs or multiple sclerosis, would make excellent 'listeners' for those afflicted with the same illness.

In addition, and as a further protection for patients, given the evidence of Loftus *et al.* (1997) about implanting ideas, it seems essential that anybody who offered treatment by listening—either a 'traditional' counsellor or a listener—should by law be obliged to give their patients a short resume of their social beliefs, religious affiliations, political party membership, sexual preferences or any other material that might unconsciously influence the way they treat their patients. Just saying that counsellors are 'non-judgemental' is fatuous. We are all judgemental. In the strange, one-sided conversation that occurs in a counsellor's office, patients have a right to know something of the person they are talking to. Counselling will resist such reforms. Or worse it will gloss them over with a set of mission statements about 'commitment to change'—but do nothing.

The future

The profession will be forced to change. It is hard to make predictions but it is reasonable to assume that one of the most potent forces to affect counselling in the future (as it will all professions) will be the information revolution.

The internet of the future, linked to domestic TV screens and offering far faster connectivity and download times, will pose an enormous problem to counsellors— and to others selling talking treatments. In 10 years' time it will be as easy to consult a counsellor on the web in London, as it will be a Reike practitioner in Santa Barbara or a tarot reader in Moscow. Such global consultations will be in 'real time', opening an enormous unregulated market in cheap personal advice. In addition, bizarre digital 'avatars', computer simulacrums of attractive-looking human beings programmed with a set of life-like responses, will make their appearance. Ideally suited to simple 'counselling' and mimicking many of its fundamental techniques, they will operate by using open-ended questions, echoing the final words of a patient's sentence, as well as programming themselves with the patient's Christian name from their credit card. Mary: 'I am worried about Jim'. Avatar: 'Why are you worried about Jim, Mary?'

Most people will know avatars are not real, but they will be as addictive as 'Doom'. It is amusing to think of a world where an argument with your children or a disagreement with the bread toaster can be resolved at the flourish of a remote control and a swipe of a credit card. The huge wall TV screen in your kitchen lights up: 'This is June, your virtual domestic minor incident counsellor. How can I help you?' After talking to such a creature glowing on your kitchen wall, the real thing—a flesh and blood NHS counsellor—will seem something of a disappointment!

As all professions rely on a monopoly, usually one of certification, the only way that 'flesh and blood' counsellors are likely to hold their competitive edge against the internet is by entering the market for the sale of medical certificates, especially within the NHS. Just as British GPs have only survived because they have a monopoly on access to specialists—except in an emergency you cannot obtain an NHS specialist's advice without a GP's letter—so counsellors will find they will need a regulatory role in society in order to make themselves indispensable. Apart from their own internal standards 'industry' they might, for example, offer certificates of 'social health' for employment, for work in the caring professions or, as in the case of Britain's adolescents, become psychological 'lollipop men' (renamed of course 'teen-crossing patrol attendants') regulating the transition from childhood to adulthood. The right to be unhappy, to dissent, to remain perversely ill, nasty, solitary, obsessed, sexist, deluded, visionary, to be guilty, greedy or horrible will then be threatened by mental hygienists. Only a 'prescribed' happiness will be on offer: of uniform emotions, actions and thoughts. This prescription, however, is written on water.

Fortunately human beings show an inexhaustible capacity for guile, self-delusion and dissimulation—qualities that, along with our knowledge of good and evil, are of immense evolutionary advantage. As a result 'chats' rarely work and formalized chats work least of all. As the reckless Mr Toad in *The Wind in the Willows*—a Rogerian case of badly adjusted social attitude if there ever was one—declared on emerging from a long, reproving chat in Badger's study for stealing bright red motor cars:

> Oh yes, yes, in *there*! I'd have said anything in *there*. You are so eloquent dear Badger, and so moving, and so convincing and put all your points so frightfully well—you can do anything you like with me in there and you know it. But I've been searching my mind since, and going over things in it, and I find I am not a bit sorry or repentant really, so it is no earthly good saying I am; now is it? (Graham 1988).

References

Allen, R.E. (ed.) (1990) *The Concise Oxford Dictionary*, 8th edn. Oxford University Press, Oxford.

Ashurst, P.M. and Ward, D.F. (1983) *An Evaluation of Counselling in General Practice. Final Report of the Leverhulme Counselling Project.* Mental Health Foundation, London.

Bisson, J.I., Jenkins, P.L., Alexander, J. and Bannister, C. (1997) Randomised controlled trial of psychological debriefing for victims of acute burns trauma. *British Journal of Psychiatry*, **170**, 78–81.

Boakes, J. (1995) Repressed memories. *Lancet*, **346**, 1048–1049.

Boot, D., Gillies, P., Fenelon, R., Reubin, Wilkins, M. and Gray, P. (1994) Evaluation of the short term impact of counselling in general practice. *Patient Education and Counselling*, **24**, 79–89.

Bravesmith, A. (1999) Counselling in Primary Care. Routledge, London.

Chambers (1984) *Jean Jaques Rousseau.* Chambers Biographical Dictionary. Chambers, Edinburgh.

Christenson, A. and Jacobsen, N.S. (1994) Who (or what) can do psychotherapy? *Psychological Science*, **5** (1), 8–14.

Churchill, R., Dewey, H., Gretton, C., Duggan, C., Chilvers and Lee, A. (1999) Should general practitioners refer patients with major depression to counsellors? A review of the evidence. *British Journal of General Practice*, **49**, 737–743.

Eysenk, H.J. (1991) *Freud Fifty Years On*. University of Leeds Review No. 33. University of Leeds, Leeds.

Fonagy, P. and Roth, P. (1998) *What Works for Whom?* Guilford Press, New York.

Friedli, K., King, M., Lloyd, M. and Horder, J. (1997) Controlled assessment of non directive psychotherapy versus routing general practitioner care. *Lancet,* **350**, 1662–1665.

Graham, K. (1988) *Wind in the Willows*. Victor Gollancz, London.

Harvey, I., Nelson, S.S., Lyons, R.A., Unwin, C., Monaghan, S. and Peters, T.S. (1998) A randomised controlled trial and economic evaluation of counselling in primary care. *British Journal of General Practice,* **48**, 1043–1048.

Hemmings, A. (1997) Counselling in primary care. A randomised controlled trial. *Patient Education and Counselling,* **32**, 219–230.

Hobbs, M., Mayou, R., Harrison, B., and Worlock, P. (1996) A randomised controlled trial of psychological debriefing for victims of road accidents. *British Medical Journal,* **313**, 1125–1136.

Hoyle, S.F. (1994) *Home is Where the Wind Blows*. University Science Books, Mill Valley CA.

Laverty, P. (1993) A counsellor in every practice? *British Medical Journal,* **306**, 2–3.

LeFanu, J. (1999) *The Rise and Fall of Modern Medicine*. Little Brown & Co., London.

Lipian, M. (1988) Fading reveries repressed memory madness in the UK. *Lancet,* **351**, 00–00.

Loftus, E.F. (1997) Creating false memories. *Scientific American,* **272**, 51–55.

McCord, S. (1978) Counselling and accountability. *Journal of the British Association of Counselling,* **00**, 14.

OPCS (1980) *National Morbidity Statistics*. Office of Population Census and Surveys, London.

Pendergrast, M. (1997) *Victims of Memory*. Harper Collins, London.

Pope, H.G. and Hudson, J.L. (1995) Can memories of childhood sexual abuse be surpressed? *Psychological Medicine,* **25**, 121–126.

Rogers, C.R. (1961) *On Becoming a Person. A Therapist's View of Psychotherapy*. Houghton Mifflin, Boston (published by Constable, London in 1967).

Stein, D.M. and Lambert, M.S. (1984) On the relationship between therapist experience and psychotherapy outcome. *Clinical Psychology Review,* **4**, 127–142.

Strupp, H. and Hadley, S. (1979) Specfic versus non specific factors in psychotherapy? A controlled study of outcome. *Archives of General Psychiatry,* **36**, 1125–1136.

Sunday Times (2000) Government pledge for teenage mentors. *Sunday Times,* 30 January.

Terraine, J. (1980) *The Smoke and the Fire. Myths and Anti Myths of War 1861–1945*. Sidgwick & Jackson, London.

Totton, N. (1999) The baby and the bathwater: professionalisation in psychotherapy and counselling. *British Journal of Guidance and Counselling,* **27** (3), 313–314.

Wessely, S., Rose, S. and Bisson, J. (1999) Systematic review of brief psychological interventions for the treatment of immediate trauma related symptoms and the prevention of PST. *Cochrane Database* (http://www.cochrane.revabstr/ab000560.htm).

Acknowledgment

I am grateful to the Social Affairs Unit for permission to use my 'Mr Toad Anecdote' from report No. 20. 'Magic in the Surgery' (Harris 1994 p. 35).

Chapter 7

Counselling across social, sexual and ethnic differences

Ali Zarbafi

Introduction

In this chapter I shall look at how 'differences' across ethnic, gender and class categories rear their heads in the context of primary care. Primary care is a setting in which the nature of the work and the range of patients pose constant challenges to counsellors and other primary health care team members, both in their work with patients/clients and with each other. I shall reflect on some of these challenges before discussing how we respond to 'difference'.

The primary care setting

The 'atmosphere' in a general practice surgery is often one of a very tangible urgency. This is not surprising given the work involved. Staff are faced on a day-to-day basis with illness and death. Loss, disappointment, impotence, a fear of not knowing, a need to know, hope, joy and relief are all feelings shared by the doctors, nurses, health visitors and receptionists, as well as the patients. Anxiety stems from the bewildering range of physical and non-physical complaints presented at the practice.

In this setting, the GP is the 'gatekeeper'. By this I mean the key decision-maker, who either treats the patient or decides where the patient should go for tests or more specialized help. As the GP has very little time, there is a sense of speed. The short time spent on individual consultations, and the medical model, which prioritizes checking for physical symptoms for any complaint, *defends the doctors from being overwhelmed and thus contains their anxieties* and enables them to work effectively.

The difficulty with this way of working is that there is very little time for exploration, for allowing oneself to be puzzled, to not know. The patient is also not really able to give their story or thoughts on what may be troubling them. So a surgery is a place where patients may experience themselves as objects rather than subjects. Contemporary working practices mean that doctors, unlike the community doctor of old, spend more time prescribing than relating (for a classic definition of institutional defences in surgeries see Wiener & Sher 1998, pp. 161–163). The degree of 'objectification' of patients will vary between practices and individuals. It is important to remember that a practice exists in a geographical location with its own history and sense of belonging. In many areas, generations of families become familiar to the practice and vice versa and so a sense of community and the development of local knowledge become very important to the way the doctor and the practice in general treats the patient. This also affects how the patient relates to or sees the practice. For many patients the practice surgery is a very important place that they have known for a long time, even all their lives, and they do not feel objectified in the way described above, but feel it is a place which actually knows them. In a time when faith in both social services and the Church has declined, the general practice has or can become not just a place of medicine, but also of community, of belonging and of some form of leaning post unavailable elsewhere. It is ideally located to deal with key issues in people's lives, to do with loss, frustration, rage, mourning, joy, etc. This can require a co-ordinated and sometimes very practical response. So one finds that a practice is a networked organization, with midwives, nurses, counsellors and social workers working together, as well as letters going off to lawyers, the Department of Social Security, housing departments, and so on.

However, one of the modern trends, especially in city practices, is that there is a higher turnover of registered patients, combined sometimes with a larger size of practice. A doctor in such a practice will spend a great deal of time seeing people s/he does not know, or does not remember due to lack of time, and who have no substantial history of attachment to the practice. This is likely to be experienced as a loss by the doctor and the practice staff, especially the receptionists, as their need to belong to their local population and a yearning for familiarity is undermined.

In this context, there can be a growing alienation between the surgery and its patient list. This point is illustrated by the attitude towards 'home visits'. In my experience, in a South London fundholding practice with 20 000 patients, some doctors look at 'home visits' as a huge inconvenience. They generally have no idea whom they may be visiting and, being overworked, they have lost touch with their sense of being part of the community in which they work. In a small surgery in West London, however, the single Asian doctor who knows many of her patients makes many home visits, sometimes up until midnight, and this gives her a more intimate rather than alienating sense of the work.

It is in the context of growing alienation that it is most likely that unconscious use is made of socially available stereotypes, in order to defend the practice and doctor against being overwhelmed. With black and Asian patients, as well as refugees, gays and patients with disabilities, these available stereotypes kick in immediately. Class stereotypes can also be powerful. If a patient is particularly inarticulate or extremely articulate, the doctor's approach can vary from patronizing the patient, to giving too much time to a patient who is similar to them or displays characteristics that the doctor admires. Through the use of stereotypes, the members of the primary health care team are shielded from uncertainty, their own limitations and the limitations of medicine.

On the other hand, the vast practical experience accumulated within the team and the face-to-face contact with patients can facilitate the challenging of stereotypes, as they are constantly undermined in individual interactions. Issues around responding to difference, yet avoiding the dangers of stereotyping, are obviously very important for the primary health care team, including the counsellor.

The counsellor

The counsellor can provide an extension of the doctor's care for his or her patients, as well as an attempt to contain the difficult, sometimes intangible anxieties the patient brings, the doctor feels and the surgery is awash with. The counsellor can negotiate the relationship between the unconscious, uncertainty and certainty (generally a defence) by introducing observations and thinking which may lead to some clarity. This role is initially carried out in relation to the patient, but in time the counsellor can extend it to the doctors, receptionists and other staff and to meetings of the doctors and the whole primary care team. The counsellor works 'slowly' compared with the speed of other things going on in the practice. S/he does not rush around. S/he waits for the patient and for others if necessary. S/he may sit and think about a patient after they have left, write notes in a thoughtful way, wait for the next patient while remembering the session before or reading the doctor's letter. Even when one is working on very short contracts, the time one has as a counsellor is much greater than is available to anyone else in the surgery culture.

A practice which uses counsellors may be showing by its acceptance of this difference an understanding that one-off, hopeful and quick answers, provided for example by medication, on their own are not adequate to deal with all the complex feelings and worries with which modern-day patients are faced. However, even within the counselling provided in primary care, the emphasis on 'brief therapy', sometimes with a limit of six sessions, may be seen as inappropriately searching for the 'quick fix', failing to take sufficient account of the differences between the needs of different individuals.

The context I have laid out is important in recognizing the vast array of people who may come to see a counsellor within a surgery. Looking across my own caseload in the last eight years working in primary care, I have seen patients from numerous ethnic backgrounds, gay and lesbian patients, and patients from a whole range of income groups and social classes. Our counselling team, comprising four counsellors for most of that time, has itself become quite well balanced by representing a broad cross-section of ethnicity, gender, sexuality and class.

Being faced with 'difference'

The broad question here is to do with how counsellors can feel challenged by a patient who is 'different' to them. The main 'differences' that come to mind are ethnicity, disability, gender, sexuality and class. The next question is 'who is worried about the difference?' Is it the counsellor, the patient, the doctor or the nurse? This is followed by 'what is the worry and why?' All these questions are relevant whether it is the counsellor, for example, who is feeling threatened by a same-sex gay patient who acts in a seductive manner towards them, or it is a patient who is denigrating the black or Asian counsellor by making comment about how the country is over-run by 'foreigners'. These situations are challenging for both counsellor and client, but if appropriately handled they may lead to a new perspective for both (see Gordon 1996 for one perspective on difference).

Clinically speaking, however, 'difference' challenges one's own identity and cosy assumptions. To avoid difference generally means an inability to deal with the world unless it is an extension of one's own self. To be challenged by difference is to get to know oneself, as one has to discover one's own difficulties and limitations. For example, many people from other cultures in the world have a completely different view of elders, the meaning of love and marriage, dirt and cleanliness, dreams, family, etc. All these important areas of life have been culturally defined over hundreds of years in different societies and cannot be reduced to a Western notion of cultural and psychological reality (see Farhad 1999 for a perspective on identity).

I remember a Sudanese man who once told me that in Islam dreams are the work of the devil and one prays to avoid dreams. Should we try to free this man from his delusions or is he describing a significant and culturally important concept, which needs to be thought about, understood and elaborated? Another woman from Egypt who was having difficulties in her arranged marriage was not concerned about love in the passionate individual sense, but about correct behaviour in the family and her husband respecting her in the way she respected him. Is she in denial or is she describing a fundamental assumption about marriage being primarily about honour, duty, respect and responsibility in her culture?

In many non-Western cultures the self is not as individualistically defined and is more located in the context of community and traditions, but this does not mean that the person is less 'individual' than someone raised in a Western tradition. An Indian woman having difficulty with her authoritarian husband and stepmother cannot be simply seen as 'undifferentiated', but needs to be asked how she can regain her place in her family according to her own traditions.

Case history A: Kate

I remember when I had my first lesbian client that I felt quite apprehensive. How could I, a man, help someone who saw her natural partner in life to be a woman? I felt excluded and also had a stereotype in my head that she would believe that men are not good enough for her or may even hate men. She came about a relationship with her partner, which was very violent. This only aggravated my fear that I would be no good and she would 'spit me out'. The other fantasy I had was that as my name is Iranian, she would expect me to be intolerant of homosexuality. I half expected and hoped that she would not turn up.

So I had a lot of baggage to take into the session. The client turned up on time, looking like a stereotypical hard lesbian and I sunk further into my inadequate 'Woody Allen man' frame of mind, waiting to be rubbished. However, Kate, an Irish woman, hardly noticed me and poured out her worries about her behaviour and her relationship. I learnt from her that she was struggling to relate to her partner in a way that was not destructive, as well as trying to understand why she lost control so easily. It became clear that she hated herself for 'disappointing' her family because of her sexuality and so she took any uncertainty in a relationship as a confirmation that she was unworthy and unlovable. She was like a desperate child with parents who did not really connect to her. I recognized that my main concern before the sessions was also one of not connecting with her and of not being able to be of any use to her. However, rather than recognizing this as a common male fear in relation to women, the fact that Kate was a lesbian meant that I had a social container or stereotype to which I could attribute all these worries. In other words, it is not just the client's projections and one's 'countertransference' which needs to be kept clearly in view, but also how these fantasies can be easily supported and solidified by social stereotypes.

Most stereotypes, whether racist or sexist, generally underline some attributes at the expense of others, thereby drawing an extreme picture. Descriptions like 'they like music, are lazy, criminal, sexually hungry' and so on, which many white people apply to black people, clearly constitute a description of a figure who is not 'conscious' but 'unconscious' and at the mercy of instincts and desires. These are characteristics which exist in all human beings but are projected on to black people. Many black people have internalized this image of themselves and one of the tasks of therapy may be to look at this internal image. Given the historical nature of this stereotype over hundreds of years and the widespread practice of racism, some black patients may find it impossible to work with a white counsellor although I have never personally come across this.

However, in cases where this is so, the counsellor needs to be sensitive to the request for a counsellor from an ethnic background acceptable to the client, as to persevere may be abusive. If there is resistance, it will usually show itself at some point and the counsellor needs to take it seriously, both as a projection and as a real issue that exists in the society and world they live in. The counsellor needs to look at the power issues that exist in the counsellor–patient relationship and how these affect the way the patient sees themselves and how they operate in the world.

Similarly, if a woman does not want to see a man because of a history of sexual abuse that wish needs to be respected. The same issues can be worked through or looked at with a woman counsellor. A strict Muslim woman or man may also only want to see a counsellor of the same sex. This also needs to be respected.

On the other hand, if a white patient does not want to see a black or Asian counsellor this is clearly both the expression of a personal terror and the overt operation of a convenient, sometimes unconscious social stereotype. This is being used defensively to stop the patient from looking at themselves or their 'shadow self' and maybe exploring aggressive feelings. If the counsellor is part of a team it may be useful for the patient to see someone similar to them in order to explore these very feelings. It may, however, become clear that the patient cannot tolerate any ambivalence, is unable to reflect and therefore may be unsuitable for any insight-orientated counselling. Generally, as with any projection, it is important to work with it as the client may be exploring something very difficult.

A black colleague of mine pointed out that black people see white people as cold, too intellectual, 'uptight' and not in touch with their feelings. This is an image of someone 'disconnected' or frightened of his or her unconscious. Again, what is being described is an extreme image, but it serves a purpose as it describes those attributes from which black people have historically been excluded, as well as their anger at being first the slaves and then the subjects of white people.

Case history B: Sharon

A number of years ago I saw a young black woman (Sharon) in her mid twenties who was having difficulties at work. All the colleagues with whom she had worked for quite some time had left due to difficulties in the organization and now she felt like the odd one out, excluded by the new staff and fearful. Her sleep was restless and she felt anxiety in her stomach and had recently had a panic attack. These were all new feelings for her and she did not understand where they had come from. Relating the story of her life she told me that she had been adopted at the age of two. Her white adoptive mother always told her what a beautiful little girl she was: a cute little black girl with a big smile—rather like a doll, I thought.

Sharon's mother already had four other children of her own and was also a child-minder. 'The house was always full of children and as I become older I became chunkier and bigger boned—much bigger than my mother expected and so she lost interest in me.' In telling me the story she remembered her feelings of being left out, alone and the odd one out. After a few sessions, she had a particularly poignant dream. 'I am in my flat, except that my front room is full of my mother's old furniture. None of my furniture is there. I go on to the balcony for some air as I am confused, when suddenly the balcony gives way for a split second and I feel panic and my heart starts racing.' It became clear that some of her feelings about her place in her family and her own image of herself were being relived, through projection of these into her work situation. In many ways, Sharon's life linked very clearly to the history of black and Asian people who are seen in a particular way by white people and then dropped when they fail to live up to those stereotyped expectations. It also shows very well the difficulties that can arise when an individual's specific identity is weakened by this experience.

Case history C: John

An example of how a patient can stereotype the counsellor and reject what s/he represents was brought to me quite sharply with another client, John, who was a white 'biker'. He was sent by the doctor and arrived very reluctantly. He was in a relationship with a woman where both drank heavily. They had had an argument and she had taken his little girl away from him claiming he was violent. He was distraught and suicidal. He was a very tall, leather-clad, tough-looking guy, with various earrings and tattoos and long hair. We could not have been more 'different' in our backgrounds, lives and looks. I felt like a completely boring, dull, establishment figure, who must seem to him to have 'sold out'. He pointed this out to me straight away and started challenging me. 'How can YOU help ME? How could YOU possibly understand ME?'

I understood his point of view, but he had me stereotyped as a representative of everything he had always shunned and escaped from. I was a boring settler and he was a free spirit, servant to no one. 'I can just get on my bike and ride. Nobody tells me what to do. How can you understand that? I bet you've never even been on a bike!' It became clear that I represented 'society', which had taken away his daughter, as well as his parents who had put him in a children's home. I reminded him of his inability to really trust anybody to be on his side. His anger with me was also another way of describing how frustrated he felt with himself, his mistakes, his lack of foresight and his inability to think clearly. He rejected the stereotype I represented, yet he envied what he imagined I had that he wanted. The difference between us was also the measure of the split that existed in him.

I was unable to help him and, soon after his father died a week later, he committed suicide.

The primary care team

Working with others in a primary care team also means acknowledging and dealing with difference and overcoming stereotypes. In the practice in which I work, the team, including the doctors, generally meets monthly. It is my experience that it generally takes doctors, nurses and health visitors more than two years to get used to the idea of counselling and for the counsellor to get used to working with all these health professionals, talking about patients' lives and illnesses and body parts in matter-of-fact technical detail. Initially, the counsellor may feel out of place or excluded by the others or not sure what or how much to say. However, once this difficult period is over, the team meetings tend to start reflecting the presence of a counsellor. This shows itself in how both the counsellor and the other team members start appreciating and internalizing to some extent the perspectives which each professional brings to patients. Everybody is being educated.

The presence of the counsellor also helps professionals to think about the feelings, fantasies and stereotypes they have of particular patients. They are able to discuss a patient in a less technical way and one that makes less use of rigid categories. I have often sat in a meeting where the doctor, supported by the team, feels that a patient needs to be referred to a psychiatrist. The presence of a counsellor generally means that the doctor hesitates and there is a more in-depth discussion of the individual patient, which then clarifies what should be done (see Balint 1993 on doctor–patient perceptions). The following case is an example of this.

Case history D: Hamid

Hamid is a very good example of how the practice team can feel the need to defend itself against a patient who attracts negative stereotypes and can experience a lot of anxiety about how to respond to him, medically and socially. Hamid, a 28-year-old man, was introduced into one of the meetings as a very quiet patient. The doctor described him as someone who never looked at her, worried a great deal about his bowels, had a rash on his face and wanted various fairly insignificant moles removed from his face. He had cut himself across his arms, lived alone, was not in any relationships, was unemployed and she suspected that he was an unacknowledged gay man. He was very depressed but refused medication. The male health visitor had been asked to go and see him at his flat as the doctor was worried that he may do something to himself, but Hamid refused to open the door and told the health visitor to go away. The health visitor said he felt that he needed a psychiatric visit.

The practice manager then interjected that the receptionists felt very uneasy around him, as he mumbled, wore a bomber jacket and was six foot six inches tall. I asked where he was from. People were not sure. He had a pretty rough South London council estate accent. Looking at the notes the doctor then said that he had moved around a great deal between surgeries in South London and had been at this surgery for two years. Someone suggested he was a Muslim.

The team members were feeling quite impotent and useless and were worried they had reached their own limits. For them, Hamid had become an 'unfathomable' figure who was obviously troubling everybody in one way or another. A psychiatric referral would obviously be of huge relief to the surgery, although there was doubt as to whether he would accept this and his condition was unlikely to warrant sectioning. Listening to all this I was faced with a very unappealing and puzzling figure. I asked why he was coming to the surgery and somebody said 'Maybe he wants to reach out or just talk'. Once this thought was expressed then it became clear that if this was the case he may like to see a counsellor. The doctor was relieved, as was everybody else, as they had possibly just solved a puzzle and seen a way forward. They had gone from thinking about symptoms to wondering about motivation.

A long period of counselling unravelled Hamid's circumstances and feelings, challenged many of the stereotypes about his behaviour and state of mind and helped him to be clearer about what he wanted from life. He did not need a psychiatric referral and has not been seen by the doctors since the early months of counselling.

Referring to outside agencies

In certain situations, for example with patients who may be HIV positive or patients who are refugees, problems and circumstances may seem overwhelming and too far outside the experience and expertise of the counsellor. It may be tempting to refer clients on to places like the London Lighthouse for HIV patients, or The Medical Foundation, or Nafsiyat for Refugees, or any local equivalent. However, this may not always be appropriate or necessary. Many HIV patients, for example, are confronting mortality in a very immediate way and, unless the counsellor feels that they need a supportive holistic organization geared around their needs, s/he should offer counselling as to anyone else in a similar situation. The counsellor may have to work with the stereotypes and fears that they hold. However, any client sitting opposite the counsellor is a stranger, who they must get to know.

With refugees the issues can be made more complex by various practical issues. Many refugees need interpreters, who are rarely if ever available in surgeries. So a relation may be co-opted to describe something to the doctor, maybe inadequately because of the very presence or closeness of the patient. Refugees generally also need a great deal of practical help, especially if they have just arrived and the counsellor needs to remember this. It is very easy to get captured by the 'trauma' of the refugee when actually what the individual may need in the first place, even ultimately, is to get on with life and to get to know his or her way around their new country. If it is impractical for the counsellor to offer help with this, then it may be more helpful for the refugee to be referred to an organization able to offer welfare advice, help with writing reports to lawyers, and so on, as well as counselling.

In some counselling organizations it is possible to work with refugees using professional interpreters. In primary care, this is generally impractical as it requires a budget which is not usually available. However, if interpreters can be used in a surgery then they must be accredited or trained interpreters with a track record. The role of interpreters needs to be taken much more seriously, with proper training and a code of practice. There are many horror stories about 'amateur' interpreters being brought in, who find themselves overwhelmed by the material, or tell the client to pull him or herself together, or embellish answers and so on. Not taking the profession of interpreting seriously is another way of not taking patients who are 'different', in having language difficulties, seriously.

However, even professional interpreters may not be the answer. Language is the primary container and describer of one's subjectivity and if an individual is struggling, they may have a clinical need to express themselves in their original language. Even for those who can speak English as their second 'learnt' language, some things may get lost or not get described in the new language, which is more of the head (learnt) than the heart (felt). Few surgeries have the ability to cater for language differences and so a specialist agency, which can communicate with patients in their original language, may be useful.

On the other hand, it is also important not to assume that a person is not prepared to work in a broken second language, as in some cases the original language may also be their psychological prison. The new language may give them a new freedom to express themselves.

Conclusions

General practices offer access to counselling to many people who would otherwise not have such an opportunity. I have in this chapter concentrated, through my case examples, on patients who experience themselves as alone, outside, disconnected, angry and desperate. We live in times where communities, especially in cities, can often seem to be absent, and where the burden on the individual is great. A practice can be a place where feelings of exclusion, alienation, difference and isolation are brought regularly and where the surgery staff and the patients have to face the consequences of these and attempt to challenge them. In acknowledging and respecting difference, yet challenging the stereotypes and prejudice often associated with these, counsellors can contribute to the ability of the practice to care equally for the diverse range of its patient population.

References

Balint, E., Courtenay, M., Elder, A., Hull, M. and Julian, P. (1993) *The Doctor, the Patient and the Group*. Routledge, London.

Farhad, D. (1999) The meaning of boundaries and barriers in the development of cultural identity and between cultures. *Psychodynamic Counselling*, 5 (2), 161–171.

Gordon, P. (1996) A fear of difference? Some reservations about intercultural therapy and counselling. *Psychodynamic Counselling*, 2 (2), 195–208.

Lees, J. (1997) An approach to counselling in GP surgeries. *Psychodynamic Counselling*, 3 (1), 33–48.

Wiener, J. and Sher, M. (1998) *Counselling and Psychotherapy in Primary Care*. Macmillan, London.

Chapter 8

Experiences of the counselled: the client's perspective

Jane Keithley and two clients

Introduction

The first part of this chapter discusses what is known about the views of users of counselling services and the implications of taking client perspectives into account. The second part is a synthesis of two reflections on counselling, written by clients from their own experience.

Clients and counselling in primary care

During the 1990s, access to counselling became part of the range of services offered in many general practices, largely as a result of GPs' perceptions of the benefits it could bring to their practices, rather than patient demand. However, previous evidence suggested support for provision of such services, both from clients and from the population generally (Keithley 1982; Thomas 1993).

From the clients' point of view, there are obvious reasons for locating counsellors in primary care. Many people 'medicalize' their emotional and relationship problems. It is estimated that between 10% and 33% of consultations include such emotional problems (Gray 1988; Goldberg 1995). Thomas (1993) found that over half of a sample of people consulting their GP said that they had felt the need to talk to an 'independent counsellor' during the previous three years. A 1992 MORI poll reported that 80% of respondents saw counselling as an appropriate way of helping people with depression (cited in Curtis Jenkins 1995). The accessible, free and non-stigmatized nature of primary care services, the high respect in which GPs are held and cultural beliefs about how best to tackle such problems all contribute to people approaching members of the primary care team. The team is likely to be aware of many of the problems and life changes of patients. A counsellor can also sensitize other team members to the emotional problems behind some patients' somatic symptoms (Papadopoulos & Bor 1995).

Even GPs with counselling expertise may encourage their patients to seek counselling help from someone else. It could be difficult for 'patients' to become 'clients', presenting medical issues (which the GP is expected to investigate, diagnose and treat) and emotional difficulties (for which a very different counselling response is appropriate) to the same person in the same context (Cocksedge 1989; Rowland *et al.* 1989). A study of patients with emotional problems who did not raise these during a consultation, found that this was often because they perceived that the GP had insufficient time, lacked interest or could do nothing to help (Cape & McCulloch 1999). Most evidently, consultations lasting five or 10 minutes offer little scope for exploring complex circumstances and feelings, compared with hour-long counselling appointments.

Some studies have asked counselling clients about the advantages of providing counselling in primary care (for example, Keithley 1982; Thomas 1993; Corney in Corney & Jenkins 1993; Booth et al. 1997b). They report overwhelming support for such a service, even from those who have not personally found counselling to be of help. If counsellors are members of the primary care team, clients may be more confident that different aspects of their care are fully co-ordinated, and that they are being referred to someone who is known and trusted by their GP, so ensuring confidentiality and lessening their apprehension. The surroundings are familiar, usually geographically convenient and not labelled as specifically for those with emotional or relationship problems, so avoiding stigma or embarrassment. Prompt referral and the fact that the service is free have also been reported as advantages. It is interesting to compare these comments with those reported from individuals referred from primary care to a community mental health team (Wakefield et al. 1998). The length of waiting times, changes in staff, inadequate support after discharge and concern about being seen entering the team base were all highlighted as concerns.

However, reservations have also been expressed about providing counselling in this setting and are, in some respects, an alternative interpretation of the features seen as advantages. Referral to a known and trusted counsellor is also likely to mean restricted choice for the prospective client. A general practice may offer anonymity in the sense of not being identified solely with one service, but the proximity to the clients' homes and the increased likelihood of meeting people they know threaten anonymity. Professionals collaborating and co-operating in care could be seen as a threat to confidentiality. It could also mean that if there is a breakdown in their relationship with one professional, it is difficult for them to make a 'fresh start' with another. However, it seems to be doctors and counsellors who are most concerned about confidentiality (Monach & Monro 1995). Clients tend to view sharing information between counsellor and GP as a matter of course and a positive benefit (Keithley 1982; Thomas 1993).

It has been suggested that clients who are 'prescribed' counselling may lack motivation or feel resentful at being 'passed on' (Heisler 1979; Booth et al. 1997c). There is little evidence to substantiate this, although as studies tend to be of those who accepted the referral, we do not know the views of those who rejected counselling. Some studies have suggested that many clients of primary care counselling would not have sought counselling elsewhere (Waydenfeld & Waydenfeld 1980) and that some initially reluctant or sceptical individuals eventually report benefits (Keithley 1982).

Individuals often come to counselling with little idea of what kind of help to expect, or with inappropriate expectations (Thomas 1993; McLeod 1990). A referral to counselling through primary care could prepare individuals for their initial encounter with the counsellor, ensuring they have realistic expectations (Marsh & Barr 1975; Waydenfeld & Waydenfeld 1978). However, it does seem that referrals often include little guidance and patients would welcome more explanation from the GP (Keithley 1982; Thomas 1993).

Clients on counselling: process and outcomes

A growing number of studies have sought to evaluate counselling, in primary care and in other settings, but there is considerable disagreement as to their usefulness and validity (see Chapter 5). Here, we shall focus on the evidence in relation to client views.

One way of seeking clients' views is to ask about their satisfaction with the service they received, and its general helpfulness. They can rate themselves on predetermined scales designed to measure change. Or they can specify their own goals and aspirations and rate how far these have been achieved. A common difficulty, particularly in primary care, is that the clients, their problems and the counselling 'product' which is on offer, are so variable. Rather than asking what views clients have of counselling, we should be asking more specific questions about 'what can the views of clients tell us about what works, for whom, in what circumstances?' (Roth & Fonagy 1996).

Client views about the general helpfulness of counselling in primary care have attracted considerable scepticism, partly because they are so positive as to be of little use as a discriminatory measure. Waydenfeld and Waydenfeld (1980) found that almost all of the 47 clients who returned questionnaires reported counselling to be of some help. Spiers and Jewell (1995) reported that of 85 patients who completed their questionnaire, over 90% found their counselling experience helpful and a similar proportion said they would seek counselling help again. However, there is some evidence that satisfaction ratings can discriminate between client views of counselling and other responses to their psychological problems. The Edinburgh Primary Care Depression Study found that patients rated counselling from a social worker more positively than drug therapy prescribed by a psychiatrist, cognitive behaviour therapy from a clinical psychologist or routine GP care (Scott & Freeman 1992). It was also the only form of treatment that more than a small minority would definitely want again should their depression return.

However, doubts about the validity and reliability of overall satisfaction and helpfulness measures run deeper than their apparent optimism. They have been criticized for being too general, for reflecting more on how a service is delivered than its outcome, and for asking clients to rate something without being aware of alternatives (Ruggeri 1994). Scott and Freeman (1992) found no relationship between the high value placed on counselling and its effectiveness compared with other treatments. In addition, in any mental health services, client views risk being perceived as being related to their problems, unreliable or even part of an illness itself.

However, a spirited and persuasive case has been advanced for taking account of client satisfaction. Most fundamentally, where clients have choice, services that produce widespread dissatisfaction are unlikely to survive due to high drop-out rates, a failure to engage with the help offered and a lack of recommendation to others. There is also evidence that client views differ from those of service providers: on expectations of the service, its nature and its outcomes. Service monitoring cannot thus rely on provider reports alone (Keithley 1982; McLeod 1990; Ruggeri 1994). Patten and Walker, in their study of the expectations of marriage guidance clients, sum this up: 'The consumer's view is a 'voice to be heard'... which is ignored at the peril of inappropriate referrals, disappointed clients and frustrated counsellors' (Patten & Walker 1990, p. 38).

Dismissing the importance of client satisfaction is also contrary to the principles of 'user-led services'. For counsellors, 'insight into the way it looks from the other chair' (McLeod 1990) may improve their practice, or at least their awareness of the importance of communicating clearly, at an early stage, the kind of help that counselling can and cannot offer.

'Satisfaction' may be related to process rather than outcome, but in counselling, process and outcome are likely to be inextricably entwined (Booth *et al.* 1997a, pp. 51–68). Ruggeri (1994) argues that satisfaction, especially long term, is an important although not the only variable in the quality and effectiveness of care. He suggests how to maximize the usefulness of satisfaction measures. In particular, measures should offer more options than a 'satisfied/not satisfied' dichotomy, and should acknowledge that 'satisfaction' is multidimensional: it can incorporate quality of care, accessibility, cost and the physical environment, for example. Qualitative studies of client views on counselling can uncover a complex picture. When I asked primary care counselling clients 'Did counselling help you at all?', just over half gave an unequivocally positive response, about one-quarter expressed mixed feelings and one-fifth reported no help (Keithley 1982). However, when asked to expand on this initial response, almost all clients expressed a complex mixture of feelings, which was very inadequately conveyed by a unilinear concept of helpfulness–unhelpfulness. Most expressed both reservations and positive aspects, and the initial response was often misleading. This suggests the advantages of adopting an in-depth, qualitative approach rather than relying on simple answers to simple questions.

McLeod (1990) summarized research evidence on the aspects of their counselling experiences that clients have found most helpful. Most frequently mentioned are factors likely to be common to all forms of counselling: a chance to talk to someone with an interest in their problems and who understands, encouragement and reassurance, the instilling of hope, an increase in self-understanding and emotional release. Counsellors, unlike GPs, can offer a substantial period of uninterrupted time. Interestingly, many clients also mention 'advice', although McLeod suggests they may have a very broad definition of what 'advice' includes. Several studies have found that personal liking for the counsellor, the degree of rapport, trust, respect and goodwill, are important, although not sufficient, for 'successful' counselling as perceived by clients (Keithley 1982; Hunt 1985; McLeod 1990).

However, a lack of practical help and 'advice' in counselling seem to be the principal sources of client dissatisfaction. In the studies quoted above, some found it difficult to see how 'just talking' could tackle their problems. Others reported counselling as helpful, but the benefits as 'wearing off' over time. This supports Ruggeri's (1994) argument that client studies should assess long-term as well as short-term satisfaction with counselling.

Ruggeri notes that even studies of something as subjective as 'client satisfaction' rely heavily on instruments and measures generated by professionals. This is also true of more specific studies of counselling outcomes. Many of these include 'clients' views', but usually as self-ratings of clients on predetermined, standard instruments for measuring quality of life or psychological health. So, for example, Boot *et al.* (1994, cited in Papadopoulos & Bor 1995) conducted a 'before and after' study of two patient groups, using the General Health Questionnaire. The results showed that the group who had received counselling from qualified counsellors for acute psychological problems improved more than those who had been advised by their GP. On the other hand, Scott and Freeman (1992), using a well-established depression rating scale in their study of treating depression in primary care, found little evidence that specialist treatments, including social work counselling, were more clinically effective than routine GP care. In addition, they had much higher costs.

Booth *et al.* (1997b) argue that many of these standard measures, especially if developed for use in mental health services, are inappropriate for counselling clients, who come with a wide range of problems and rarely fit into standard diagnostic categories. They suggest clients should set their own goals and define their own problems against which to judge outcomes. Their study of 51 clients of counselling in 15 general practices used one standard measure (a quality of life scale), but also asked clients to describe helpful and unhelpful events after each counselling session and, at the end of counselling, to rate progress on their own previously specified goals and problems. The high drop-out rate (over half) from their research has to be borne in mind, but they argued that for most clients, counselling helped to tackle their problems and achieve their goals.

However, perhaps more interesting are the goals that clients specified. The vast majority sought 'change'—in feelings, attitudes, behaviours, situations and relationships. Almost half hoped to improve their 'understanding', while around one-fifth wanted the opportunity to express their feelings to someone. The helpful aspects of therapy most frequently mentioned were 'reassurance', 'problem solution', 'involvement' and 'insight'. The authors also suggest, in line with some other studies (Llewellyn 1988; Rogers *et al.* 1995), that there are differences between counsellors and clients in their objectives and criteria for success. Clients tend to specify problem-solving and simple forms of help, whereas counsellors are more concerned with the aetiology of the problem and its transformation through insight.

The validity of client and counsellor perceptions of 'success' in counselling is increasingly under scrutiny with the move to 'evidence-based health care' (see Chapter 5). This move has contradictory implications for the value placed on listening to clients. On the one hand, service-user views can be seen as a legitimate and important part of the evidence base that should replace the individual views and unsubstantiated clinical judgements of service providers. On the other hand, the 'gold standard' is still widely held to be the randomized controlled trial (RCT); a model which fits uneasily with the qualitative, often subjective, data associated with concepts like 'client satisfaction' or 'helpfulness'. In the messy world of primary care, it is also difficult (and undesirable) to simulate the controlled environment, with the manipulation of one variable, to which RCTs aspire. Failure to challenge the ideal of the RCT could mean devaluing client views in favour of 'harder' data.

Listening to clients: a more radical agenda?

Listening to client views, however valuable, does not give service users, let alone the wider public, a say in the aims, methods or outcomes of such an exercise. A more radical move would be to involve clients- and potential clients—in decisions about the provision, planning, setting up and monitoring of counselling services in primary care. This would give users a proactive role, rather than simply responding to questions which service providers decide to ask them. This has not been evident so far. The rapid growth in primary care counselling in the 1990s is widely associated with the spread of GP fundholding (see Chapter 4), but not in response to demands from practice populations, or to fundholders canvassing patients' views.

The NHS has no strong tradition of democratic accountability, nor of user participation. When health services are 'free', offer little choice and are provided by highly skilled, high status professionals, they tend to operate in a paternalistic fashion, led by the interests of the providers rather than the users (Hogg 1999). However, recent governments have attempted to increase the 'choice', 'voice' and involvement of users. Public involvement means that decisions are more likely to reflect people's preferences, concerns and values; produce services better suited to local needs; and be credible in the eyes of users and the general population. Even unpopular decisions are more likely to be accepted if local people feel that they have been listened to and if the reasons are fully explained (Barnes 1997). Involving the public can thus be in the political interests of those making health care decisions as well as in improving service quality.

However, in the NHS, such involvement has been mostly indirect. The perceived importance of 'expertise' in decisions about health care has given an important mediating and 'championing' role for representatives or 'agents' of users: Health Authorities and, increasingly, primary care organizations (PCOs). These agents have been charged with identifying and taking account of user views in the commissioning of services. In the early 1990s, the 'Local Voices' initiative (NHS Management Executive 1992) aimed to ensure that local people's views were part of the assessment of health care needs carried out by Health Authorities. More recently, PCOs have become key players in commissioning services, including counselling, and are expected to engage the local population in commissioning decisions (Department of Health 1997). It is not yet clear how they will take on this task. Are they most likely to assume that the GPs' close clinical contacts with individual patients, together with their professional status and expertise, enables them to speak and make decisions on our behalf?

The use of agents complicates the issue of who is the 'consumer' of counselling services in primary care. Rather than seeking to directly involve clients or practice populations in developing and evaluating counselling services, the providers will increasingly need to address PCOs, responding to their views and preferences if they are to persuade them to commission counselling services on behalf of direct users (see Chapter 4). Hopefully, these views will be influenced by clients, and also by the broader practice populations. However, this is by no means self-evident and these developments may do little to improve democracy in decision-making in health care and thus in counselling in primary care.

Mixed feelings: personal accounts of counselling

The second part of this chapter draws on personal accounts by Sheila and Maureen (not their real names). Both are articulate graduates, one in her forties and the other in her late thirties. Neither are 'typical' clients: indeed, no such creature exists. However, their reflections on counselling convey something of what it feels like to be 'on the receiving end'. As far as possible, their words are left to speak for themselves.

Routes to counselling

Sheila experienced counselling as an undergraduate, when her GP referred her to a student counselling service, and more recently, when she referred herself to a counsellor based in a general practice of which she was not a patient. She talks about why she (or others) thought counselling might be helpful. While she was a student:

> Within the space of six months, three members of my family (all in their own ways very important to me) had died and a long-term relationship had ended. The black clouds of depression gathered over my head and I would find myself, for no apparent reason, washed by feelings of misery and hopelessness. My concentration went, my work was suffering. I was overwhelmed by feelings of anxiety about my parents—I was convinced that they too would die and rang them every day just to make sure they were still alive. I didn't seem to be able to do anything and there seemed little point in continuing my own existence when I couldn't work and everyone I cared about was leaving me. Physically, I felt permanently 'unwell'—I had one cold after another and even my bones felt tired.

After two visits for help with physical symptoms, and some ineffective antidepressants, her GP suggested counselling. Her response was ambivalent:

> Whilst I was unimpressed by the effects of the antidepressants and unsure about taking any other drugs... I was also wary of going to see a counsellor. Other students, who were known to be seeing the counsellor, were felt by 'the rest of us' to be the inadequate ones, the ones who couldn't cope, the ones who had 'cracked up'. These were not labels I would readily apply to myself.

Eighteen years later, Sheila again found herself suffering difficulties:

> These were a result of a combination of several factors including an accumulation of stress built up during my previous employment, the grieving process associated with leaving that work behind and relationship difficulties rooted in childhood experiences. Other than severely disrupted sleep patterns, I had no obvious physical symptoms to focus on this time around. Instead I was beset by feelings of guilt, failure and confusion.

However, this time she did not turn to her doctor:

> I clearly recognized that my problems could not be solved by the medical profession directly. My reluctance to take drugs had increased over the years and my own experience (both at work and personally) had told me that what I needed was counselling.

Her own general practice did not offer a counselling service, so following a recommendation from a (counsellor) friend, she contacted a counsellor who worked in a nearby medical centre, but who could also provide a service on a sessional fee basis for individuals who were not patients of the practice.

Maureen's route to counselling has been very different:

> I was given the opportunity to attend counselling by my employers. I work as a social researcher in a university... and, because of the sensitive and stressful nature of my current study, there was funding within the research proposal for counselling.

It was envisaged that counselling could strengthen her ability to cope with the extent of death and dying to which the research project was likely to expose her. However, she too had mixed feelings:

I didn't think of myself as the type of person who went to counselling. I come from a working class family where discussion of difficult issues is discouraged. Although not stigmatizing in the sense of being shameful, going to counselling would be seen by my family as self-indulgent and a matter for jokes rather than serious consideration as a source of help.

Both women took a while to decide to make their first counselling appointment. Maureen (characteristically!) engaged in some 'research':

In the course of trying to come to a decision, I talked to three counsellor friends. I spoke to two nurses in the palliative care teams I work with, who refer people to counsellors. They recommended some books, but I didn't feel I had the time to read them. I sent off to the British Association of Counsellors for information sheets, which I didn't find very helpful, because they assumed a higher level of knowledge than I possessed, and for a list of local accredited counsellors.

Sheila focuses on the difficulties around making her first appointment:

I dithered and pondered and felt myself lapsing into the state of high anxiety which had taken me to the doctor in the first place. Eventually, in desperation, I made the appointment via the student union office. This in itself was a difficult task, as I felt that everyone would know what I was doing, a feeling which was reinforced by the location of the counsellor's office. It was situated in a corridor, nowhere near the medical centre, the door was clearly labelled, there was nowhere to hide—if you were in that area the chances were that you were seeing the counsellor.

Her second experience, arranging to see the counsellor in a general practice, was very different:

Making the appointment was straightforward and my first visit to the practice felt very comfortable, although I was on unfamiliar territory. I reported to the desk just like any other 'patient', sat with everyone else in the waiting room and was collected by the counsellor after a short wait. It all felt very simple—there was no feeling of being particularly identifiable and the atmosphere in the medical centre was very relaxed.

In contrast, Maureen received counselling at her counsellor's home and suggests that a general practice setting may not suit everyone:

I never feel at ease in any health care settings and would have found it difficult to attend sessions in the impersonal rooms of a GP's surgery.

Experiencing counselling

So how do these women describe their experience of counselling?

Visiting the counsellor was a very positive experience. I saw the counsellor over a period of about three months for about an hour a week. We talked through the issues which confront anyone who has suffered bereavement and she helped me to find ways of getting back to work. It felt good to be able to unload my problems on to someone who clearly understood how I felt and who didn't seem to mind when I spent a large part of the session in floods of tears. Physically I felt much better—less prone to coughs, colds, headaches and cold sores and much less 'weary'. Mentally, I gradually began to feel much more capable of dealing with things myself and developed a much more positive perspective on life—and death.

It was several months before I felt really well. However, I feel that this episode of counselling was definitely beneficial in the long term. For example, a couple of years later there were two more deaths in the family—I felt much more able to deal with that situation and although I grieved, this was a positive process, not a disabling one. I also felt more confident about making relationships with people—I had a much more philosophical outlook, valuing what I had rather than fearing loss. (Sheila on her first experience of counselling.)

After 10 hour-long sessions with a counsellor 18 years later, Sheila again feels substantial benefits:

Even in the short-term, I have shifted from a situation where I was incapacitated by my mental state, to one where I can face the future not only with equanimity but with a reasonable degree of confidence.

Maureen describes in detail some of her early impressions—and bemusement— when she started counselling:

During the initial sessions the counsellor's strict adherence to the one hour limit struck me as very strange in contrast to her apparently intent interest in me during the hour. Looking back I can now see it as part of the negotiating and marking out of this new counselling relationship and process. At the time, having but little knowledge of counselling and its ways, I was merely bemused by this and many other aspects of our sessions together. It would have been helpful to have been given clearer information, both before I began and during the early sessions so that I could have better understood what was intended to happen in them. I still don't know, but they now feel as if they were a preparation for the later sessions of counselling 'proper', in that they allowed a focus and format for the counselling sessions to emerge from the topics that I brought up in these early sessions and the ways in which I was approaching them.

She continues:

As someone whose job depends on my ability to enable other people to talk to me whilst I attend carefully to them, I found the enforced role reversal in the counselling sessions intensely frustrating and difficult to accept. In the early sessions I also found myself feeling quite powerless, despite the client-centred and client-driven rhetoric of counselling, since the counsellor seemed so much in control of both the setting and the ground rules of the process. She seemed to have firm boundaries of time and behaviour, to which I was expected to conform, and the process demanded that I divulge difficult and intimate information about myself and my work without the counsellor taking any similar risks.

Maureen describes what happens in the sessions:

The sessions have varied in their nature although they are constant in being driven by the topics and issues that I decide to raise. They are always in the same place and with the same person and so, unlike many consultations with health professionals, they easily build, one upon the next and can pick up and develop continuities, themes and contrasts from earlier sessions. The sessions mostly take the form of me talking whilst the counsellor listens. She never interrupts but waits until I have come to a stop and then either sums up, interprets or questions what I have said, generally with an emphasis upon my feelings in connection with that topic. Undoubtedly the most remarkable part of the experience for me has been realizing the power of being truly listened to and heard. Perhaps I mean being heard with not just the other person's ears, but also with their hearts and minds. This has resonance with my work, because the people I interview frequently comment that health professionals don't really listen to them and can't seem to hear what they are trying to say. When it happens, it is a very powerful experience and complete within itself, i.e. there is no need to do anything beyond the listening; simply being heard is enough in itself.

Despite this, Maureen is more ambivalent than Sheila about the helpfulness of counselling:

Has it helped? Since I did not go into it with any very clear aims or expectations, this is quite difficult to answer. I suppose what I was looking for was the opportunity to talk to an outsider on a predetermined and regular basis about issues that arose from my work because I thought that this would help to make me feel better and to enable me to carry on with the job. I had come to accept that there could be value in talking to a professional outsider, as the only available source. It was certainly apparent to me that death was not a subject with which many of my usual sources of support—family, friends, colleagues—were particularly comfortable, quite apart from the risk of breaching the boundaries of the confidentiality promised to the participants in the research.

The second side to the arguments given to me in support of counselling was that you could speak more freely because you would be speaking to someone whose own emotions you didn't need to worry about. I was less convinced by this. Counsellors and their clients are only human after all and humans do care about one another. In therapeutic relationships also I want an emotional component to the care, not merely professional competence, and consider any 'problems' that this form of the relationship might occasion more than compensated for by the consequent strength of that working relationship.

The sessions have given me the time and a safe place and person with whom to explore and express my feelings about my work and myself. By having the chance to tell my story and then to reflect on it, features of it that were implicit may be made explicit and examined, or its implications can be explored and ways of dealing with them considered. The counsellor can often provide a different perspective on my story and thus enable me to view events in a different light or to consider other ways of addressing problems. She also encourages me to see and value my own strengths and to have the confidence to make use of them.

As the research progresses, I feel more hopeful, self-confident and self-accepting, with more insight and self-awareness and equipped with better ways to solve problems and make decisions that I feel happy with. It is hard to know how much of that to attribute to the counselling and how much to other changes and influences. However, I do continue to attend the sessions and to value both the time I spend in them and the continuing insights that I take away from them.

To sum up, my initial feelings of reluctance and scepticism have been largely overcome during the course of my counselling, although I still retain some reservations. Armed with my present experience and knowledge, I would now feel more confident about making use of counselling support in the future.

Counselling in a primary care setting

Sheila sees a number of advantages in locating counsellors in primary care, including ease of initial access:

The most difficult step to take in approaching a counsellor is the first one—making an appointment. The location of the counselling service within the medical centre made the process much easier—it felt no more difficult than making an appointment to see a doctor or nurse. The medical centre felt welcoming, comfortable, anonymous and safe. Going to the doctor is, in itself, an acceptable thing to do—no one expects to be told why you are there and, in a busy medical centre, there are lots of people that you could be there to see.

Counselling provided as part of primary care is also often free for the client and both Sheila and Maureen identified finance as a potential barrier to access:

As a community development worker, I am very aware of the need for counselling services. The lack of such services, free at the point of delivery, generates a number of difficulties, not only for community development staff, but for a wide range of people employed in areas of disadvantage. (Sheila)

I am sure I would not have considered going had I had to pay for myself. It would have seemed too much money to be taking from our family finances to spend just upon myself and for no guaranteed outcome. (Maureen)

Adequate information about the availability and nature of a counselling service is also identified as crucial:

Deciding to go to counselling would have been helped by the provision of better pre-counselling information, both in order to allow me to make a more informed choice about whether or not it would be a suitable source of support and to enable me to make better use of the sessions once I began. I would recommend that people who are thinking about going to counselling for the first time be provided with good quality information, in a suitable format. They should have the opportunity to discuss what can be expected from counselling and how to make best use of it—both in each session and over the whole course. In addition they should be clear about what they themselves will have to be prepared to do/feel, how that particular style of counselling works, what it might be able to achieve and what the ground-rules of the counselling relationship are. It would also be helpful to see any agreed policies or codes of practice and to clarify the nature of confidentiality within counselling. (Maureen)

Sheila argues that the potential in primary care for making the service more widely known and understood is not fully realized:

People who do not visit their doctors regularly may be unaware of precisely what services are provided at their practice. It is important that the availability of a counselling service, including a brief explanation of how it can help, is widely publicized. Unless such information is mailed out it will only be available to people who go to the surgery.

Those involved in introducing or managing counselling services in primary care should also reflect on two other comments from Maureen. She writes about the three-way relationship between her employer (who 'referred' her to counselling as a GP might), the counsellor and herself:

I often felt that it would be difficult to refuse the offer of counselling, because of the implications for my working relationship with my employers. Once at the sessions, I often felt that there were, to coin a phrase, three of us in the relationship, and wondered about who was working for whom, to what end and what the implications were for the boundaries of confidentiality.

Finally, she makes a plea for choice for those seeking counselling:

It is important to provide a choice of location, counsellor and counselling style, to suit a range of individual circumstances, rather than to seek for one, blanket solution.

Primary care has many attractions as a location for counselling services, but Maureen warns us of the dangers of assuming that it should be *the* location.

References

Barnes, M. (1997) *Care, Communities and Citizens*. Addison Wesley Longman, Harlow.

Booth, H., Cushway, D. and Newnes, C. (1997a) Evaluation of counselling in primary care: how can research be made more useful for practitioners? *Counselling Psychology Quarterly*, 10, 51–68.

Booth, H., Cushway, D. and Newnes, C. (1997b) Counselling in general practice: clients' perceptions of significant events and outcomes. *Counselling Psychology Quarterly*, 10, 175–187.

Booth, H., Goodwin, I., Newnes, C. and Dawson, O. (1997c) Process and outcome of counselling in general practice. *Clinical Psychology Forum 101*, **March**, 32–40.

Cape, J. and McCulloch, Y. (1999) Patients' reasons for not presenting emotional problems in general practice consultations. *British Journal of General Practice*, 49, 875–879.

Cocksedge, S. (1989) GPs should not counsel long term. *Journal of the Royal College of General Practitioners*, 39, 347.

Corney, R. and Jenkins, R. (1993) *Counselling in General Practice*. Routledge, London.

Curtis Jenkins, G. (1995) Effectiveness in counselling services: recent developments in service delivery. *Counselling in Primary Care Trust*, 1, 7–12.

Department of Health (1997) *The new NHS: Modern, Dependable*. HMSO, London.

Goldberg, D.P. (1995) Epidemiology of mental health disorders in a primary care setting. *Epidemiologic Reviews*, 17 (1).

Gray, P. (1998) Counsellors in general practice. *Journal of the Royal College of General Practitioners*, 38, 50–51.

Heisler, J. (1979) Marriage counsellors in medical settings. *Marriage Guidance*, **March**, 153–162.

Hogg, C. (1999) *Patients, Power and Politics: from Patients to Citizens*. Sage, London.

Hunt, P. (1985) *Clients' Responses to Marriage Counselling*. Research Report No. 3. National Marriage Guidance Council, Rugby.

Keithley, J. (1982) *Marriage counselling in general practice*. PhD thesis (unpublished), University of Durham, Durham.

Llewellyn, S. (1988) Psychological therapy as viewed by clients and therapists. *British Journal of Clinical Psychology*, 27, 233–237.

Marsh, G.N. and Barr, J. (1975) Marriage guidance counselling at a group practice centre. *Journal of the Royal College of General Practitioners*, 25, 73–75.

McLeod, J. (1990) The clients' experience of counselling and psychotherapy: a review of the research literature. In *Experiences of Counselling in Action* (Mearns, D. and Dryden, W., eds). Sage, London, pp. 1–19.

Monach, J. and Monro, S. (1995) Counselling in general practice: issues and opportunities. *British Journal of Guidance and Counselling*, 23, 313–325.

NHS Management Executive (1992) *Local Voices. The Views of Local People in Purchasing for Health*. Department of Health, London.

Papadopoulos, L. and Bor, R. (1995) Counselling psychology in primary health care: a review. *Counselling Psychology Quarterly*, 8, 291–303.

Patten, M.I. and Walker, L.G. (1990) Marriage guidance counselling: 1. What clients think will help. *British Journal of Guidance and Counselling*, 18, 28–39.

Rogers, D., McLeod, J. and Sloboda, J. (1995) Counsellor and client perceptions of the effectiveness of time limited counselling in an occupational counselling scheme. *Counselling Psychology Quarterly*, 8, 221–231.

Roth, A. and Fonagy, P. (1996) *What Works for Whom? A Critical Review of Psychotherapy Research*. Guildford, New York.

Rowland, N., Irving, J. and Maynard, A. (1989) Can general practitioners counsel? *Journal of the Royal College of General Practitioners*, 39, 118–120.

Ruggeri, M. (1994) Patients' and relatives' satisfaction with psychiatric services: the state of the art of its measurement. *Social Psychiatry and Psychiatric Epidemiology*, 29, 212–227.

Scott, A. and Freeman, C. (1992) Edinburgh Primary Care Depression Study: treatment outcome, patient satisfaction and cost after 16 weeks. *British Medical Journal*, 304, 883–887.

Spiers, R. and Jewell, J.A. (1995) One counsellor, two practices: report of a pilot scheme in Cambridgeshire. *British Journal of General Practice*, 45, 31–33.

Thomas, P. (1993) An exploration of patients' perceptions of counselling with particular reference to counselling within general practice. *Counselling*, 4, 24–30.

Wakefield, P., Read, S., Wilson, F. and Lindesay, J. (1998) Clients' perceptions of outcome following contact with a community mental health team. *Journal of Mental Health*, 7, 375–384.

Waydenfeld, D. and Waydenfeld, S. (1978) *Counselling in the General Practice Setting*. North London Marriage Guidance Council, London.

Waydenfeld, D. and Waydenfeld, S. (1980) Counselling in general practice. *Journal of the Royal College of General Practitioners*, 30, 671–677.

Chapter 9

Counselling and young people

Gillian Turner and Joan McSloy

Introduction

Young people present to primary care with a variety of issues for which counselling may be useful (Sawyer & Bowes 1999). However, young people may not attend primary care services because of concerns about lack of confidentiality, power and control. Within this chapter, we outline a framework for effective counselling with young people with the aim of enabling young people to make informed decisions. This framework acknowledges the unique position of young people in society and the power imbalance between young people and adult professionals. The practicalities of providing an accessible service to young people within primary care are described as well as information about other support systems available to young people.

Young people in context

Young people are variously defined as youths, teenagers, adolescents, children and young adults. The age range of 'young people' is accepted as 13–25 years within UK youth work, 10–25 years in the USA and 10–18 years by the Department of Health in the UK. In some arenas such as fashion, beauty and sport, youth is idealized, but more usually young people are portrayed as difficult, disruptive, unpredictable and irresponsible. This image, often portrayed in the media, is inaccurate and discriminatory. Young people are usually under the control of adults in the family, in schools and within other institutions. Politically and legally young people have limited rights.

The Children's Act 1989 was a major step forward in defining the child's needs as paramount and suggesting young people should be involved in decisions affecting them. The UN Convention on the Rights of the Child (United Nations 1989) ratified by the UK in 1992 defines the rights of children and young people to education, health care and freedom from abuse. Article 12 stresses the importance of involving young people in issues affecting them. Consultation with young people has occurred in health-related research and service development (Cohen & Emanuel 1998), but there is more experience of consulting and involving young people within local government (Willow 1997). 'Empowerment' of young people is a key ingredient in effective health promotion with this age group (Health Education Authority 1998; Social Exclusion Unit 1999). Although this is broadly accepted, working with and sharing power with young people can be threatening to adult professionals (Lansdowne 1995). There are conflicting societal attitudes about how much autonomy a young person should have alongside the 'duty' to protect that young person (Alderson 1995; Alderson & Montgomery 1996). Children's and young people's rights are now acknowledged, but advocacy by adults on behalf of young people remains more common than young people speaking out on their own behalf and being heeded (Lansdowne & Newell 1994).

Young people's health

Young people have hitherto been wrongly assumed to be a healthy group who do not use health services. Recent studies have shown that 91% of teenage young women and 83% of teenage young men visit their GP in any year with most attending two or three times each year (Donovan *et al.* 1997). Young people tend to use primary care for physical complaints, respiratory symptoms, musculoskeletal problems and skin complaints (Macfarlane & McPherson 1995). This is in stark contrast to the morbidity and mortality data for this age group and young people's own assessment of their major health concerns. The commonest cause of death among teenagers in the UK is injury and poisoning including suicide (Department of Health 1994). The commonest reason for admission to hospital is orthopaedic trauma for young men and termination of pregnancy for young women (Henderson *et al.* 1993). Morbidity related to mental health, sexual health and the use of substances all appear to be increasing (McMiller & Plant 1994). However, young people in general do not access primary care to seek help with these issues (Gregg *et al.* 1998). GP consultations with young people are significantly shorter than with their older counterparts (Jacobsen *et al.* 1994). Health professionals often feel uncomfortable in consultations with young people who may themselves feel awkward. This can result in less productive consultations and missed opportunities for health promotion. Training for professionals in communication skills with young people, exploring the assumptions adults make about young people and addressing the specific needs of particular groups of young people can improve the welcome a service gives to its young users (McNulty & Turner 1998; Sanci *et al.* 1999). Brook Advisory Centres and the Loudmouth Theatre Company provide good training programmes suitable for primary care teams (see 'Useful contacts' below).

Young people consider their health holistically, aware of the influence of their circumstances and the way they feel on their behaviour and their physical health (McNulty & Turner 1998). Family and peer relationships, educational achievement and aspirations are all important aspects of a young person's well-being. Information alone does not ensure healthy behaviour. Young people, like adults, often need an opportunity to explore feelings, pressures and anxieties in order to be able to adopt healthy behaviours, for example in the areas of sexual health or substance use (Aggleton 1996).

Developing services accessible to young people

There are many barriers preventing young people accessing services. There is always a power difference between adults and young people. When the adult is also a professional, informed, highly paid service provider, the power difference can be detrimental to a consultation and to effective counselling. There is a danger that the young person views service providers and parent as allies. There can also be a 'culture' difference between young people and adults, which all members of a team should be aware of in order to make young people feel as welcome as possible.

Most services are run by adults primarily for adults. Young people are expected to conform to an adult setting and not cause discomfort or embarrassment to the adult users of the service otherwise they are denied access to the service. A glance at most waiting areas will confirm this view. In many services young people are expected to attend with their parents. Even when this is not the case many young people remain unaware that they could attend alone and this needs active publicity to young people, with reassurance regarding confidentiality. Displaying a confidentiality statement in the waiting area is helpful (Appendix 1). Child and Adolescent Mental Health Services and Social Services provide services for young people only with the knowledge and consent of their parents. The reasons for this are clear from the perspective of service delivery, but this can be a significant barrier to young people seeking help around particular issues. Some young people need to explore issues independently before they can develop strategies for involving their families. Others are in situations where the most positive way forward for the young person is to seek solutions without the involvement of their family. This possibility is rarely acknowledged or catered for.

Primary care staff who work with families often communicate with parents about the health of their children. This can continue inappropriately and unhelpfully as the young people become older. Young people should be considered as patients in their own right, enabled to attend independently of their parents and be given the opportunity to consult alone when they do attend with family members. All too often health professionals unconsciously identify with parents, communicating with them more easily and creating the situation of two adults in powerful positions (parent and doctor) discussing the problem of the less powerful young person. This can be disrespectful and disempowering, sometimes increasing antagonism between a young person and their parents. Developing the skills to engage directly with young people, to gain their perspective on a health-related situation and tap into their motivation for any change is an important skill. However, the skills of individuals are only one ingredient in an accessible service for young people. All members of the team require training in young people's needs, respecting confidentiality and welcoming all young people. Good practice must be established and deliberately maintained rather than depending on the skills of individual staff.

The critical factor is a respectful attitude towards young people by all members of the team. Consideration of young people as service users by providing young people's magazines, a range of music in waiting areas, and a range of posters and leaflets can all make young people feel more welcome. Involving young people specifically in consumer satisfaction work is important. A less formal atmosphere is experienced as more welcoming by people of most ages but informality should not be confused with an unprofessional or poor standard of service. The principles of respect for, working with and welcoming all young people should be integral to the organization within which young people's services are provided. Otherwise the quality of a young people's service will gradually deteriorate.

Services have to be experienced as 'safe enough' for young people to use them. Confidentiality is a critical part of this sense of safety. In addition, young people need to be able to protect their privacy, their reputation and their control of situations in order to experience a service as safe (McNulty & Turner 1998).

Confidentiality

Assurance of confidentiality is the most important factor in enabling young people to access health services (McPherson 1996; Ford *et al.* 1997; McNulty & Turner 1998). Confidentiality is an issue of control, a crucial issue for young people and vital within the counselling process—possibly in particular for young people with specific issues such as experience of abuse or low self-esteem (Daniel 1997). Legally and professionally, it is clear that the duty of confidentiality owed to a young person is as great as to any other person (British Medical Association 1993). The Children's Legal Centre has explored the nuances of this in practice and is a useful resource (Children's Legal Centre 1992) (see 'Useful contacts' below).

Confidentiality for young people is based on their experience of trusting the person they are seeing, an example of 'who you are, not what you are'. Recent research into confidentiality and young people, where young people were the co-researchers, identified that 'for young research participants confidentiality was inextricably linked to trust, secrecy and loyalty. In the counselling relationship, trust and confidentiality do not come from detailed explanations of what can be offered. In the eyes of the young person trust has to be demonstrated and indeed earned by the counsellor. Trust will come when young people and their rights are respected and they are valued and respected' (McSloy 1998, p. 82).

Most young people are not aware that primary care is confidential except in exceptional circumstances such as disclosure of serious harm. Young people's primary concern is that their family, teachers or friends might find out the content of their consultation. Most young people understand why confidentiality would have to be broken if an individual was suffering or at risk of harm including serious self-harm. If other agencies must be informed, for example following child protection guidelines, this must be explained to the young person before information is shared. It is helpful if phone calls sharing information can be made in the presence of the young person as this appears to lessen their sense of loss of control (McNulty & Turner 1998).

Recent research found that 74% of young people aged 12–18 years thought that their GP could inform their parents of their consultation against their wishes (Kari *et al.* 1997). Unfortunately current practice in primary care is patchy. Incredibly some practices still display notices that patients under 16 years will not be seen without a parent present (Brook Advisory Centres 1996). Young people's knowledge of their rights is increasing and it can be expected that a young person will take legal action against a practitioner who denies their legal right to confidentiality.

Sadly, young people's own experience may reinforce their view that primary care is not confidential for young people, particularly those young people under 16 where the GP may know the young person's parents. Young people who have experienced breaches of confidentiality often share this with their friends. This news can spread rapidly among young people and may undermine any growing confidence young people have in services (McNulty & Turner 1998). Uncertainty about confidentiality is a major barrier preventing young people accessing primary care with sensitive issues and may well explain why most young people consult about purely physical concerns. A confidentiality statement, reassuring young people about the confidential nature of consultations in primary care, while stating clearly the limits to confidentiality, should be displayed in waiting areas and consultation rooms (Appendix 1). A more detailed statement of the confidentiality policy of the counselling service should be available for young people to take away so that they are fully informed before deciding to embark on counselling (Appendix 2). All members of the primary care team require training and reminders about how to maintain the confidentiality and trust of young people to ensure that the confidentiality statement is followed in practice by the entire team. For young people to feel safe using a service the practicalities of ensuring their confidentiality must be considered, including how appointments are made, who else is in the waiting room and the possibility of computer screens being visible to parents.

There can be a tension between offering a confidential counselling service to young people and communication between the adult professionals involved in that young person's life. In our experience, routine communication from the counsellor to the young person's GP, social worker or teachers is detrimental to the counselling relationship with that young person. If information is to be shared it should be with the consent of the young person. This may need to be explored further when establishing a service in primary care as many referrers expect feedback.

Different workers, disciplines and agencies can offer different levels of confidentiality. Young people need to know this in order to make informed choices about where to seek help. Young people may choose to access services where they can retain anonymity for certain issues when they fear loss of control. Services within the voluntary sector can often offer more flexible, confidential services and are an important part of the choices young people should have (Rayment 1994).

Management of confidentiality

The House of Lords ruling in the case of Gillick (1985) had the effect of permitting doctors to provide medical treatment to children under the age of 16 years, without parental consent, where they were found by the doctor to be competent ('Gillick competent'). The Children's Legal Centre has reviewed recent case law and feels that this has limited the effect of the Gillick ruling. They advise that this ruling should not be viewed as giving automatic rights to professionals to offer confidential advice, treatment or counselling to young people under 16. For example, they feel it is unlikely that a young drug user or young person with a history of mental illness would always be classified as Gillick competent and therefore have the right to access confidential services without parental consent.

The reality of counselling with young people around highly sensitive and personal issues is that a significant proportion of what they confide could fall within the 'at risk' category, depending on the interpretation or understanding of the counsellor and the policy and practice of the organization. Risk-taking behaviour is an acknowledged characteristic of adolescence (Jessor 1998). In the main, young people survive the risks that they take and often learn from them (just as adults do!). If an adult were to breach confidentiality on every occasion that a young person described an 'at risk' situation then regular breaches would occur. Pertinent examples are child abuse and drug use.

For example, a 15-year-old young man wants to share his feelings and experiences of sexual abuse with a 'professional' and definitely wants confidentiality maintained. A voluntary project could decide it was in his best interests to maintain his confidentiality and work with him towards getting out of his abusive situation. The project may follow the practice of solicitors and state legal privilege, i.e. no duty to rescue in public law. Certainly there is no statutory duty to pass on information given to them by a young person.

The same young man could disclose the same information to a teacher who would have to act upon the information, follow local authority guidelines and breach confidentiality almost immediately. Failure to adhere to local authority child protection guidelines is not a criminal offence, but could lead to disciplinary action. If the young man were to approach his doctor with this disclosure, he could generally be afforded the time to express his feelings in confidence. The doctor may allow the space and time for the young man to prepare himself before the information is passed on following child protection guidelines. Counsellors attached to primary care may face particular difficulties in this area. Operating from within the British Association of Counselling code of practice and Gillick guidelines, a counsellor can offer high levels of confidentiality to a competent young person. However, he or she may still experience difficulties in maintaining the confidentiality of a young person in certain situations. For example in the case of a young person known to the practice to be a drug user, other professionals may expect to be given information on the 'client' by the counsellor.

Given the Children's Legal Centre's view that young drug users may not be viewed as Gillick competent, could they access confidential counselling without parental consent? Clearly young drug users do access confidential counselling through GP surgeries and projects are specifically established to meet this very need. Some professionals argue a commonsense view, stating that each situation should be addressed individually. The Standing Committee on Drug Addiction (SCODA) take this commonsense approach one step further. In their publication *Building Confidence* (1994), as well as suggesting the individual approach, they also stress the importance and need for close supervision and strong management support when working with young people around drug issues. SCODA sends clear signals of the sensitivity and complexity of maintaining confidentiality in these circumstances.

Counselling young people

It is widely accepted that the outcome of any counselling intervention is determined by the relationship between the counsellor and client with self-determination as a prerequisite (Bond 1993). When young people choose to access counselling they generally have the belief that they will get help to solve problems or will receive direction or advice. It is interesting to note young people's perception of counselling as advice-giving. They expect that the counsellor will have knowledge concerning their specific problems and will be understanding, caring and supportive (Gibson-Kline 1996). However, whether or not a young person seeks help depends on the perceived benefits of doing so and also the perceived threat of negative consequences which might result from seeking help. For example in relation to drug use, fear of police and other statutory involvement has been found to be a significant deterrent with regard to seeking help (Darke *et al.* 1996).

There is still stigma attached to 'going for counselling' and the whole concept of counselling is alien to many people within our communities. Young people have to overcome these barriers and also the general attitude that their difficulties may not be as serious as those of adults (Lansdowne & Newell 1994; Franklin 1995). Adults usually define their own problems, but young people often have their problems defined by the adults around them. Adults tend to be aware of the behaviours that cause concern or disturbance to adults rather than what is actually causing distress to the young person. The question 'who's problem is it?' can be illuminating.

What are adults' expectations of counselling for young people? Many adults are unaware or confused about the nature of counselling as compared to advice, support or other interventions. We know that parents are most likely to seek professional counselling for their children when the young person's behaviour is posing problems for themselves (Raviv *et al.* 1992). We are aware from first-hand experience that teachers, social workers, health professionals and other adults refer young people for counselling for a diversity of reasons or behaviours. These can include perceived antisocial behaviour, bullying, violence, disruptive behaviour, non-attendance at school and non-conformity to societal norms. We recognize that this list is by no means exhaustive and accept that many professionals 'encourage' young people to attend counselling out of genuine concern for their welfare. Yet, where does encouragement end and coercion begin? Are we expecting young people to come out of counselling as more 'reasonable', responsible and well-behaved citizens, conforming to adult-determined norms? If young people still display what society defines as antisocial behaviour do we then perceive counselling as having failed or the young person as having failed? Client satisfaction and long-term outcome measures may be the only useful measures by which a counselling service for young people should be evaluated.

Bond (1992) suggests that two distinctive systems of ethics and practice are in use by counsellors working with young people in education which are informative for counsellors within primary care. The integrated model assumes that the institution's goals are comparable with the client's goals, emphasizes the counsellor–institution relationship as the primary ethical perspective and sees the counsellor's primary responsibility as promoting the well-being of the institution through their work with clients. In contrast the differentiated model assumes that the counsellor will meet the institution's goals by respecting client autonomy and emphasizes the counsellor–client relationship as the primary ethical perspective. The relationship between counsellor and young person exists in the context of the issues of power, authority and control and the ethos of the institutions within which young people function. The family, primary care and indeed the health service can be considered as institutions in this regard. Counsellors working in primary care need to discuss with other team members the model which informs their work with young people.

Providing counselling to young people needs to improve their psychological well-being in the short and longer term. Receiving professional counselling from a trained adult may confirm a young person in the role of passive recipient. This can foster dependency on professional help for emotional issues rather than normalizing emotional support within friendships and family relationships. The process of seeking and receiving help needs to be empowering as far as possible and not reinforce a young person's sense of being powerless.

With the notable exception of peer-counselling initiatives (Cowie & Sharpe 1996), counselling is carried out by adults. Yet young people may be resistant to adult interest or concern for their behaviour or distress, and suspicious of the adult's motivation. The issues young people choose to address in counselling can be different to those issues that cause concern to the adults around them for which they are referred (McNulty & Turner 1998). Whether we are the referrer for, or provider of, counselling we need to address and explore these issues and recognize the potential that exists both within and without the counselling relationship for adults to retain power and control inadvertently or deliberately.

The position of young people in society and the reality of their relationships with adults and the actual limits of their choices (e.g. housing, money) must be understood before counselling is undertaken. Knowledge of the legal and ethical framework is essential, but as important are experience of working with young people and an understanding of the realities of young people's lives.

Counselling skills are useful for anyone working with young people from whatever discipline. However, young people are not the same as adults. Skill in counselling adults is not automatically transferable to counselling young people. The style of counselling may need to be more flexible to be appropriate for some young people, such as shorter sessions, a less formal, more interactive style or a reminder to attend with another 'chance' to attend after not attending. There must also be clarity about the difference between using counselling skills and offering formal contracted counselling. A different level of skill, experience and supervision is needed. Supervisors must provide counselling expertise and knowledge and have experience of young people's issues. Unfortunately there are few opportunities to train in counselling young people specifically. We have found standards for professionals offering formal counselling to young people helpful (Appendix 3).

Support for young people

The provision of counselling for young people within primary care should be developed with knowledge of other support available to young people. These include young people's relationships with each other, families, pastoral care within schools, youth workers, young people's centres, 'drop-ins', issue-based projects and multiagency 'one-stop-shops' aimed at young people.

Peer relationships become increasingly important during the teenage years. Good, reciprocal emotional support among friends is an important part of emotional well-being. Many young people share important worries and concerns with their friends rather than with adults. Friends are, therefore, an important support network for young people. Peer education and peer support acknowledges the importance and skills of young people in supporting one another (Cowie 1999). It also has the considerable benefit of normalizing the help-seeking process and increasing self-esteem of the peer helpers (Turner 1999).

There are an increasing number of 'one-stop-shop' facilities designed exclusively for and sometimes with young people. These centres offer a range of health-related services, some with a particular focus on counselling. Two notable examples of good practice are End House in Durham and Streetwise in Newcastle upon Tyne, where extensive evaluations have demonstrated the success of both projects (see 'Useful contacts' below). End House received the Smith Kline and Beecham Health Impact Award in 1999, described as 'succeeding in making a real difference to the health of its community often working from moderate resources'. The judges particularly acknowledged that young people found the one-stop-shop approach accessible.

Specialist facilities such as these often grow out of the voluntary sector, where local people take action in their own communities. Best practice seems to result when statutory agencies offer real support such as finance, staff or other resources and decision-making remains at the local level. In the case of young people's centres local decision-making should mean the active involvement of young people at all levels and stages. In reality, some services consult with young people on a regular basis, whilst others go further by ensuring that young people are represented in staffing, management and service delivery. Equal partnerships between young people and adults appear to be the key to success. The rhetoric is easy. The practice is more difficult.

Ironically, offering exclusive services for young people can lead to the exclusion of young people from mainline and majority services. Many one-stop-shop facilities face endless struggles for financial security. Funding packages are often short term, constantly undermining the work of the projects that in the meantime have raised the expectations of young people. There is a need for flexible responsiveness but unsustained short-termism is unethical. In our efforts to offer specialized counselling and health-related services to young people, are we compartmentalizing and segregating young people's issues? Are we failing to address the real issue of why young people do not feel comfortable accessing 'mainstream' counselling and health-related services? Are we socially excluding young people from major resources and the mainstream? 'Young people are not all the same and not a different species' (McNulty & Turner 1998).

Organizational issues

Counselling can play a part in promoting the health and well-being of young people now and the adults they will become. However, providing counselling services alone will not solve the increasing prevalence of psychosocial problems among young people. Social change is required, increasing the respect and power young people have and tackling inequality and social exclusion. To reduce inequalities and achieve equality of access it is necessary to target resources and services to young people with particular issues, and to 'vulnerable young people' without stigmatizing. Services must focus on the great strengths of young people rather than develop a perspective of 'young people as problems'. Actively and meaningfully involving young people in service development, decision-making and audit is one way. Young people need to be involved in the evaluation of any counselling service provided for them, determining appropriate outcome measures in partnership with adult service providers and commissioners.

Primary care trusts now have responsibility for commissioning services for their population. A long-term commitment to sustained intervention for young people's well-being is needed, guarding against a series of poorly evaluated, disjointed pilots and projects. A multiagency response, ideally led by young people, is needed to tackle the underlying issues of inequality, exclusion and young people's lack of political voice.

References

Aggleton, P. (1996) *Health Promotion and Young People.* Health Education Authority, London.

Alderson, P. (1995) *Listening to Children: Children, Ethics and Social Research.* Barnados, Basildon.

Alderson, P. and Montgomery, J. (1996) *Health Care Choices: Making Decisions with Children.* Institute for Public Policy Research, London.

Bond, T. (1992) Ethical issues in counselling and education. *British Journal of Guidance and Counselling,* **20,** 51–63.

Bond, T. (1993) *Standards and Ethics for Counselling in Action.* Sage, London.

British Medical Association (1993) *Confidentiality and People Under 16.* Guidance issued jointly by the British Medical Association, General Medical Services Committee, Health Education Authority, Brook Advisory Centres, Family Planning Association and Royal College of General Practitioners.

Brook Advisory Centres (1996) *What Should I Do? Guidance on Confidentiality and Under 16s for Community Nurses, Social Workers, Teacher and Youth Workers.* Brook Advisory Centres, London.

Children's Legal Centre (1992) *Working with Young People—Legal Responsibility and Liability.* Children's Legal Centre, Colchester.

Cohen, J. and Emanuel, J. (1998) *Positive Participation: Consulting and Involving Young People in Health-related Work.* Health Education Authority, London.

Cowie, H. (1999) Peers helping peers: interventions, inititatives and insights. *Journal of Adolescence,* **22,** 433–436.

Cowie, H. and Sharp, S. (1996) *Peer Counselling in Schools—a Time to Listen.* David Fulton Publishers, London.

Daniel, S. (1997) *Confidentiality and Young People. Working Together, Conflict, Contradictions, Chaos or the Best Interests of Young People?* Centre for Social Action, de Montfort University, Leicester.

Darke, S., Ross, J. and Hall, W. (1996) Overdose among heroin users in Sydney, Australia: responses to overdoses. *Addiction,* **91,** 413–417.

Department of Health (1994) The health of adolescents. In *On the State of the Public Health 1993.* HMSO, London, pp. 74–112.

Donovan, C., Mellanby, A.R., Jacobson, L.D., Taylor, B. and Tripp, J.H. (1997) Teenagers' views on the general practice consultation and provision of contraception. *British Journal of General Practice*, **47**, 715–718.

Ford, C.A., Millstein, S.G., Halpern-Felsher, B.L. and Irmin, C.E. Jr. (1997) Influence of physician confidentiality assurances on adolescents' willingness to disclose information and seek future health care: a randomised controlled trial. *Journal of the American Medical Association*, **278**, 1029–1034.

Franklin, B. (ed.) (1995) *The Handbook of Children's Rights—Comparative Policy and Practice*. Routledge, London.

Gibson-Kline, J. (1996) *Adolescents: from Crisis to Coping—a Thirteen Nation Study*. Butterworth–Heinemann, Oxford.

Gregg, R., Freeth, D. and Blackie, C. (1998) Teenage health and the practice nurse: choice and opportunity for both? *British Journal of General Practice*, **48**, 909–910.

Health Education Authority (1998) *Promoting the Health of Children and Young People—Setting a Research Agenda*. Report of a HEA expert working group chaired by Henrietta L. Moore. Health Educaction Authority, London.

Henderson, J., Goldacre, M. and Yeates, D. (1993) Use of hospital in-patient care in adolescence. *Archives of Disease in Childhood*, **69**, 559–563.

Jacobsen, L.D., Wilkinson, C.E. and Owen, P. (1994) Is the potential of teenage consultations being missed? A study of consultation times in primary care. *Family Practice*, **11**, 296–299.

Jessor, R. (ed.) (1998). *New Perspectives on Adolescent Risk Behaviour*. Cambridge University Press, Cambridge.

Kari, J., Donovan, C., Li, J. and Taylor, B. (1997) Adolescents' attitudes to general practice in North London. *British Journal of General Practice*, **47**, 109–110.

Lansdowne, G. (1995) *Taking Part. Children's Participation in Decision Making*. Institute for Public Policy Research, London.

Lansdowne, G. and Newell, P. (eds) (1994) *UK Agenda for Children*. Children's Rights Development Unit, London.

Macfarlane, A. and McPherson, A. (1995) Primary health care and adolescence. *British Medical Journal*, **3111**, 825–826.

McMiller, P. and Plant, M. (1994) Drinking, smoking and illicit drug use among 15 and 16 year olds in the United Kingdom. *British Medical Journal*, **313**, 394–397.

McNulty, A. and Turner, G. (1998) *Not Just a Phase We're Going Through: Final Report of the Northumberland Young People's Health Project*. North East Datagraphics, Ashington.

McPherson, A. (1996) Primary health care and adolescence. In *Adolescent Health* (Macfarlane, A., ed.). Royal College of Physicians, London, pp. 33–41.

McSloy, J. (1998) *Confidentiality and young people—a descriptive ethical enquiry*. MA thesis, University of Durham, Durham.

Rayment, B. (1994) *Confidential—Developing Confidentiality Policies in Youth Counselling and Advisory Services*. Youth Access, London.

Raviv, A., Maddy-Weitzman, E. and Raviv, A. (1992) Parents of adolescents: help seeking intentions as a function of help sources and parenting issues. *Journal of Adolescence*, **15**, 115–135.

Sanci, L.A., Coffey, C.M., Veit, F.C., Day, N. and Bowes, G. (1999) Evaluation of a program in adolescent health care for family physicians designed according to evidence-based practice in continuing medical education: a randomised controlled trial. *Journal of Adolescent Health*, **24**, 81.

Sawyer, S.M. and Bowes, G. (1999) Adolescence on the health agenda. *Lancet*, **354** (Suppl. 2), 31–34.

Social Exclusion Unit (1999) *Teenage Pregnancy—Report by the SEU*. HMSO, London.

Standing Committee on Drug Addiction (1994) *Building Confidence—Advice on Confidentiality Policies for Drug and Alcohol Services*. Standing Committee on Drug Addiction, London.

Turner, G. (1999) Peer support and young people's health. *Journal of Adolescence*, **22**, 567–572.

United Nations (1989) *UN Convention on the Rights of the Child*. HMSO, London.

Willow, C. (1997) *Hear! Hear! Promoting Children and Young People's Democratic Participation in Local Government*. Local Government Information Unit, London.

Useful contacts

Brook Advisory Centres (offers training to primary care staff). Telephone: 0171 833 8488.

Children's Legal Centre, University of Essex, Wivenhoe Park, Colchester, Essex CO4 3SQ. Telephone: 01296 873820.

End House Young People's Centre, 92a Claypath, Durham DH1 1RG. Telephone: 0191 383 1414.

Loudmouth Theatre Company (offers training) Contact Chris Cowan, telephone: 0121 446 4880; e-mail: info@loudmouth.co.uk

Streetwise, Groat Market, Newcastle upon Tyne NE1 1UQ. Telephone: 0191 230 5400.

Appendix 1

Confidentiality

All of the members of our practice team know that confidentiality is important for people using the service. Young people in Northumberland have said that this is particularly important for them.

Even if you are under 16, you have a *right to privacy* and you can speak to a nurse or doctor in complete confidence, about any issue.

The only exception to this is if the health professional believes that keeping something confidential puts you in danger and at risk of serious harm. This is an extreme situation, and if they need to have support from another worker, they will discuss this with you. *In all other circumstances, we will not pass on information about your visit to anyone else.*

Northumberland Young People's Health Project, 1998

Appendix 2

Confidentiality policy of the counselling service

The counselling service recognizes that confidentiality is of the utmost importance to young people using the service, and is therefore essential to the effective running of the whole service. A 'service user' means anyone approaching the service for help, support, information, advice or counselling.

A young person who uses the service has the right to be confident that information given to the counsellor will not be shared with anyone else within or without the counselling service. Anything the young person chooses to divulge will be kept confidential unless it is the express wish of that person that the information be passed on.

Limits to confidentiality

There are certain exceptions to these rules of confidentiality; i.e.

(a) If the counsellor believes you are at risk of significant harm, or that you may seriously harm another person. 'Significant harm' means impairment of a young person's health or development (physical, intellectual, emotional, social or behavioural).

(b) Any disclosure involving abuse cannot be kept confidential. Abuse can be physical, mental or sexual, and means that the young person is not being treated or respected in the way that he or she would wish to be. It could be making the young person feel sad, hurt, lonely, frightened, etc.

Referral from a third party

Sometimes the young person is referred to the counselling service by someone else; e.g. a member of the teaching staff. Unless the limits to confidentiality apply, information will not be shared with this third party unless the young person gives their full and informed consent.

Where the young person has referred himself or herself, the counsellor will not divulge this to any third party unless the limits to confidentiality apply.

Sometimes the young person will request that information is shared with a third party. The counsellor has an obligation to ensure that the young person knows what is being divulged and to whom, and to make clear the consequences of disclosure.

Based on Draft Model Policy from SCODA
(From McNulty & Turner 1998)

Appendix 3

Standards for counsellors at Northumberland Young People's Health Project sessions

A distinction is made between staff and young people using 'counselling skills' in their formal or informal contacts with young people during health sessions and members of staff offering 'contracted counselling' and advertising themselves as 'counsellors'. Many staff will have received basic counselling skills training and of course use of these skills informally is encouraged whenever this is appropriate.

Standards for formal contracted counselling:

1 Counsellors be appropriately trained to a minimum standard of Certificate in Counselling, preferably a postgraduate Diploma, recognized by the British Association of Counselling.

2 A written statement of the meaning and limits of confidentiality within the counselling situation will be given and explained to each young person before entering into formal counselling. Counsellors must maintain confidentiality appropriately within the multidisciplinary team of the Young People's Health Session and particularly act appropriately regarding child protection concerns according to Northumberland Child Protection Committee Guidelines.

3 Each counsellor to take responsibility for receiving adequate and appropriate supervision according to British Association of Counselling guidelines (two hours monthly) by a recognized and suitably trained supervisor. Counsellors are encouraged to find a supervisor with experience and skill in counselling young people.

4 Counsellors should adhere to the BAC Code of Ethics and Practice for Counsellors and undertake to continue working within this code.

5 Each counsellor to take responsibility for collecting basic monitoring data of clients attending for counselling including basic demographic data and referral topic, and encouraging clients to complete client satisfaction questionnaires. Both these documents should be returned to the Northumberland Young People's Health Project office for compilation and analysis.

6 Counsellors are strongly encouraged to attend multidisciplinary training organized by Northumberland Young People's Health Project. Counsellors will receive the regular information mailings from the Northumberland Young People's Health Project.

7 Counsellors should be particularly aware of the legal, ethical, social and psychological issues relevant to counselling young people under the age of 16.

8 Counsellors are encouraged to remain in contact formally or informally with other counsellors offering a service to young people in Northumberland.

(From McNulty & Turner 1998)

Part 3

Counselling problems

Chapter 10

Psychiatric disorders

Kevin Gournay

Introduction

Mental health services had been cited as priorities for action within various policy documents throughout the 1990s. However, when the Blair Government was elected, these services remained in a state of impoverishment, and the staff within them had very poor morale. In 1998, the first National Service Frameworks in health care were set up, intended to improve quality and reduce unacceptable variations in health and social care delivery. Mental health and coronary heart disease were the first two priority areas and the National Service Framework for Mental Health was published in late 1999 (Department of Health 1999). For the first time this policy framework went beyond mere rhetoric, as it set out a real programme for action, underpinned by some new resources and set out within the context of different priority areas. Central to the framework was the setting of standards in five areas, each standard based on evidence and knowledge, supported by service models and examples of good practice. Altogether, there are seven standards in the five areas, and two of them explicitly focus on primary care and access to services for anyone who may have a mental health problem. Thus, the specific targeting of primary care and mental health should lead to unified action across all groups involved in providing services to primary care. These groups range from charitably aided self-help organizations, through counsellors, general practitioners, social workers and mental health professionals, including psychologists, nurses and psychiatrists.

This chapter will consider how psychiatric disorders should be targeted within primary care and examine some of the problems which, for the moment, mean that services are provided in a very haphazard and idiosyncratic fashion. However, prior to setting out the picture of psychiatry in primary care, it is very important to discuss one of the underpinning features of the mental health services of the future, i.e. evidence-based medicine.

The importance of evidence-based medicine in future mental health services

The National Service Framework highlights the importance of two initiatives—the National Institute for Clinical Excellence and the Commission for Health Improvement. The National Institute for Clinical Excellence is essentially responsible for defining best practice, and with it the evidence which underpins this. The Commission for Health

Improvement provides a mechanism for ensuring that all service providers come up to acceptable standards. Implicit in the work of the National Institute for Clinical Excellence is the principle that everything that we do should be underpinned by evidence. This will mean that no longer will patients be subject to the idiosyncratic approaches of individual professionals using dubious methods, but they will be entitled to receive the best possible treatment, based on sound evidence. The current gold standard for defining what is effective is the randomized controlled trial. In turn, this standard is now accepted as a central currency for all policy initiatives around evidence-based medicine. Furthermore, the worldwide Cochrane Collaboration will be the main mechanism for examining the efficacy and relative efficacy of treatment approaches. This collaboration provides a method for aggregating the evidence of all published trials in each area and takes account of the quality of that evidence. Therefore, the methodology used in Cochrane reviews recognizes that there are good quality and poor quality randomized controlled trials. The systematic reviews commissioned for the Cochrane Collaboration provide best evidence in a format that is understandable to all. The Cochrane Library is now available on CD-ROM in every professional library across the country and thus any professional can access what is known about treatments and various conditions. Perhaps even more importantly, patients are now able to access the same evidence via the internet and all clinicians now know (and some fear) the patient who comes armed with Cochrane print-outs. Although this is seen by some professionals as a negative aspect of the information explosion, it seems clear that the future will see a general public much more versed in evidence and with increasingly sophisticated knowledge of matters which were previously only known within professional domains.

What are the implications of such an approach for the counsellor, community psychiatric nurse or psychologist in primary care? The answer is that they are profound and wide-ranging. Already the National Service Framework is being implemented so that educational programmes for the workforce are underpinned by evidence of efficacy of treatments from randomized controlled trials. There is also an expectation that the commissioning of services will be led by the principle of whether the service has proven efficacy. Thus, to take a hypothetical case, if a primary care group wishes to provide a service for people with panic disorder with agoraphobia, it will expect that those providing the service will use the best evidence approach, i.e. behavioural and cognitive behavioural treatment. It will not wish to purchase the psychodynamic therapies which have no evidence to support their use in this condition. Along with the evidence-based approach will come the need to be more precise about diagnostic category, and here traditional psychiatric models of mental distress seem to have won the day. Evidence-based medicine brings with it the need to define precisely the condition to which treatments are applied and, therefore, the diagnoses found in the *International Classification of Diseases* and the *Diagnostic and Statistical Manual* of the American Psychiatric Association will become the central descriptors of mental health problems.

The mental health professional workforce

It has become absolutely clear that the mental health workforce has major problems dealing with those with the most serious and enduring mental illnesses. A wide range of policy documents have long recognized that mental health professional workforces are overstretched and that there are difficulties providing even the most basic of inpatient and community services. Recently the Clinical Standard Advisory Group Depression Committee (Department of Health 2000) published a report on care and treatment of people with depression across the UK. This demonstrated very clearly that services for people with depression are patchy to say the least, and in some areas of the UK there is virtually no access for the general public to psychological treatments. It is common for people to wait months for an assessment, and thereafter be provided with a very limited number of treatment sessions. This work is perhaps the best recent example of the impoverished state of mental health services.

Also during 2000, the government set up a workforce action team, whose job is to develop a strategic plan for strengthening the mental health workforce. This team (of which this author is a member) comprises a very wide range of individuals from both health and social care, and there is a more adequate representation from traditionally under-represented groups, including patients, and a range of 'non professionals', including counsellors. Although the number of psychiatrists has increased over the years, there are still just over 2000 psychiatrists employed in the adult mental illness field in England and the ratio of psychiatrists to GPs is approximately 1 : 12.5. (Goldberg & Gournay 1997). To compound the problem further, more than 10% of consultant psychiatrist posts remain unfilled.

With regard to community psychiatric nurses (CPNs), the last census (Brooker & White 1997) revealed that in England there are approximately 8000. The Mental Health Nursing Review, carried out at the beginning of the 1990s (Department of Health 1994), suggested that the focus of these nurses should be on those with serious and enduring mental illness. One of the reasons for making this recommendation was the fact that in 1990 CPNs were increasingly moving towards primary health care and work with people with adjustment disorders, anxiety and depression, using counselling techniques. At the same time, the focus of CPN work was moving away from people with schizophrenia. This led to a situation where 80% of people with schizophrenia in the community had no services from a community psychiatric nurse. The Mental Health Nursing Review recommendation has led to CPNs focusing their efforts more on the needs of people with schizophrenia and other serious and enduring illnesses, within the context of community mental health teams. However, a substantial number of CPNs continue to work in primary care, often assuming counsellor roles. Arguably, using CPNs in this fashion is not only to the detriment of people with schizophrenia but, as research shows, is also a squandering of a precious public resource (Gournay & Brooking 1994, 1995).

The third significant group of mental health professionals is clinical psychologists. Again there are relatively small numbers in the British system. Although there are some 3000 clinical psychologists on the register of the British Psychological Society, many of these are not employed in direct clinical work with patients. For example, some of those with a clinical qualification work in other areas such as educational psychology, research, teaching or management. Furthermore, a small but significant number of clinical psychologists are engaged in whole-time or part-time private practice. The point also needs to be made that many clinical psychologists have not received training in evidence-based therapies such as cognitive behaviour therapy. These individuals may have only received training in the psychodynamic and psychoanalytic therapies which are arguably redundant in this era of evidence-based approaches.

The fourth group of mental health professionals to be considered are nurse behaviour therapists. These nurses have received full-time training in behavioural and cognitive behavioural therapy and there is considerable research which testifies to the clinical and cost-effectiveness of their approach (Gournay 1999). The training of these nurse therapists began because of a recognition that there was only a very small workforce with skills in behaviour therapy to target people with conditions known to be responsive to this approach (e.g. agoraphobia, obsessive compulsive disorder, simple phobias, sexual problems). At the present time there are approximately 250 whole-time equivalents in clinical practice across the UK and a substantial majority of this workforce targets its efforts toward people in primary care settings (Gournay et al. 2000). Nevertheless, with each therapist treating about 70 patients per year (to completion), the numbers of people who can benefit from such treatment by nurse therapists remains fairly small.

Indeed, if one calculates the total number of nurses, psychologists and psychiatrists trained in cognitive behaviour therapy and makes the assumption that each whole-time therapist would treat approximately 70 patients per year, the entire mental health workforce will treat between 50 000 and 75 000 patients per year (Goldberg & Gournay 1997). If one sets alongside this figure the numbers of people who at any one time suffer from disorders known to be responsive to cognitive behaviour therapy, the picture becomes daunting to say the least. Based on reliable epidemiological research (Marks 1987) we know that there may be some 300 000 people suffering from panic disorder with agoraphobia, 500 000 people suffering from obsessive compulsive disorder, 500 000 people suffering from severe social phobia and so on. We are thus faced with a situation where mental health professionals need to concentrate their efforts on a very sizeable and needy population with schizophrenia and other serious mental illnesses. However, this workforce is also expected by some to provide treatment for people with more widespread conditions such as anxiety, phobias and depression. Thus, to paraphrase Michael Shepherd and colleagues (Shepherd et al. 1966), the central (and most realistic) requirement for the improvement of mental health services is not a large expansion of psychiatric agencies, rather a strengthening of primary care teams. Prior to examining the ways in which the primary care team may be assisted to meet the challenges that ubiquitous mental health problems provide, it is perhaps important to set out the template for treating various mental disorders which are likely to be seen in primary care. Although this template is arbitrary, it does at least provide a starting point for planning services and developing models of practice.

Severe mental disorders

Severe mental disorders such as schizophrenia, bipolar disorder, severe eating disorders and severe personality disorders are usually referred to community mental health teams and current mental health policy probably means that people with these disorders will continue to receive their specialist care from these teams. However, there is little doubt that primary care services have to accept some of the burden of care. For example, we now have evidence that depot medication is increasingly prescribed, and administered by primary care staff (Gray *et al.* 1999). We also know that these patients have considerable physical health needs which demand increased attention from GPs (Fox & Goldblatt 1982). Primary care staff will continue to have substantial involvement in these ways.

Disorders which respond to both pharmacological and psychological treatments

This group contains people with depression, states of generalized anxiety and depression, panic disorder and obsessive compulsive disorders. While most of these cases can be managed effectively by the primary care team, community mental health services will need to act as a resource for consultation and also ensure that members of the primary care team are appropriately skilled. As noted above, there is a great shortage of expertise necessary to deliver the psychological treatments which are known to be effective with these conditions and, therefore, it is likely that for the foreseeable future we will need to rely on drug treatments. However, we know that drug treatments are often compromised because of poor psychological and pharmacological management skills by the GP. On a more optimistic note, there are now a number of training initiatives (e.g. Gask 1999; Tylee 1999) which have set out to address these issues by targeting both GPs alone and via total team training efforts of all personnel involved.

Disorders where the treatment of choice is a psychological approach

This group includes simple phobias, post-traumatic stress disorder, chronic fatigue syndrome, anxiety states, somatization disorder and mild to moderate eating disorders. These conditions can become chronic without treatment, and often lead to very considerable handicap, which belies a relatively benign initial presentation. By and large, the psychological treatment modalities which have greatest efficacy are behavioural approaches for phobic disorders (Marks 1987; Gournay 1989) or cognitive behavioural treatments for other conditions (Roth & Fonagy 1996; Deale *et al.* 1997). There seems little reason why, with the presence of appropriately trained staff, these conditions should not be treated in primary care. Only a very small minority of patients should ever really need to seek help in specialist mental health services.

Those conditions which tend to resolve spontaneously

This group includes perhaps the majority of people who present at GPs' surgeries with complaints of anxiety, depression, sleeplessness, bereavement and unexplained medical problems. The majority of people with such symptoms will indeed be subject to considerable distress, but their symptoms are usually short-lived. There is a vast array of epidemiological evidence which suggests that such symptoms are usually linked to life events of one sort or another, and could be grouped under a generic heading of adjustment disorder. The difficulty with this group of people is that the presenting symptoms are often of such severity that the GP may make a referral for counselling or other psychiatric treatment. However, if one does nothing for the patient, it is likely that, in a large majority of cases, the distress will resolve over a few weeks. One major difficulty with this group is that it is sometimes difficult to prospectively identify the minority of patients whose symptoms will not remit (Gournay & Brooking 1994). For example, when patients are referred to and receive counselling, the patient and the counsellor, and then the GP, usually attribute any improvement to counselling, rather than to the course of time and natural events. This, perhaps, is one of the main reasons why treatments which fail to show any significant results within rigorously conducted trials continue to have credibility among the general public and, indeed, professionals.

The above grouping is, of course, arbitrary, but serves to demonstrate that it is possible to consider rational ways of defining health service priorities for action. One of the difficulties with previous mental health policy was that planning was left to the vagaries of individual professionals and, during the Thatcher era, to the forces of the internal market. In turn the market was driven by demand rather than real need or, indeed, hard evidence.

Future developments in primary care

What then can be done to strengthen mental health initiatives in primary care? At one level the answer to this, of course, lies in public policy. The National Service Framework is welcome, in so far as it recognizes the disparate nature of mental health services. For the first time we have policy which is linked to a set of actions, and there is now evidence of a government initiative prepared to make a really concerted attempt to draw together the various strands of an approach. The framework sets out, within the context of a 10-year programme of a range of initiatives, to 'join up' thinking, so that, rather than being seen as two separate parts of a National Health Service, the primary care team and secondary mental health services work much more in unison. Future initiatives, such as the commissioning of mental health services by primary care groups and trusts will, undoubtedly, help this process, while workforce initiatives which are all inclusive and transcend professional boundaries will also be helpful.

It has to be said at this point that while multidisciplinary education and training involving, not only professionals, but workers from the voluntary sector and people with non-professional backgrounds is much talked about, the rhetoric is not matched by reality. Unfortunately, there is still a great deal of tribalism and many training programmes are currently 'ring-fenced'. For example, the nurse therapy training programme noted above can only be accessed by registered mental nurses; clinical psychology training is completely separate from all other training initiatives in therapeutic approaches; and the mental health training initiatives for GPs and psychiatrists are separated, not only from the other non-medical professions, but from each other. At the present time there are some modular multidisciplinary postgraduate programmes, notably at the universities of Sheffield, Birmingham and Middlesex. These programmes educate and train doctors, nurses, psychologists and others with therapeutic approaches; however, they are, unfortunately, in the minority. Public policy initiatives which are currently developing in the slipstream of the National Service

Framework should lead to the confluence of the currently separate education and training monies. Such unified education funding should lead to the burgeoning of more truly multidisciplinary initiatives. In turn, other changes such as giving nurses authority to prescribe will help to blur boundaries even further. Nevertheless, it needs to be said that the tribalism which continues to separate various professions (and those from non-professional backgrounds) is largely in the hearts and minds of individual practitioners. Perhaps modular multidisciplinary undergraduate education is the long-term answer. However, this model will take many years (if ever) to achieve.

Future training initiatives

Nurses are the most numerous group in the British NHS and there are currently 637 000 nurses, midwives and health visitors registered with the United Kingdom Council for Nursing, Midwifery and Health Visiting (UK Central Council 1999). In primary care the most numerous group are practice nurses and, at the present time, there may be 20 000 in post in the UK. Recent research (Gray *et al.* 1999) has shown that practice nurses, *de facto*, carry out a wide range of mental health tasks. However, they are largely undertaking these roles without any substantial training. There are currently a number of initiatives under way to train practice nurses in the detection and management of common mental disorders (Gournay 1999). It seems clear that practice nurses could do a great deal more not only to recognize mental health problems, but also to assist the GP in the monitoring and maintenance tasks, which should accompany treatment by medication, and also in providing some of the simpler brief psychological treatments. Similarly, there is some evidence to suggest that health visitors have a major role in the detection and management of postnatal depression (Holden *et al.* 1989). As with practice nurses, this substantial group of professionals could be mobilized to undertake some treatment and management tasks for this needy group, who clearly do not currently receive the services that they require.

There is little doubt that the nurse therapy model described above is very useful. However, it also seems clear that we need to deliver training in evidence-based approaches to much larger numbers of nurses and others. Many clinical psychologists employed in the British NHS have not received formal training in cognitive behaviour therapy and, therefore, the retraining of some members of this workforce may be an important priority. In turn, a very large number of counsellors (from various backgrounds) who are employed in the primary care sector could also be a target for retraining. There is little doubt that the future NHS will have little place for individuals using approaches not based in sound experimental evidence. Therefore, many of the psychodynamic, psychoanalytic and more esoteric psychotherapies will wither (in the public sector at least).

One of the most important future developments will be the new workers in mental health in primary care, which was announced as part of the NHS plan published in late 2000. This proposal forms part of a package of measures designed to strengthen primary mental health care. The government has set aside 27 million pounds to train and employ these workers in primary health care trusts. The overall aim of this initiative is to ensure quicker access to more effective treatment for common mental disorders, and with that comes the need to provide information to the general public about treatment and referral. These workers will be trained to deliver brief evidence-based techniques, such as cognitive and behavioural therapies; however, they are likely to come predominately from a non-health professional background and, possibly, many of them will be new graduates in psychology and social sciences. The government does not intend that this group should replace counsellors or other primary care staff as the initiative is centred on augmenting the existing workforces.

Finally, the information technology revolution has brought with it an array of computerized treatment programmes, mostly centring on cognitive behaviour therapy (for a brief review see Marks 1998). These computer programmes usually need a little professional input by way of making an initial diagnosis and then introducing the patient to the technology. The results of research on this new way of delivering treatment is very impressive and there are now well-tried and tested computer programmes for phobic anxiety, obsessive compulsive disorder, depression and other common mental disorders.

Implications for counsellors

The first four years of the Labour Government elected in 1997 arguably produced more changes in mental health policy than ever before. There is no doubt that these changes will have a major impact on counsellors. The training and practice of counsellors will undoubtedly need to emphasize the importance of evidence-based approaches, and the need to look critically at theoretical frameworks. With the advent of new workers in mental health in primary care, who will largely be from a non-health professional background, there will probably be a shift in emphasis away from mental health professionals. It is at long last now being recognized that even if the mental health workforce could be substantially enlarged (and the prospect of this is very doubtful), people with common mental disorders, who are in need of skilled intervention, will never be able to meet their requirements from a small band of doctors, nurses and psychologists. However, the counselling profession obviously represents an enormous resource. Government has recognized a need for the efforts of all those who provide mental health interventions to be much more focused. Hopefully counsellors will be increasingly involved in the development of strategy at a local level, and the primary care trusts will in future be the primary vehicle for the development of local policy. Overall, therefore, the counselling profession will need to adapt to evolving, evidence-based theoretical frameworks, and new skill sets. However, in addition, the counselling profession will need to become more cognisant of health policy and at local level individual counsellors will need to become more politically active in asserting the importance of the counselling role in primary care.

Conclusions

The new century has started with the recognition that mental health in primary care is in a state of disarray. Only a relatively small number of people receive appropriate treatment for their condition and new public policy has had to develop structures which will provide equity of access to evidence-based treatment for all who need it.

Mental health services, and mental health professionals in particular, will clearly never be able to provide a comprehensive approach to mental health problems in primary care. The role of the mental health services will be to provide treatments for the most severely ill patients and to assist in strengthening the skills of the primary care team. Future training initiatives should be targeted to all professions, but nurses are the most numerous and obvious group for training attention. New technologies will provide self-help treatments that will augment other initiatives. However, it must be stated, with great emphasis, that the overall task of dealing with mental health problems in primary care is truly Herculean in its dimensions.

References

Brooker, C. and White, E. (1997) *The Fourth Quinquennial Survey of Community Psychiatric Nurses in England and Wales.* Department of Nursing Monograph. University of Manchester, Manchester.

Deale, A., Chalder, T., Marks, I. and Wesley, S. (1997) Cognitive behaviour therapy for chronic fatigue syndrome: a randomised controlled trial. *American Journal of Psychiatry,* **154,** 408–414.

Department of Health (1994) *Working in Partnership: a Review of Mental Health Nursing.* HMSO, London.

Department of Health (1999) *The National Service Framework.* HMSO, London.

Department of Health (2000) *The Report of the Clinical Standards Advisory Group on Depression.* HMSO, London.

Fox, A. and Goldblatt, P. (1982) *Longitudinal Study—Socio-Demographic Mortality Differential.* LA No. 1, 1971–1975. HMSO, London.

Gask, L. (1999) A course in mental health skills for general practitioners in Manchester. In *Common Mental Disorders in Primary Care: Essays in Honour of Professor Sir David Goldberg* (Tansela, M. and Thornicroft, G., eds). Routledge, London, pp. 171–182.

Goldberg, D. and Gournay, K. (1997) *The General Practitioner, the Psychiatrist and the Burden of Mental Health Care.* Maudsley Discussion Paper No. 1. Institute of Psychiatry, London.

Gournay, K. (1989) *Agoraphobia: Current Perspectives on Theory and Treatment.* Routledge, London.

Gournay, K. (1999) The future role of the nurse in primary mental health care. In *Common Mental Disorders in Primary Care: Essays in Honour of Professor Sir David Goldberg* (Tansela, M. and Thornicroft, G., eds). Routledge, London, pp. 92–102.

Gournay, K. and Brooking, J. (1994) Community psychiatric nurses in primary care: a randomised controlled trial. *British Journal of Psychiatry,* **165,** 231–238.

Gournay, K. and Brooking, J. (1995) The CPN in primary care: an economic analysis. *Journal of Advanced Nursing,* **22,** 769–778.

Gournay, K., Denford, L., Parr, A.-M. and Newell, R. (2000) Nurses in behavioural psychotherapy in the UK: a 25-year follow-up. *Journal of Advanced Nursing,* **32** (2), 343–351.

Gray, R., Parr, A.-M., Plummer, S. *et al.* (1999) A national survey of practice nurse involvement in mental health interventions. *Journal of Advanced Nursing,* **30** (4), 901–906.

Holden, J., Sagovsky, R. and Cox, J. (1989) Counselling in general practice settings: controlled study of health visitor intervention in the treatment of post natal depression, *British Medical Journal,* **298,** 223–226.

Marks, I. (1987) *Fears, Phobias and Rituals.* Oxford University Press, Oxford.

Marks, I. (1998) Computer aids to self treatment of anxiety. *Progress in Neurology and Psychiatry,* **12** (2), 35–37.

Roth, A. and Fonagy, P. (1996) *What Works for Whom? A Critical Review of Psychotherapy Research.* Guildford Press, New York.

Shepherd, M., Cooper, B., Brown, A. and Kalton, G. (1996) *Psychiatric Illness in General Practice.* Oxford University Press, Oxford.

Tylee, A. (1999) Training the whole primary care team. In *Common Mental Disorders in Primary Care: Essays in Honour of Professor Sir David* Goldberg (Tansela, M. and Thornicroft, G., eds). Routledge, London, pp. 194–208.

UK Central Council (1999) *The United Kingdom Central Council for Nursing, Midwifery and Health Visiting: Annual Statistics.* UKCC, London.

Chapter 11

Substance misuse

Pip Mason

Introduction

Many of the health problems that prompt patients to visit their GP or practice nurse are related to smoking, heavy drinking or misuse of medication or illicit drugs. Sometimes brief advice from the GP can be enough to encourage and enable the patient to change his or her lifestyle (Russell *et al.* 1979; Wallace *et al.* 1988; Saunders *et al.* 1991; Anderson & Scott 1992; Babor & Grant 1992). However, many people, due to the entrenched nature of the habit and due to elements of physical addiction find it very difficult to change without more intensive help. Others do not want to change or are ambivalent about it. They drink, smoke or take other drugs for important reasons, are attached to this behaviour and feel resistant to having change imposed upon them. It is in this context that some general practices have been exploring the potential role of counselling.

There are three main categories of situations regarding substance misuse counselling in primary health care. The first is when a patient requests help for a substance misuse problem because s/he believes it to be a problem and wants to reduce the harm and/or change the drug use. Resolution of the difficulty will probably involve a mixture of counselling, advice, medical treatment and education.

In the second type of situation a health professional wants the patient to change the substance use because it is contributing to a health problem or concern. In such a situation, although the counsellor has the client's best interests at heart, the starting point of the intervention is the counsellor's wish for the patient to change, not the patient's wish to do so. Again a cocktail of counselling, advice, medical treatment and education may be appropriate but with different measures of each, with an initial goal, not of changing the behaviour but of engaging some motivation to consider change.

In the third type of situation a patient asks for help in dealing with a family member's substance misuse. The patient may be requesting help to change not his or her own behaviour but someone else's. The first stage of such an intervention will be to reframe the goals to make them realistic. Counselling to help the patient cope with, or change, his or her own responses to the substance misuser will be appropriate and may be accompanied by advice on coping strategies. Provision of information may help to inform the process.

Most of the substance misuse counselling projects that have been established and evaluated in primary care relate to alcohol problems. Alcohol agencies, especially in the voluntary sector, have been concerned to improve their links with primary care and to increase the accessibility of their counselling services. Recent policy developments in smoking in the UK (Department of Health 1998) are associated with increased interest in the provision of more intensive support for smokers trying to quit. Primary care is a focus for some of these developments (K. Lewis, personal communication regarding the Help to Quit project). Models developed in these fields are likely to have relevance for other forms of substance misuse and, of course, many patients use and experience difficulties related to their use of more than one type of substance.

Key concepts

Dependence

There is considerable academic debate around the concept of dependence or addiction. There is not space in this chapter to go into the debate, and it is not necessary to resolve it in order to work effectively with people with substance use problems. Below are some facts and working assumptions that are helpful in considering the type of assistance someone will need in order to change a substance misuse habit and the role counselling can play.

Sometimes a person's nervous system adapts to the continued presence of a psychoactive drug

This process is referred to as neuroadaptation or 'physical addiction'. Some drugs have a greater potential for this than others. For example it is rarely, if ever, seen in cannabis users but is frequently a factor in smoking and in benzodiazepine use. Sudden withdrawal from a drug to which one's nervous system has adapted can produce a variety of symptoms, ranging from the highly unpleasant and inconvenient (such as the irritability and loss of concentration people often experience on giving up smoking) to the dangerous (such as delirium tremens when recovering from alcohol). Controlled withdrawal using reducing doses of the drug itself or other substitute medication makes this process more manageable. Counselling can help people develop other coping strategies and manage their anxiety during withdrawal.

Human beings are purposeful and use substances to meet needs and fulfil functions in their lives

Changing substance use can expose otherwise unmet needs in a person's life. For example, a person who uses alcohol to relax may find it difficult, after cutting down, to unwind at the end of the day without a drink. Counselling is a very appropriate way to help people to identify the functions of their drug use and the new skills and activities they will need to maintain change. Sometimes drugs are used to mask deep-seated difficulties and counselling around the function of the drug use will lead into other counselling areas, such as bereavement, sexual abuse or relationship problems. Occasionally drug use masks mental illness and the need for medical or other treatment is only discovered when the drug use changes.

Changing habits is difficult

Aside from the chemical properties of the substance, the associated pattern of behaviour can be difficult to change. Substance use may also be an established part of group behaviour, the functioning of the family system or of social rituals. Cognitive behavioural counselling (see below) can assist in breaking habits or replacing them with other 'countering' behaviours. Teaching assertion or other social skills may be required to resist pressure from others.

Stages of change

Regardless of the degree of dependence on the substance, people changing addictive behaviours go through certain stages. Prochaska and DiClemente (1986) have described these stages and the related processes. Figure 11.1 is adapted from their work.

Precontemplation describes the stage when a person has either never considered changing or has thought about it but is not really interested. The precontemplator can see plenty of reasons for continuing drug use and not enough reasons to change. Possibly there are, as yet, no problems resulting from the drug use. If there are problems the precontemplator does not recognize that they are linked with or related to the drug use. Sometimes there are severe problems, clearly linked with the drug use, but the benefits the drug confers or the functions it fulfils are too important to pass up.

Contemplators, on the other hand, are aware that there would be benefits from changing and/or that their current behaviour is harmful. However, they are not yet ready to make the decision to change. At this stage people are weighing up what they would gain by changing against what they would lose.

People in *determination* are poised on the brink and preparing to change. They may be ready to hear suggestions about how they might go about it.

The *action* stage is dynamic. Help may be needed with detoxification, finding alternative ways to meet needs and changing other behaviour patterns that are associated with the substance use.

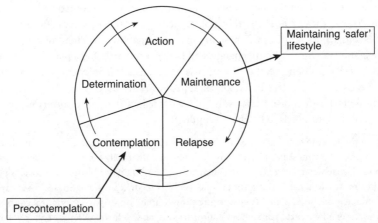

Fig. 11.1 Stages of change (adapted from Prochaska & DiClemente 1986).

It is an old adage that anyone can stop drinking or smoking but 'staying stopped' is more difficult. The *maintenance* stage can be a struggle for years before the person begins to feel that the substance misuse is no longer a problem lurking in the wings but a former problem that is now resolved.

Most people who change an addictive behaviour have at least one *relapse*. Changing an addictive behaviour is best seen as a process, not a single event, and many people try several times before maintaining change. It is possible to learn from each unsuccessful attempt and move on to contemplate having another go, with the benefit of having past experience on which to draw.

Counselling is clearly appropriate for supporting and empowering clients who are in the stages of determination, action or maintenance. In relapse, counselling may be helpful in enabling the client to come to terms with and learn from the experience and to make another attempt. Other forms of counselling can help engage and maintain motivation or facilitate problem-solving and these may be appropriate for contemplators or precontemplators.

Methods

The most effective treatments for alcohol and other drug problems include counselling. The counselling methods that have been proven to work are those which are designed to 'set in motion a self-directed process of change' (Miller *et al.* 1998). Typically they are more structured than some counselling methods used in other areas while still relying on high quality empathy and a client-centred approach. It is well established in the area of alcohol problems that brief counselling (one to four sessions) is effective compared to no treatment or being placed on a waiting list (Bien *et al.* 1993), and counselling designed to engage motivation (motivational enhancement therapy) is effective over only three sessions (Project MATCH Research Group 1997). This makes substance misuse counselling a very practical option within the context of busy general practices.

Changing a behaviour such as smoking, drinking or other drug use requires the client both to believe that such a change would be worthwhile (outcome expectancy) and to believe that he or she will be able to achieve it (self-efficacy) (Rollnick *et al.* 1999). Counselling approaches therefore focus on enabling the client to explore how important it is to him or her to change, and then on constructing a plan for how to go about it with confidence. Substance misuse is seen as a learned behaviour that helps meet needs, and cognitive behavioural approaches are used to develop alternative coping skills. Heather and Robertson (1997) describe the range of interventions the alcohol counsellor needs to be able to conduct:

> If counsellors are to be equipped to deal effectively with the broadest range of problem drinker, ... they must be able, not only to listen empathetically but to act as adviser, role models, coaches and environmental engineers. They should be able to run a social skills training session, carry out a functional analysis of drinking, negotiate targets and drinking guidelines, plan a cue-exposure programme, draw up a behavioural contract between drinkers and their spouses and/or friends, and so forth. Otherwise they will be limited in the number of people they can effectively help.' (p. 189)

Motivational approaches

A helpful way of conceptualizing motivation is as a set of scales, weighing the pros and cons of changing. There is no such thing as an unmotivated *person*, but some people have more motivation to continue their substance use than they do to change it. Continuing any sort of substance misuse involves the person taking action, and it frequently costs them money and effort. Therefore it is not appropriate to see precontemplators as passive or apathetic. Rather, as they see it, they have too many reasons to continue as they are and they do not consider change worthwhile. Motivation changes over time and between situations, as the scales are seen to tip one way or another. Factors that give more weight to the reasons for change include:

1 Receiving new information about the damage substance misuse causes or about the benefits of change.

2 Being able to see the personal relevance of general information about substance misuse.

3 Changes in a person's value system or priorities.

4 Being able to see that change is really possible as well as desirable.

Motivational interviewing is a style of counselling originally described by William Miller (1983). It seeks to address the ambivalence felt by those considering or attempting change and to manage constructively the resistance that people show when someone else appears to put pressure on them. In order to use this approach effectively, the counsellor requires all the basic skills of active listening, empathy and a non-judgemental approach and to be able to use them within a framework of specific, deliberate strategies to engage motivation. Motivational interviewing is best learned from a skilled practitioner and trainer, and most alcohol and drug training units provide courses. Miller and Rollnick (1991) provide a good source for reading about the approach. Some key concepts are:

1 The conceptualization of motivation not as a personality trait, but as an interpersonal process. Denial is seen not as inherent in the alcoholic or addicted individual but as a product of the confrontative ways in which counsellors sometimes choose to interact with people with substance misuse problems.

2 The balance metaphor for motivation. People feel two ways about change, recognizing some problems relating to the substance use but also having reservations about doing anything about it. The process of motivational interviewing can be seen as enabling the client to acknowledge this ambivalence and reappraise the possible benefits of change.

3 Skilful use of empathy and affirmation to enable the individual to feel empowered and motivated towards positive action to take care of him or herself.

4 Strategies to increase awareness of the role and effects of substance use in the context of the client's life and overall intentions. Increasing the dissonance between the substance use and the client's important goals is a key strategy.

Rollnick *et al.* (1999) have developed a method for conducting brief consultations on behaviour change in medical settings, based on many of the principles of motivational interviewing and carried out in a spirit of negotiation rather than confrontation. This approach is very appropriate to substance misuse issues.

Cognitive behavioural approaches

Frequently people use, and continue to use, substances in order to change the way they feel. Maintaining change in the substance use will depend on finding alternative cognitive or behavioural ways to change their feelings. Cognitive behavioural approaches:

+ Analyse the patterns of events, thoughts and feelings that are associated with the substance use (functional analysis)
+ Identify the possibilities for change
+ Explore options with the client
+ Help the client to learn techniques to modify beliefs or irrational thought processes in order to change feelings and consequent behaviours
+ Develop behavioural techniques and skills to change thoughts and feelings.

An example of how a cognitive behavioural approach can help to understand someone's drinking or drug use and the possibilities for change

Mr J drinks and smokes heavily. He wants to get fitter and have more money to spend on other things so would like to give up smoking and cut down on his drinking. He is able to go through the week smoking very few cigarettes. He is not allowed to smoke in the office and tends to stay in at home for the midweek evenings. On Friday nights he goes to the pub straight from work with his colleagues. He starts out intending to drink only two or three pints and not to smoke but he soon accepts a cigarette and spends the rest of the evening in the pub drinking several pints of beer. This sets a pattern for the weekend. The events associated with this pattern (which he wants to break) are:

+ His friends assume that he will go along as usual
+ He has money in his pocket
+ He has no other plans for the evening
+ He does not drive to work, so has no constraints with regard to drink/driving.
   He thinks:
+ I've had a hard week so deserve a good night out
+ The lads will think I'm being miserable if I don't go with them
+ It's a poor sort of night out if you can't have a few drinks and a smoke
+ I'll worry about my health when the weekend's over
+ Right now I deserve to let my hair down and have fun.
   He feels:
+ Tired at the beginning of the evening

- Relaxed after the first couple of drinks
- Resentful, as if he is depriving himself, if he does not accept drinks and cigarettes.

It can be seen that there are any number of options, such as to:

- Reconsider whether it is really important to him to change and look at being alcohol and tobacco free as a reward to himself rather than a deprivation
- Change jobs to break the pattern
- Leave his money and cashpoint card at home on Fridays so that he cannot be tempted to go out after work
- Change his group of friends to a crowd who enjoy themselves without drink and cigarettes
- Plan to go away at weekends straight from work as an alternative reward for a week's work
- Learn to be more assertive at refusing drinks/cigarettes
- Take disulfiram (antabuse) so that he cannot drink at all, so that the relaxation of his self-control after a couple of drinks is avoided
- Read more to frighten himself about the health risks, to strengthen his resolve
- Develop a positive image of himself as a non-smoker and light drinker.

Some of these strategies are behavioural and some cognitive. We may consider some of them to be easier or more likely to succeed than others. Mr J will have his own views on which are most compatible with his self-image, his values and his sense of what would be possible. The counselling task is to generate options, explore them, assist Mr J in choosing between them and then to support him as necessary in taking action.

It is clear from this example that cognitive behavioural strategies are appropriate for clients who want to change, are ready to explore their difficulties in doing so, and are keen to find effective strategies.

The twelve steps model

This approach, used by Alcoholics Anonymous and Narcotics Anonymous, amongst others, is most appropriate for people who have recognized that their substance use has become a major problem in their lives and are experiencing a loss of control over it. Counsellors who use this approach are often people who have themselves had problems of 'chemical dependency' and have been trained to help others to use the methods that they themselves found useful.

A 12 steps approach has some aspects in common with all approaches to substance misuse counselling; for example 'one day at a time' is widely accepted as a useful attitude to adopt when trying to change behaviour, as is the importance of peer support. Other aspects such as learning to accept one's 'powerlessness' over the substance contrast sharply with other approaches that seek to strengthen the clients' belief that they do make choices and decisions at every stage in their substance use and can choose to act differently. (More information on this approach is available from Hazeldon Europe, PO Box 616, Cork, Ireland.)

How effective is counselling in helping people with substance misuse problems?

A variety of counselling approaches have been found to be effective when they are used specifically to address the substance misuse and issues related directly to it. Heather and Robertson (1997) describe nine ingredients in a recipe for effective alcohol counselling. These are:

- Understanding and treating drinking in context
- Problem-solving
- 'More action, less words'
- Family, friends and community involvement
- 'Make it worth their while'
- Mastering the cues
- Self-management and target-setting
- Counsellors and models
- Client choice.

In essence, Heather and Robertson's view is that effective alcohol counselling is practically oriented and maintains a focus on the possibility of change. With regard to counsellors and models, they remind us that:

> No study has ever shown professionals, whether psychiatrists, psychologists, social workers or nurses, to be any more successful at helping problem drinkers than non-professionals given a brief training in alcohol counselling (Heather & Robertson 1997, p. 189).

They emphasize that, aside from the model of counselling used, empathic, skilled counsellors are more effective than others in helping problem drinkers. This links with the concept of client choice. When offered a choice of goal (i.e. abstinence, controlled use, harm reduction) and of treatment method, clients are more likely to be attracted to seek help and the success rates tend to improve (Parker *et al.* 1979).

Bien *et al.* (1993) identify the six elements most frequently present in those brief interventions for alcohol problems that have been proved to be effective. They are summarized by the acronym FRAMES:

- *Feedback* regarding the client's personal situation
- Emphasis that *responsibility* for change lies with the client
- *Advice* to change
- A *menu* of alternative courses of action
- An *empathic* counselling style
- *Encouragement of* self-efficacy.

Miller *et al.* (1998), in their summary of the evidence for the efficacy of specific treatment methods for alcohol problems, find that the two treatments that come top of their table are the structured counselling interventions described as 'brief interventions' and 'motivational enhancement'. On the other hand, 'general alcoholism counselling' comes out relatively poorly in controlled treatment trials. Recent medication trials have tended to test the effectiveness of drug therapy as an addition to rather than instead of various 'talk therapies' and this combination seems to have some advantages.

The message seems to be that counselling for substance misuse works if it is structured, focused on the issue of motivation and change and conducted by a competent, empathic counsellor.

How well does it work putting it into primary care?

Frequently, help for substance misuse problems is seen as secondary or tertiary care. However, over the last couple of decades it has been increasingly recognized that problems relating to substance misuse can often be effectively managed by primary care and community-based services. Potamianos *et al.* (1986) conducted a randomized trial of community-based versus conventional hospital management of 151 drinkers, and concluded that treatment at the community day centre was at least as cost-effective as hospital treatment of alcohol abuse. Babor *et al.* (1986) reviewed early intervention strategies for managing alcohol problems in the primary health care setting and concluded that 'low intensity, brief interventions have much to recommend as the first approach to the problem drinker in the primary care setting' (p. 23).

Drummond *et al.* (1990) randomly allocated problem drinkers to a specialist clinic or to a GP for treatment and found that 'after an initial detailed assessment and advice session, the treatment provided by GPs is at least as effective as that from a specialist clinic with respect to improvements in drinking behaviour and alcohol-related problems' (p. 915).

Clearly, however, there are difficulties in adding any more than minimal brief advice to the heavy workload of the practitioner. There have, therefore, been recent experiments in placing specialist alcohol counsellors in general practices, to explore whether this improves patient access to and take up of services and/or raises awareness of the issue in the practice team.

Mason (1997a) evaluated one such project that placed an alcohol counsellor in three general practices for a period of two years. The counsellor (from a psychiatric nursing background) was employed, trained and supervised by the local voluntary sector alcohol counselling team, who also ran a counselling service from their own premises in the city centre. The project dramatically increased referrals from GPs resulting in 'greater numbers of people finding a route to alcohol counselling than could ever be expected through running the more traditional community-based services' (p. 216). Thirty per cent of those referred had not previously been offered help with their drinking.

Members of the practice teams felt that the service was easily accessible and that its location in the practice was an advantage. However, they would have preferred the counselling to be part of a broader pattern of services including home detoxification, and subsequent service developments were along these lines.

An audit of practice notes took place before and after the project to identify any changes in the teams' activity around alcohol screening and intervention (Mason 1997b). Comparisons were made with a control practice that had no counsellor. The presence of a counsellor was associated with considerable increases in the meaningful recording of alcohol consumption in the patients' records (i.e. specified in units of alcohol rather than described as 'heavy' or 'social'), in the identification of heavy drinkers and those with related problems, and in the frequency of doctors and nurses advising patients to cut down.

Other similar projects support these findings anecdotally and in their annual reports. There has also been interest in some of the process issues in setting up such projects (Findlay & Smerdon 1993). In common with generic counsellors in general practice, alcohol counsellors need good structures for professional support and supervision. These are usually provided through the post being managed by a community-based alcohol counselling agency. It can take time for the counsellor to become known and attain credibility within the team, especially when (as is usual) they are only there for one or two sessions per week. There is not always a suitable room available for counselling work and clear confidentiality protocols need to be set up. However, these issues are not unique to this counselling speciality.

Conclusions

Substance misuse is a complex area. The drugs used, the circumstances, methods of use, social structures surrounding use and many other factors impinge on the issue. The substance misuse itself may be a symptom of other problems.

Many types of intervention can be helpful, including advice, information, prescription of other drugs, education and counselling. An understanding of the stages of change and the nature of motivation helps to provide a structure for such complexity and eclecticism. As alcohol and drug agencies continue to work more closely with primary care teams clients are likely to have greater access to counselling as part of the care package offered in primary care.

References

Anderson, P. and Scott, E. (1992) The effect of general practitioners' advice to heavy drinking men. *British Journal of Addiction*, 87, 891–900.

Babor, T. and Grant, M. (eds) (1992) *Project on Identification and Management of Alcohol-related Problems. Report on Phase II: a Randomised Clinical Trial of Brief Interventions in Primary Health Care*. World Health Organisation, Geneva.

Babor, T., Ritson, E. and Hodgson, R. (1986) Alcohol-related problems in the primary health care setting: a review of early intervention strategies. *British Journal of Addiction*, 81, 1, 23–46.

Bien, T.H., Miller, W.R. and Tonigan, J.S. (1993) Brief interventions for alcohol problems: a review. *Addiction*, 88, 315–336.

Department of Health (1998) *Smoking Kills; a White Paper on Tobacco*. HMSO, London.

Drummond, D.C., Thom, B., Brown, C., Edwards, G. and Mullan, M.J. (1990) Specialist versus general treatment of problem drinkers. *Lancet*, 336, 915–918.

Findlay, M. and Smerdon, G. (1993) *The John Dawson Project—Short Report*. Cornwall Council on Alcohol, Truro.

Heather, N. and Robertson, I. (1997) *Problem* Drinking, 3rd edn. Oxford Medical Publications, Oxford.

Mason, P. (1997a) Alcohol counsellors in general practice. *Journal of Substance Misuse*, 2 (2), 85–93.

Mason, P. (1997b) Alcohol counselling services in general practice (part II): who uses them and how? *Journal of Substance Misuse*, 2 (4), 210–216.

Miller, W.R. (1983) Motivational interviewing with problem drinkers. *Behavioural Psychotherapy*, 11, 147–172.

Miller, W.R., Andrews, N.R., Wilbourne, P. and Bennett, M.E. (1998) A wealth of alternatives, effective treatments for alcohol problems. In *Treating Addictive Behaviors*, 2nd edn (Miller, W.R. and Heather, N., eds). Plenum Press, New York, pp. 203–216.

Miller, W. and Rollnick, S. (1991) *Motivational Interviewing*. Guilford Press, New York.

Parker, M., Winstead, D., Willi, F. and Fisher, P. (1979) Patient autonomy in alcoholism rehabilitation: II program evaluation. *International Journal of the Addictions*, 14, 1177–1184.

Potamianos, G., Meade, T.W., North, W.R.S., Townsend, J. and Peters, T.J. (1986) Randomised trial of community-based centre versus conventional hospital management in treatment of alcoholism. *Lancet*, 2, 797–799.

Prochaska, J.O. and DiClemente, C.C. (1986) Towards a comprehensive model of change. In *Treating Addictive Behaviors. Processes of Change* (Miller, W.R. and Heather, N., eds). Plenum Press, New York, pp. 3–27.

Project MATCH Research Group (1997) Matching alcoholism treatments to client heterogeneity: Project MATCH post-treatment drinking outcomes. *Journal of Studies on Alcohol*, 58, 7–29.

Rollnick, S., Mason, P. and Butler, C. (1999) *Health Behaviour Change, a Guide for Practitioners*. Churchill Livingstone, Edinburgh.

Russell, M.A.H., Wilson, C., Taylor, C. and Baker, C.D. (1979) Effect of general practitioners' advice against smoking. *British Medical Journal*, 2, 231–235.

Saunders, J.B., Reznik, R.B., Hanratty, S. *et al.* (1991) *Early Intervention for Harmful Alcohol Consumption*. Paper submitted to the Advisory Committee of the Research into Drug Abuse Programme. Department of Community Services and Health, Canberra.

Wallace, P.G., Cutler, S., Brennan, P.J. and Haines, A. (1988) Randomised controlled trial of general practitioner intervention in patients with excessive alcohol consumption. *British Medical Journal*, 297, 663–668.

Chapter 12

Chronic illness and disability

Simon Parritt

Introduction

There are estimated to be around 50 billion disabled people in the world and whilst the majority of these are in the developing world, in the UK there are around eight million or 12% of the population. The primary care system is often the most frequent point of contact and on-going medical support for many disabled people and, with the growth of counselling within primary care, it is important that counsellors become familiar and comfortable working with this client group. As part of this they should also ensure that they are aware of the wider issues that face disabled and chronically ill people, as well as having explored and reflected upon their own attitudes, beliefs and feelings towards disability and chronic illness in all its presenting forms.

As with any other client population, there is a great diversity within the group. Counsellors are always on their guard against labelling and emphasize that their clients are unique individuals. In addition, definition and identity as a disabled person can be difficult both for the counsellor and often the client. The general provision of accessible counselling available to or taken up by disabled people is difficult to quantify. Few reports or studies identify this group, unless the disability is linked to mental illness, when statistics are collected within a service. This is partly because classification itself is problematic.

The World Health Organization (1980) has defined disability as the deficits in performance of activities as a result of physical impairment. So we might refer to clients having a physical or sensory *impairment*, but being *disabled* by their environment, physical or attitudinal. Johnston (1996) builds on this in a model that conceptualizes physical impairment as the deficits in structure or functioning of some part of the body and social handicap as the deficits in social functioning. This model, however, lacks the broader perspective of the lived experience of disabled people themselves. Counsellors need to guard against adopting a model based upon 'able-bodied assumptions of disability' (Oliver 1983, p. 61). Oliver sees this not just as a question of semantics, but a challenge to find new ways of operationalizing 'the concept of disability based upon the notion that disability is a social creation.' (p. 66). When working in primary care, where the referring or lead health professional is normally a GP, there can be a particular difficulty in seeing beyond the medical model, especially for able-bodied therapists whose own internalized working model of disability might not have been explored or examined in their supervision or training. It is also worth reflecting upon how the counsellor's own internalized response to a disabled client is similar or different when working with clients with mental illness, physical disability, learning difficulties or cognitive impairment.

The attitudes and experiences of therapists working with disabled clients are of central importance. The notion that there is a particular technical skill or knowledge base that counsellors need to learn in order to work with disabled clients is largely untrue, and of less importance than empathy and a personal understanding of their own attitudes and internalized model of disability. There is also considerable empirical evidence to suggest that people avoid social interaction with ill or disabled people because they find it difficult and distressing (Davies 1961; Goffman 1963; Dunkel-Schetter & Wortman 1982; Mills *et al.* 1984). Evidence also suggests that friends and family avoid those who become depressed as a result of their illness or disability and that this is also true of health professionals (Frank *et al.* 1986). In the light of such research, counsellors may also share similar feelings that will impinge upon the therapeutic relationship and approach. This is an area that should be explored with a supervisor who has a good understanding of the issues and perhaps has a disability themselves, though this may be difficult due to the small number of suitably qualified disabled counsellors.

In addressing disability and chronic illness together there are several problems, as whilst a client might be willing to see themselves as 'suffering from' a chronic illness they might not want or accept the label of being a disabled person. This division exists also within counsellors themselves who, when asked to identify the number of their clients who are disabled, will report none or a very low number (Parritt & O'Callaghan 2000). Many clients with chronic conditions that can be disabling, such as diabetes, epilepsy or arthritis are not perceived as disabled people by themselves, their family or society.

Another obvious, but often neglected fact is that having a disability is not the same as being ill. Whilst a client might, for instance, be visually impaired, they are not ill and the impact upon their well-being largely depends on how accessible society and the physical world are to them. This is equally true of a wheelchair user who is healthy and whose main concerns are integrating with the social and economic life of their own world, rather than illness or disease. Understanding this distinction and working with the client's actual lived experience is essential. The use of language often demonstrates the underlying assumptions and it is common to hear someone being referred to as 'wheelchair bound' as opposed to a wheelchair user. The implication is clearly the notion of imprisonment. Similarly, looking at how the term 'suffering from' is used in terms of disability can also reveal much about underlying assumptions and beliefs concerning the origin and attribution of suffering.

Counsellors working in primary care equally may see disabled clients who are also ill or unwell in a variety of ways. The danger for both the client and counsellor is to be unclear about, or not separately assess, the relative impact of impairment, health, culture and the socioeconomic environment in which they live. Having an understanding of the social model of disability (Finklestein 1981; Oliver 1983; French 1993) and how it relates to counselling offers one path through the often uncharted waters that counsellor and client have to travel in order to avoid pathologizing the disability. This is perhaps an area that distinguishes working with this client group from others, but also has much in common with the kinds of issues and approaches that are relevant when working cross-culturally.

A predominantly biomedical model has been the basis for the development of services for disabled people and has focused upon active physical treatment, with very little understanding of the psychological and sociopolitical experience of living as a disabled person. Where medicine has failed to 'cure' or 'repair' a person, interventions are aimed at helping clients 'come to terms' with their disability, which can all too easily mean accepting a new, lesser role and usually reduced status in society. They are in danger of becoming the passive recipients of care, charity and sympathy from others. Counsellors need to be alert not to collude with this narrow 'rehabilitation' framework. There are obviously economic and physical access barriers, but it is also worth considering how the philosophy that underpins many counselling or psychotherapeutic approaches within the statutory health care system may compound this constrained and negative approach.

Counselling by its very nature concentrates upon the individual, couple or family and looks to the individual within this perspective to find insight or change. Philosophically it might be argued that for most clients this is an adequate reflection of the constraints of the fuller experience of living within a complex modern society. However, where disability is a factor, counsellors cannot ignore the reality that many situations and opportunities for change are not within the immediate control of their client or their current support systems.

Take as an example a young wheelchair user in their early twenties with cerebral palsy and communication difficulties, who is referred because of being desperately unhappy as they cannot find a boyfriend or girlfriend. The reality of this client's life may be one of social exclusion and poor educational opportunities. The counsellor should not minimize the difficulties of meeting and finding a sexual partner. The origin of the young person's distress and unhappiness is as likely to be located in social attitudes and social and economic opportunities as in the client's impaired physical functioning. Sexuality and disability may offer a counsellor the greatest challenge and insights into their own preconceptions of what disability means for them. Disabled people may come to feel unattractive in every sense of the word, neither expecting nor deserving of physical love and affection and feeling unable to give anything to others of value.

This reveals the way in which stereotypes and discrimination operate both within clients themselves and counsellors. To be a disabled person is to be by default identified as part of a low status, dependent group and few people voluntarily opt to join such a group. In fact, many high profile successful people with disabilities say in interviews that they do not see themselves as disabled, revealing perhaps their own internalized negative model of disability and distancing themselves from other disabled people's experience. Unlike other minority groups, being disabled is a group to which anyone may become a member at any time in their lives. In America the disabled community often refers to able-bodied people as TBAs—temporarily able bodied. Why is this important? Because it emphasizes the arbitrary nature of the distinction between disabled people and others in the formers' on-going experience of social exclusion and discrimination that over time can undermine and corrupt self-esteem and personhood.

As counsellors it is thus important to understand the distinction between the impact upon the client of the physical illness or impairment and the disabling effects of discrimination. A client may present with a range of psychological difficulties, but it is important not to pathologize the disability itself.

There has been a tendency in the past to allow ideas and models of loss to be the primary model by which counsellors conceptualize disability and illness. Any loss of function is an important and traumatic experience, especially during or following such things as a spinal cord injury or stroke. However, the on-going and traumatic shift of an individual into the world of disability, benefits and social services can be as traumatic, if not more so, than the physical impairments themselves. Counsellors working with this client group should be prepared to familiarize themselves with the reality of living with a chronic illness or disability. This familiarization ought not to be in terms of what might be termed the 'tragedy model', but more in terms of the social exclusion and discrimination that their clients are likely to encounter in their everyday lives. This will free the counsellor to listen with a greater depth of understanding to the presenting problem for its aetiology and subsequently to work more sensitively with the client on a way forward. For example, when someone is referred with the commonly used phrase 'not coping with his or her disability', the counsellor is more open to asking her or himself, 'Coping with what aspect of the lived experience?' and listening to the client's answer.

The consequences of living with a disability or illness can be profound. Social status, income, power, respect, employment and social contact are just some of the factors which may be affected. Whilst multiple sclerosis, for instance, may have certain physical effects such as mobility problems or fatigue, the psychological impact of this is perhaps not as great as the consequent loss of job, or the impact that becoming a disabled person has upon the client's immediate social circle. As counsellors we constrain ourselves very often to a model or theory which places responsibility upon the individual. We need to beware of this particularly when dealing with disability, as social and economic factors are fundamental in why such a client may seek or be referred for counselling.

The most difficult and challenging, but interesting, aspect of working in this field arises from the need to address both the external social circumstances that clients encounter and the internal psychological consequences. Both involve consideration of contradictory responses to what the client can and ought to challenge and what needs to be adjusted to and accepted. The external realities of the lives that clients lead have considerable emotional and psychological impacts upon them. This needs to be distinguished from assessing and helping clients incorporate and deal with the reality of the actual impact of the impairment itself and the consequent inability to function in certain areas without the assistance of others such as carers, personal assistants or enablers.

The first meeting with a client is critical as it offers both the client and the counsellor to lay the foundations for the therapeutic alliance. Clearly different doctors and counsellors have different arrangements for dealing with referral criteria. The first and important issue to consider is that GPs might see a client with a disability as primarily in need of medical support and not see the value of psychological interventions.

Therefore, widening the primary care team's understanding of how and what counselling has to offer disabled people is important. It is perhaps more likely that a patient with chronic illness will be referred as a consequence of problems in coping with their increasingly difficult situation and changes in lifestyle that such conditions as diabetes or heart disease might impose.

Stage of the onset of disability

Whilst it is obviously true that each person is an individual and that each person's experience of being or becoming disabled is unique, there are certain considerations which may have a significant influence. For instance the stage in life at which an individual becomes disabled may determine the issues of most relevance to consider within the therapeutic relationship.

Childhood years

For those with congenital disability their identity at birth is as a disabled person. This has implications for their experiences growing up as a disabled child and the restrictions and discrimination they may face. Many will have spent periods away from home in hospital undergoing medical treatments. A familiarity with health professionals may influence the client's attitude towards the counsellor, seeing him or her as another person who is going to treat them. Parents' attitudes to having a child with a disability can operate in many ways, from denial to overprotection, and the client's sense of autonomy and independence may be greatly affected later in life as a result and therefore may be a significant factor to be examined. For those educated in segregated schools, the level of education was and can still be poor. Experiences of living and dealing with relationships may be limited, as the 'normal' stages of adolescence may not have been possible. The individual experience of growing up as a disabled person should be explored in the early assessment stages of counselling. Whilst there is likely to be a common thread amongst most congenitally disabled clients, the individual interpretation of experience and their immediate support and family environment will have had a major influence on their current experience.

There can also be a case for counselling the parents, but this is sometimes a difficult issue. Understandably, most parents are concerned with pressing for information, practical help and access to services for their child. It is all too easy for professionals to see parents' anger and sometimes resistant attitudes as requiring counselling due to their 'inability to accept' their child's disability. This may be pathologizing what is appropriate anger with poor access to services, support and treatment. In a typical example, a parent was referred as 'not coping' with her child's profound and terminal disabilities. She was described as angry and aggressive, refusing to accept respite placements and a change in medication. It was important here to acknowledge that the client had been 'sent for counselling' and that she may not want or need counselling. In effect the client was fighting and pushing for her child to gain access to the best available services. She was well informed about medications, the impact upon her child and the circumstances of the respite home. The key was acknowledging her feelings as real and founded not in a pathological resistance to the approaching loss of her child, but in a long and bitter experience of struggling for support and seeking the 'best' for her child in a competitive environment for resources. The client felt both heard and supported and was later able to negotiate in a way that those who referred her found rational, but none the less discomforting for themselves. Later, and in her own time, this client was able to accept further counselling and look at the impending separation and loss, as her son needed hospice involvement. This is an example where adopting a social model perspective is not always a comfortable place for the counsellor who is part of the multidisciplinary team.

Adolescence

Adolescence can be a particularly difficult time in anyone's life. The way adolescence and disability interact varies according to whether the person has been disabled from birth or becomes disabled during adolescence, as the result of a particular event or a long-term condition becoming evident. In either of these circumstances, there is the earlier experience of having been accepted as a 'normal' member of society and family. There are, therefore, two levels that might be useful to examine and explore. The first is the change of identity and the second is the altered functional ability as a result of the impairment. Late adolescence can be a particularly challenging time for anyone and becoming disabled at this stage significantly compounds those challenges. Counsellors can find disentangling the issues of adolescence from disability a difficult task. On the other hand, this is also a time of identify formation and experimentation and this can work in a positive way, enabling the client to establish a positive self-identity as a disabled person.

Early adulthood

In early adulthood, the impact of becoming disabled is often to curtail a life which has only recently been embarked upon. Job, profession, friends, pastimes and personal relationships, all newly established or being established, must be reassessed and changed, if not abandoned. Impairment itself may prevent an individual from continuing to play a certain sport or hold a particular job. Whilst disabled sports or support to return to employment is often possible, it is hard for some individuals not to see this as second best, due to prejudices which are already part of the individual's internalized concept of disability as dependent and worthless. Establishing oneself as a member of the community must suddenly be renegotiated and assessed. Many people negotiate this in a successful and self-affirming way, but this may not always be the case. Seeing a client in the early stages of this process may afford some opportunity to lay the foundations for later. However, it should be borne in mind that for many disabled people the counsellor can be seen as yet another intrusion into their autonomy and privacy. Coming to terms with disability can be a constant struggle with the intrusion of others, especially professionals, into their lives. The counsellor may not only add to the number of occasions for this struggle to take place, but may be experienced as a unique type of threat to someone's mind and emotional life. Understanding this dynamic is essential if the therapeutic relationship is to succeed in helping the client. Even if the client arrives for counselling many years later, it is still of great importance that the counsellor should understand and find a way to support and respect these concerns, even if the person concerned has no insight into this aspect of their resistance.

Middle years

The middle years are the time when many people will present themselves for counselling. The onset of a disability at this stage has the obvious impact of changing the client's social role, or at least threatening to do so, in the case of chronic illness or progressive conditions. Family concerns and a person's relationship with their partner will often be paramount once the initial diagnosis or rehabilitation has been carried out. It may be easy for the counsellor to fall into the trap of attributing the presenting issue, such as depression or anxiety, to the onset of the illness or disability. The reality may be very different and distinguishing between existing predisposing factors and the contribution of disability or impairment itself is perhaps the primary task. Marital and sexual difficulties can be a major factor in many people's lives and having a disability may compound these problems.

Older age

Most people who are disabled are older people. Whilst old age is not a disability or illness, as we age we often acquire different impairments and it is perhaps unusual for a person to reach the end of their life without experiencing some disability and/or chronic illness. One of the inequalities and discriminations that older disabled people face is a special kind of invisibility. Disability can be perceived as an inevitable part of growing older and whilst having a spinal cord injury at 59 might be perceived as traumatic, requiring a major life shift, if it occurs at 65 the person will not receive the same level of financial or social support. Once again these issues compound the counsellor's task in identifying areas where clients' distress or difficulty can be improved. There may be the loss of role as a grandparent or spouse, or perhaps work which has been enjoyed beyond the official retirement age. Counsellors should familiarize themselves with the issues of counselling elderly people, use that knowledge in conjunction with the previously mentioned issues of disability and recognize that the two can compound and interact with each other.

People who reach old age are by definition survivors and have a wealth of life experience and skills, many of which will be valuable in adapting to their new situation. Equally, many of these skills might serve to impede the counselling process and rehabilitation. For instance, a person's view of carers who offer support through social services may well be one of gratitude, apologizing for 'being a burden'. For someone who might have cared for others, both within the family and outside, in paid employment or in a voluntary capacity, becoming the recipient of care and support can be a major difficulty. This is often accentuated by professional workers' attitudes to the older person, unwittingly treating them as dependent, almost child-like. Combating this environment which the individual encounters outside the counselling room is problematic, as counselling only occupies a short time compared with the impact of clients' other contacts in their day-to-day life as a disabled or chronically ill person in receipt of care. Reframing and combating ageism within the client themselves may be a major part of the process, before or at the same time as addressing any issues around the impairment or illness. Intimate relationships and sexuality are also areas which are not afforded the same attention with the older client as with other age groups. Disability will not always impact upon these areas, but it is important for counsellors to be aware of and assess them for all clients. They should not neglect the needs and feelings of the elderly person, for whom the impact of their loss of privacy or intimacy with a partner can have far reaching emotional and psychological impacts.

The example of Mrs B illustrates the challenge of understanding these impacts. Mrs B was referred because she was perceived as being depressed following a stroke. She had been admitted to hospital and eventually discharged home to the care of her GP. Despite the fact that she had a very obviously close relationship with her husband of 58 years and they had shared a bed all their married life, no one had addressed her feelings about being provided with a single bed downstairs. The practicalities of managing the stairs and home care services were the primary concerns. Mrs B and her husband felt grateful for all the help and assistance they were offered. It was only after the counsellor had explored the relationship dimension that the loss of physical closeness and intimacy was identified as a major factor in the client's depression and that it was not just a consequence of the stroke.

Specific knowledge

No counsellor can know everything about all illnesses and disabilities that are likely to present in their practice. However, this is no reason to either avoid clients or claim not to possess the necessary skills or knowledge. Many disabled people who have had their disability for some time, are likely to be the experts on their own bodies and medical condition. Counsellors should never be afraid to say they do not know, or to ask the client to explain something that is important for the counselling process. However, there is a responsibility on counsellors to inform themselves as and when they can. Many disabled and chronically ill people spend their lives educating others in various aspects of their lives as disabled people. Doctors and other health professionals often take a medical history again and again and in the end clients will be adept at reeling out their medical history, even if they may privately resent having to do it yet again. So the principle should be for counsellors to inform themselves of the general issues and ask about specific individual issues. Each client with multiple sclerosis will experience the impact of it differently, both psychologically and physically, but there are a range of effects such as fatigue of which counsellors should be aware.

The counsellor's role

Given the special issues which may confront disabled clients, counsellors will be faced with reconsideration of their boundaries and role. Keeping appointment times and regular attendance can be of great significance for many clients and counsellors. Whilst this still may be relevant for disabled clients, the factors which prevent clients attending, such as chronic fatigue or variable health, should always be considered and allowed for. Equally, reliance on such services as Dial-A-Ride or other disability transport provision can make adherence to strict times difficult, if not impossible. This is not an issue of client resistance or avoidance, but a sociopolitical issue of discrimination. It is a good example of the loss of independence and access which disabled people live with every day of their lives.

Another contentious issue is that of advocacy. Counsellors may be asked by the client, or officially requested to make statements in support of clients' attempts to improve their autonomy or access to services. Working in primary care is to be part of a team and the counsellor may be the only member of that team who has knowledge of a patient's whole life. To the team, the counsellor's client is a patient and semantics are sometimes important. The word 'patient' has many meanings. Being patient is often what is required of a disabled person. The counsellor will need to be clear why and to what purpose a client requests them to act as their advocate and be fully supported in supervision. It may be that, unlike other clients, there are special circumstances where this is appropriate depending upon the counsellor's personal and professional stance.

Conclusions

There is nothing unusual or special about disabled people and those living with a chronic illness except that they have impairments or health problems that may be functionally limiting and living with these may be made easier with counselling support from time to time. It would be unreal to suggest that being a disabled person is only difficult because of society's attitudes and barriers. There can be pain, fatigue and loss of functions which are, in themselves, for most people difficult and unwanted. However, it is also true that the social and environmental factors greatly compound and in some instances create more distress and pain than the physical impairments themselves. Counsellors who work with individuals with a disability or a chronic illness need always to be aware of these factors.

References

Davies, F. (1961) Deviance disavowed: the management of strained interactions between the visibly handicapped. *Social Problems*, 9, 120–132.

Dunkel-Schetter, C. and Wortman, C.B. (1982) The interpersonal dynamics of cancer: problems in social relationships and their impact on the patient. In *Interpersonal Issues in Health Care* (Friedman, H.S. and DiMatteo, M.R., eds). Academy Press, New York, pp. 60–100.

Finklestein, V. (1981) To deny or not to deny disability. In *Handicap in a Social World* (Brechin, A., Liddiard, P. and Swain, J., eds). Hodder & Stoughton, Sevenoaks/Open University Press, Milton Keynes.

Frank, R.G., Wonderlich, S.A., Corcoran, J.R., Umlauf, R.L., Ashkanazi, G.H., Brownlee-Duffeck, M.B. and Wilson, R. (1986) Interpersonal response to spinal cord injury. *Journal of Social and Clinical Psychology*, 4, 447–460.

French, S. (1993) Disability, impairment or something in between? In *Disabling Barriers—Enabling Environments* (Swain, J., Finklestein, V., French, S. and Oliver, M., eds). Open University Press, Milton Keynes/Sage, London.

Goffman, E. (1963) *Stigma: Notes on the Management of Spoiled Identity.* Prentice Hall, Englewood Cliffs, NJ.

Johnston, M. (1996) Models of disability: challenging the WHO model. *The Psychologist,* 9 (5), 205–210.

Mills, J., Redgrave, F.Z. and Boyer, K.M. (1984) Reducing avoidance of social interaction with a physically disabled person by mentioning the disability following a request for aid. *Journal of Applied Social Psychology,* 14, 1–11.

Oliver, M. (1983) Social work with disabled people. Macmillan, London.

Oliver, M. (1993) Re-defining disability: a challenge to research. In *Disabling Barriers— Enabling Environments* (Swain, J., Finklestein, V., French, S. and Oliver, M., eds). Open University Press, Milton Keynes/Sage, London.

Parritt, S.W. and O'Callaghan, J. (2000) Splitting the difference: an exploratory study of therapists' work with sexuality, relationships and disability. *Sexual and Relationship Therapy,* 15 (2), 151–169.

World Health Organization (1980) *International Classification of Impairments, Disabilities and Handicaps: a Manual of Classification Relating to the Consequences of Disease.* WHO, Geneva.

Chapter 13

Problems of interpersonal relationships

John Eatock and Tim Bond

Introduction

This chapter considers the interpersonal aspects of providing counselling in primary care. It opens by considering the significance of relationships in this setting. The sections that follow consider different challenges faced by the counsellor. The first section will consider the counsellor's own relationship with the primary health care team, especially the GP, and the referral process. The rest of the chapter will look at some of the relationship problems that commonly present to the counsellor working in primary care. Throughout the chapter we have referred to the person coming for counselling as the 'patient'. We are well aware that the person is, properly speaking, always the doctor's 'patient' and the counsellor's 'client', but solely for the sake of consistency, we have decided to use the name generally given to those availing themselves of the services offered in primary care.

Interpersonal relationships are an inescapable feature of most aspects of work in primary care. They have the potential for supporting or undermining the work of the practice in many different ways. Good working relationships between colleagues enhance personal and professional satisfaction by supporting the development of coherent and high quality services. Poor personal relationships can fracture the delivery of services, induce high levels of stress and ultimately lead to the collapse of services or the practice itself. The quality of relationships between colleagues has an impact on the relationships between staff and patients. Staff who are confident that they are being appropriately supported and challenged by colleagues are much better placed to offer appropriate support and challenge to patients. There are also less opportunities for those patients who are so inclined to undermine relations between team members. Any service that is required to work with the full range of the population requires considerable personal and interpersonal resilience, especially when the service is provided to people impaired by illness or other difficulties. The situation is further complicated by the fact that many of the problems that patients present concern their own interpersonal relationships with parents, partners, children, colleagues, neighbours and others. Estimates vary because the figures are so dependent on the diagnosing clinician's awareness of the significance of relationship difficulties as a source of the patient's problems or symptoms. However, relationship difficulties are a major feature in those patients who present exclusively psychological problems, as well as the 30–40% for whom psychological problems are a significant component of the reason for consulting the clinician. The current trend to transfer services away from hospitals to direct provision in the community has the effect of increasing the primary health care worker's involvement with informal carers and their relationship with the patient, often in very demanding circumstances.

Although interpersonal relationships are an inescapable feature of work in primary care, they are not necessarily the primary focus of concern for all members of the team, nor do all members have equal expertise in responding to difficulties in relationships. The introduction of counselling into general practice primarily stemmed from recognition of an unmet need that adversely affected patient health and secondarily was intended to assist the general functioning of the primary care team. Typically, the first counsellors to be appointed to primary care were specialists in relationships who had been trained by the National Marriage Guidance Council, now known as Relate (Marsh & Barr 1975). The training and background of counsellors has widened beyond specialists in intimate relationships working within a psychodynamic tradition to counsellors from a wide variety of backgrounds. However, one of the core features of most approaches to counselling is giving attention to the therapeutic relationship as an essential component of the work (Horvath & Geenberg 1994; Clarkson 1995; Feltham 1999). The emphasis on understanding and working through particular types of relationship in counselling training contrasts with medical training, where the emphasis is inevitably on understanding the scientific basis of medical knowledge and its implications for treatment. The scientific basis of medicine can encourage a detached and depersonalized style of relating to others in order to accomplish systematic observation, diagnosis and treatment. This can leave doctors ill equipped to construct the kind of relationships and insights required to respond to psychological problems in general and patients' interpersonal difficulties in particular. Medical training is sometimes criticized for neglecting this aspect of general practice (West 2001). Increasingly many doctors and nurses interested in the interpersonal dimensions of health care seek supplementary training as part of their continuing professional development. The Balint groups are a long-standing example of how some doctors have sought to redress this need. Supplementary training in counselling skills is another way of developing improved relationship skills and is an increasingly widespread practice. The addition of counsellors to the primary care team extends the capacity to respond to many different aspects of interpersonal relationships.

Most patients are seen individually. In these circumstances it is easy to lose sight of the complex of relationships that surround the consultation. When patients present in primary care, they not only present with themselves and their needs—bringing with them the whole gamut of their own relationships—but they also place themselves within another system and network of relationships that is as complex as their own. The doctor and every member of the primary health care team, and indeed the whole health care system, impact on the life (and health) of the presenting individual, for better or worse. Within this system there is likely to be the counsellor in primary care who is also within a web of relationships. This web is not constant and may be on the brink of change. If, as seems likely, counsellors in primary care cease to be self-employed individuals (as many were during the days of fundholding general practices), then a new subsystem of the counsellor's relationships with other psychological therapy services within whose domain they may be employed will be created.

Relationships within the health care team and the referral process

Relationship of the counsellor to the doctor and primary health care team

In general, and ideally, the primary health care team is focused on the task of improving the health of patients. Just as much of counselling is said to be 'client-centred', so the primary health care team is 'patient-centred', but within the culture and ethos of primary care where for many years the 'medical model' has been paramount. More recently, there has been a trend towards a more holistic approach, or what has been termed the 'biopsychosocial' model of health that takes psychological and social factors, including patients' relationships, into account. However, the extent to which this has been adopted varies considerably because of the competing demands on the practitioner's time and the priorities of different trainings. None the less, where the biopsychosocial model operates, an opportunity is created for the counsellor to become an integral member of the team rather than merely an adjunct.

The process of introducing counselling services into general practice often challenges the preconceptions of both medics and counsellors alike. Newnes (1990), writing as a GP about the benefits of good communication with the counsellor, reported greater awareness as a doctor that the patients' problem may be emotional rather than medical. Conversely, the counsellor moved from thinking that all GPs could become psychotherapists to thinking that they should simply incorporate counselling skills and attitudes to their work with patients. This is a much more realistic expectation and provides common ground between their respective roles whilst respecting each other's specialisms. The advantage to the doctor in developing counselling skills is a greater opportunity to distinguish between the emotional and physical components of the issues presented by patients, within a style of communication that encourages the patient to be actively involved in the management of his or her own problems. Counselling skills are also a useful resource in circumstances where the clinician is breaking bad news or enabling the patient to make decisions about his or her treatment. This use of counselling skills is also helpful to the counsellor in improved referrals and the easing of communication across the professions. For patients, there is greater consistency in the type of service offered throughout the practice regardless of whether the problem is physical, emotional or a combination of both.

Reasons for referral

The reason for referring a patient to the counsellor for relationship issues is no different from the reason for referring a patient to the counsellor for any other issues.

The perception of the doctor, or any other member of the primary health care team, is that this patient may benefit from a deeper understanding of themselves and the situation that they have brought to the doctor for consultation. The doctor's medical diagnosis may not reveal any obvious physical problem or any sign of mental illness, even though it is apparent that the patient is still distressed in some way. Closer questioning by the doctor may reveal that there is some change in the patient's circumstances that may be unsettling for them.

Sue, aged 46, consults her GP over menstrual problems. During the course of the consultation she refers to a long-standing loss of libido and makes ambiguous references to her husband. The GP concentrates on the menstrual problems. When she refers to the other issues, Sue becomes tearful about an unspecified difficulty at home. The GP is aware of the full waiting room and offers a choice of making another appointment to see her or more extended opportunities to discuss the issues with the practice counsellor.

Some GPs may wish to continue this exploration with the patient along the lines that Balint advocated, realizing the potency of themselves in this encounter and its possibilities for facilitating healing. Others choose to suggest an appointment with the practice counsellor for assessment and further exploration. It may not be obvious to the referred individual that the cause of the unhappiness may be a malfunctioning relationship. Depression, anxiety, somatization, weepiness, sometimes confusion and any number of other states can be caused by relationship problems. The 'presenting problem', the initial presentation, can often mask what is really going on for the patient.

Sometimes it is the consequences of illness that creates relationship problems, for example when a previously healthy and active person becomes inactive and dependent on a partner for the first time, or the partner is experiencing negative feelings due to long-term dependence of a member of the family.

David, aged 55, seeks help due to progressive loss of co-ordination brought to a head by a series of minor accidents and difficulty swallowing. He is diagnosed as having motor neuron disease. David appears to have the emotional resources and knowledge to accept his diagnosis. His wife is devastated. She has a professional career that will conflict with her capacity to offer care. She is fearful of the possibility of David's progressive dependence on her. She is grieving over the probable loss of a long planned retirement together. She presents as experiencing panic attacks, sleeplessness and loss of appetite for the first time in her life.

It is common for partners to react differently to changes in the health of their children or parents and this can be a cause of major strain in relationships that compounds or even eclipses the process of coping with the original problem or challenge.

There are, however, other occasions when a patient will be referred. This could be when the doctor themselves, or maybe some other member of the primary health care team, or even an individual in some other part of the medical establishment (for example, a hospital department), has a difficulty with the patient at an emotional and/or behavioural level.

Sharon, aged 22, is a frequent patient who usually presents with rather vague symptoms and clearly derives unusual amounts of personal comfort from any prescriptions or sick notes.

However, when these are not forthcoming, she becomes aggressive and storms out of the practice and makes grossly unfair, but plausible, complaints to a variety of bodies creating considerable extra paperwork for the GP. Every doctor who has dealt with her becomes progressively stressed. This doctor is no exception and requires respite. After discussion with the counsellor, they agree on a way of referring the patient for counselling and how they will manage any consequential difficulties that may arise.

This may be because of some incident that has occurred in his or her own relationship with the person, some accident of diagnosis or even surgery, or an administrative error. The skills of the counsellor to assist in redressing the balance for the benefit of the patient and giving space for a reappraisal of the situation may be called upon, if the patient is so minded and the doctor believes that it may be useful. In this sort of circumstance the establishment of trust between the counsellor and the referrer is essential for the referral to be effective and helpful to all concerned.

Counsellors in primary care are aware of the strengths and frailties of the colleagues with whom they work. Over a period of time, patterns of referrals from different members of the practice can indicate that the counsellor is being used as a way of coping with something, on behalf of the referrer, that the referrer find unpleasant. In this situation, once more, that bond of trust and confidence is all the more important to prevent the possibility of a series of inappropriate patients being put on the list for counselling. Similarly, members of the primary care team may have identified strengths and weaknesses in the counsellor's responses in comparison with their expectations or knowledge of other counsellors.

Time spent on enhancing the relationship with the primary health care team, especially the doctors, is time well spent; otherwise problems will undoubtedly arise. This 'time' might include such matters as looking at mutual hopes and expectations, deciding on acceptable and efficient ways of communicating with each other and under what circumstances there would be immediate communication about the patient. Consideration of the boundaries to each others work to gain some mutual understanding is extremely important.

Any new member of the primary health care team changes the dynamic within that team and this also needs to be acknowledged and the newly aligned set of relationships adjusted accordingly. The culture of primary care may be unknown to a new counsellor and simply observing the ways of working and especially the manner in which information is passed around the team will be beneficial. Medical and health centres are busy places as they react to patient demands and many messages are given 'on the hoof' as one member of the team passes another, or happens to meet in pursuit of their own tasks. Counsellors are often used to considering reflectively 'process issues' and may not be task-orientated in the same way as, and have a different style to, other members of the team. Meetings with members of the primary health care team tend to be extremely focused to cope with the volume of business, and this may be new to some counsellors. Problems can be avoided by a good induction and the recognition that there will be a period of adjustment if the counsellor has not worked in this setting before. Of course, if the counsellor is employed by a mental health trust, or is part of a psychological therapies team, then time also needs investing in a similar way with these other colleagues.

Common relationship themes that occur in primary care counselling

Common themes concern the transitions that we all encounter during the course of our lives. They are related to the stages of human development and sometimes to societies' 'rites of passage'. The arrival of another member into the family unit (be it a sibling or the return or arrival of someone else into the household or family unit), going to or changing school or university, a marriage or new relationship, the birth or death of someone close to us, a family crisis (anything from a theft, redundancy, the illness of someone or their loss) can have differing effects on our lives and consequently on relationships with ourselves and others. How we cope with the common, and the extraordinary, events that impact on our lives affects our health at every level. The manifestation of distress can be immediate at the time when the relationship is disturbed. The distress can also manifest itself many years later, when perhaps there has been a precipitating event or incident that triggers a response. The unfinished businesses, and the emotional processes, of the past, which we did not resolve or complete, may return at a later date. Not surprisingly, most of the events of our lives involve others and our relationships. It is when they are not coping that patients decide to visit the doctor's surgery and arrive in the primary care counsellor's room as a client for counselling. Every one of the changes that befalls us involves a relationship issue that will inevitably involve loss or change, a reappraisal of self in a different situation, and the task of adjusting relationships at various levels. The usual counselling task of 'giving the client an opportunity to explore, discover and clarify ways of living more resourcefully and towards greater well-being' (British Association for Counselling 1997) always applies.

How counselling helps with relationship problems

General overview of the process

The way that counselling helps in relationship problems is, first of all, by providing a place within another relationship—the therapeutic alliance—where the problem relationship can be safely explored. This means an acceptance of the patient by the counsellor, listening to their story and the part that they have in the problem. This may mean, to a greater or lesser degree, depending on the particular theoretical orientation of the counsellor, listening carefully to the history of the relationship and the part played by the person themself in the development of the relationship. The precipitating circumstances to the problem need to be brought forth and examined. A revealing question for the counsellor to ask of themselves is 'Why has this person come for counselling at this time with this relationship problem?' The counselling will involve trying to understand what the relationship means to the individual, what hopes and expectations were placed upon it, and the placing of the relationship in the larger context, as well as seeing it from their viewpoint. Probably the first one or two counselling sessions will be taken up with this task.

As the counsellor reflects back their understanding to the patient, there may be other aspects of the problem which come to light. The purpose of all this is to facilitate the patient's perception of the situation in some psychological depth by carefully reflecting back both facts and feelings. Interventions made by the counsellor will vary according to their personal style and training but will usually follow the patient's concerns as they explore the problem. The middle phase of the counselling may move back and forth at various levels exploring issues and invariably will always have some exploration of the loss or losses that have occurred in the disruption of the relationship. There may be other aspects such as the acknowledging of pain and emotion, perhaps issues of power, helplessness or despair, developmental stages that were not completed, and possibly issues around sexuality and gender. This activity in the counselling room is often seen as therapeutic in itself as feelings are released, pain and emotion is accepted, and another person acknowledges reality as seen by the patient. As clarity is achieved, insight may come to the person as to how they may proceed. This may be enough. However, in relationship counselling the final stage usually concerns adjusting to a new situation in the relationship. This could involve ending, moving on, reconciliation with the other person, the client adapting to a new sense of self, or the acceptance of the *status quo*. Some clients will achieve these changes largely unassisted beyond the point of gaining new insights. Others may require active facilitation and possibly new knowledge or training in interpersonal skills.

When the counselling process appears to be nearing its end and achieving its mutually agreed goal, the manner of the ending can be critical.

Gina, aged 35, is grieving over the sudden death of her long-standing partner, Jill, in a car accident. She moves rapidly between grief and anger in her consultation with her GP. She experiences episodes of acute chest pains which appear to have no physical cause and she acknowledges may replicate the injuries suffered by Jill. Counselling eases the emotional turbulence and unresolved pains. Gina's major concerns are being deprived of any opportunity to communicate what her partner meant to her prior to her death and the unexpectedness of the death. Towards the end of the counselling some of the earlier symptoms return. The counsellor and Gina agreed to work together to construct a planned ending in order to avoid replicating the unplanned ending of her relationship and to maximize the restorative opportunities.

The client has come because of a disruption in the relationship, maybe even a death, and so a planned ending is a good thing. The counselling session which marks the ending of the counselling may include a review of the counselling sessions, an acknowledgement of the insight or learning that has taken place and some feedback from patient to counsellor, as well as some appreciation of the work that has been done. In other words, the ending of the counselling relationship is a model of a good ending for other relationships.

Interpersonal relationship problems—friends, family and employment

It is not uncommon for a patient to be referred to counselling because of relationship problems arising from the family situation. The process may well follow that outlined above and it is essential that the counsellor have some knowledge of family systems. Often it is the member of the family who feels most anxious about the situation who comes for help to the surgery. The patient could be the mother who feels that she cannot cope any longer with her children, the mother who has been labelled 'over anxious' at some point, or a step-parent who is finding that they are having an exasperating time with their partner's children in the new relationship. Occasionally adoptive parents come along, or those whose children have been adopted and would like to reunite with their children, or children who wish to seek out their natural parents. There are occasions when a son or daughter comes for counselling because their surviving parent is entering into a new relationship and they are finding it difficult to cope with the new situation, feeling tremendous loyalty to their deceased mother or father. There is sibling rivalry when children (sometimes now adults who have children themselves) are vying for the attention of a parent or parents. There are people coping with ageing and senile parents, who can be into early old age themselves as the population generally is living longer. Sometimes adolescents present because of demanding parents or because they feel misunderstood (see Chapter 9). There are also times when a client will present who is having difficulty because of social or cultural difference; this could be someone who is a member of a second generation minority ethnic group (see Chapter 7). The list is endless.

It is important for the counsellor to listen carefully to the story that the patient tells and also to record carefully names and the features of each relationship within the family as the story unfolds. Understanding the dynamics of the family may take some time and it is only when there has been a thorough assessment of the whole context that the counselling proper can proceed. The assessment also needs to take into account the values and norms that pertain to the family. Some counsellors may be appropriately trained to invite another member or members of the family into the sessions. This needs to be done with great care and also with impartiality. It may well be that it is 'the relationship' which would benefit from counselling and not simply the patient. However, to proceed in this manner is not always possible or desirable. It also always needs to be borne in mind that any change in the patient and their view of, or behaviour in, the relationship will have consequences which need to be carefully explored on the path to any possible changes. Insight into what is going on in the relationship and acceptance of its meaning on the part of the patient is usually important to helping the patient.

Employment relationships increasingly appear in the counselling room. Stresses caused by disciplinary proceedings, the threat of redundancy, or simply too much or too little work, as well as clashes of personalities, can contribute to difficulties with colleagues and employers. Although the context of the relationship is different, the principles and practice that inform the counselling parallel those for working with relationship difficulties in the family and social networks.

There are times when the counsellor may well feel that the wrong person is in the counselling room. The distress nevertheless is very real and can be worked with and through. There are dysfunctional families, societies and organizations. Before embarking along this into wholesale family therapy, the primary care counsellor needs to think about whether there are more appropriate services on hand to refer on to, to help with, or move in parallel to the process that may be going on in the primary care counselling room.

One area which needs special expertise is that of the sexually abusive relationship where someone has been abused as a child. There are points of law to be considered here as well as an assessment of risk. This is particularly the case when the patient is a child or young person.

Counselling couples with relationship problems

Counselling couples with relationship problems is the classic conception of relationship counselling. Derek Hill (2000) defines relationship counselling as being concerned with the 'intimate relationships between two adults'. Such relationships need not be marriages nor heterosexual. The main focus of this application of counselling is not individuals, but the system that underpins the relationship. This requires the counsellor to work in ways that are different from working individually with either of the members of the relationship. It requires communicating respect for the relationship itself as well as for both of the members of the relationship. Control of the relationship rests with its members. The counsellor works in dialogue with the relationship and as such needs to be firmly located outside it. Any changes within the system have consequences throughout the system and will impact on the partners. When working with both partners, it is easier to obtain each person's views of the impact of any change. However, in primary care it is unusual to have the opportunity to see both partners together, as consultations are more likely to be with individuals. Nevertheless, the same principle of respecting the relationship applies. When addressing relationship problems with only one of the people involved, the counsellor has to direct that person's attention to considering the consequences for the relationship as a system and for the other person. Whether working with one or more people about issues in their relationship, the counsellor's first task is to undertake an assessment.

The kind of information that the counsellor would be likely to need during the assessment process includes:

- whether there are changes the client wishes to make, and if so what they are;
- whether the counsellor and client can work effectively together, and what sort of 'contract' to offer the client (number of sessions, etc.);
- whether the referral is appropriate;
- how clients view their relationships with important figures in their lives—at home, school, work, etc.;
- their attitudes to sex, marriage and partnerships;
- any significant illnesses;
- whether a pattern or a theme or a life problem is evident;
- whether the problem envelops their whole personality;
- any previous similar episodes. (Irving 1995)

Irving suggested that it would be inappropriate to obtain this information by direct questioning and advocated less formal and freer flowing ways of obtaining it. There are two important ways in which working with couples in primary care differs from working with the classic approaches pioneered and developed by Relate and similar specialized organizations. Firstly, couples seldom present to the primary care counsellor together. One half of the relationship visits the doctor and is referred to the counsellor.

This means that the relational nature of the problem may be more disguised. Sometimes it is only after the initial session, or even later, that there is the realization by the client or the counsellor that this is really a relationship difficulty. Secondly, this is also a setting in which a wider range of problems may be presented. Some of the common themes are dealt with in other chapters, for example, sexual problems in Chapter 16, fertility and infertility in Chapter 17.

Conclusions

This chapter opened with observations about the inescapable nature of relationships in primary care and has explored some of the varied ways in which difficulties in relationships may present themselves. These difficulties can arise within the primary care team, between the counsellor(s) and the team, or form part, or all, of what is troubling patients. Sometimes difficulties in relationships may present as the unacknowledged source of physical symptoms. On other occasions relationship difficulties may be the acknowledged source of emotional or psychological distress. Sometimes the pressures of caring for someone can themselves be the source of interpersonal difficulties. It is characteristic of relationship difficulties that they rarely present as an isolated problem that is clearly separated from other aspects of the patient's life. The interconnectedness of physical, psychological and social systems justifies close collaboration between the providers of clinical and counselling expertise in the primary care team. It also follows that relationship counselling in its widest sense is a fundamental area of work for counsellors in primary care.

References

British Association for Counselling (1997) *Code of Ethics and Practice for Counsellors*. British Association for Counselling, Rugby.

Clarkson, P. (1995) *The Therapeutic Relationship*. Whurr, London.

Feltham, C. (ed.) (1999) *Understanding the Counselling Relationship*. Sage, London.

Hill, D. (2000) Couple counselling. In *Handbook of Counselling and Psychotherapy* (Feltham, C. and Horton, I., eds). Sage, London, pp. 603–611.

Horvath, A.O. and Geenberg, L. (eds) (1994) *The Working Alliance: Theory, Research and Practice*. Wiley, Chichester.

Irving, J. (1995) Interpersonal relationships and psychological problems. In *Counselling in Primary Health Care* (Keithley, J. and Marsh, G.N., eds). Oxford University Press, Oxford, pp. 101–128.

Marsh, G.N. and Barr, J. (1975) Marriage guidance counselling in group practice. *Journal of the Royal College of General Practitioners*, **25**, 73–75.

Newnes, G. (1990) Bodyguards may be better than therapy. *General Practitioner*, **15**, 54.

West, L. (2001) *Doctors on the Edge: General Practitioners, Health and Learning in the Inner-city*. Free Association Books, London.

Chapter 14

Trauma

Michael Wright

Introduction

Trauma is encountered in primary health care (PHC) resulting from a wide range of circumstances. These include transport or workplace accidents, fires, violent or sexual assaults, robberies and refugee status.

Some examples from my practice indicate the diversity of circumstances that can cause trauma. Among the people I have seen have been a train driver after a person stepped into the path of his train to commit suicide. A client I was already seeing came for a prearranged appointment a couple of days after being the first person at the scene of an accident in which four young people died. It was some weeks before she could acknowledge that the object she had seen by the roadside was a severed head.

I was asked to see a home care assistant whose mentally ill client pointed a gun at her and pulled the trigger. The gun was not real, but the trauma was. Another was a trained first aider who was unable to save the life of the person he tended. He was not prepared for the psychological impact of that death on him.

A person who visits the GP after such an experience is likely to need more than medication for anxiety, depression or sleeplessness. Medication may address some of the physiological reactions but not the psychological trauma.

Often, traumatized people think they are going mad, or that their current reactions are likely to be permanent. It is essential that the GP and other PHC professionals explain that a wide range of reactions to this abnormal experience are normal, and that in many cases these reactions will subside within a few weeks, especially with good social support from those with whom they shared the experience, and from supportive family, friends and colleagues. Unfortunately, such support is not always forthcoming, and in many cases those who are ready to provide support feel they do not know how best to help.

A skilled counsellor is likely to be able to help the traumatized person to reduce the impact of these reactions in some of the ways described in this chapter. For this, referral to the clinical psychology service, the practice counsellor (if there is one who is trained in trauma work) or a local private agency that has counsellors trained in this field, may be appropriate.

This chapter aims to give PHC professionals an overview of trauma treatments and an understanding of how traumatized people may be helped. It points to the definitions and characteristics of post-traumatic stress disorders and reactions, describes some of the principal ways of working with traumatized people, and looks at some specific implications for children and for people of different cultures. It gives most attention to debriefing.

'Debriefing' is a method that has been developed to provide early intervention. Some recent studies have questioned its value. A study commissioned by the Health and Safety Executive, and presented to the British Psychological Association's conference in 2000 suggested that its efficacy is neutral at best, and at worst damaging. Canterbury and Yule (1999) urge caution in interpreting the results of these critical studies because of the way the sample was selected, and the lack of standardized procedures across the studies. The critique chiefly focuses on situations where people in a group that has experienced trauma are obliged to take part in debriefing, often by employers who fear litigation. It is important to consider how early the intervention takes place, how much time is available for the procedure, and how carefully and thoroughly it is done. A number of studies have examined the results of debriefing only, without other counselling following.

Any psychological intervention has the potential for damage if it is done by a poorly trained person, without the informed consent of the subject, in a highly emotionally charged situation, without proper safeguards, and especially with some sense of compulsion. Debriefing is not a panacea, but it can, in the right circumstances and done well, be a very therapeutic process. For some people it will be a valuable first step in dealing with their reactions to the trauma, and they may or may not need anything more. Others may need skilled long-term counselling. Where no help is available, the effects of trauma can influence them for a very long time; 50 years or more in the case of some war veterans.

Post-traumatic stress

The symptoms of post-trauma stress have been officially recognized by the American Psychiatric Association since 1983, largely as a result of studies on the impact of trauma on veterans of the Vietnam War. Since then, the definitions of criteria for post-traumatic stress disorder (PTSD) have been modified in their *Diagnostic and Statistical Manual of Mental Disorders*, currently DSM-IV. The World Health Organization has produced slightly different criteria for acute stress reaction (ASR) and for PTSD in the tenth edition of their *International Classification of Diseases*, ICD-10. The full texts of these definitions are in Joseph *et al.* (1997). There is currently a debate on whether these criteria are broad enough to encompass the needs of many people who have traumatic experiences.

The American Psychiatric Association have labelled post-traumatic stress a psychiatric condition, yet recognize that given sufficient stress when faced with 'actual or threatened death or serious injury, or a threat to the physical integrity of self or others' (DSM-IV) almost anyone can develop PTSD. Features of this are now widely recognized as normal reactions to abnormal experiences. They have been found in adults and children of many different cultures. However, the same event may not be traumatic for everyone involved or witnessing it. Much depends upon each individual's interpretation of the experience, the impact this has on their thoughts and feelings, and their existing personality. Traumatic stress is thus 'an interaction between the person and the event' (Figley 1999).

Once post-traumatic stress reactions have become chronic, they can be extremely difficult to treat (Watson 1987). It is for this reason that a number of practitioners recommend early crisis intervention. Mitchell (1983) argues that interventions within 72 hours of the traumatic event are effective in reducing the long-term effects for emergency workers. Early crisis intervention is also recommended to support and enable emotional release in a safe supportive environment (Raphael 1986).

Early intervention with trauma

I have worked with traumas over the past 10 years, and have found that the debriefing methods developed by Dyregrov (1989), Mitchell and Everly (1993) and Raphael (1986) have provided a helpful structure for containing and exploring the event and its impact upon traumatized people. I have used a debriefing structure from two days to 12 years after the trauma, with more than 40 traumatic incidents, and have found it has produced a considerable relief of some symptoms, sometimes immediately and normally within 10 days, in all but a couple of individuals. In some cases, individuals or groups have asked for help, in other cases a decision has been made to offer this service, and invite those who were part of the experience to participate in the debrief. I anticipate that the PHC will mostly deal with traumatized individuals, rather than groups, and so I describe this process for one person. I suggest it will be valuable to have at least one person in the PHC team, or someone in private practice to call upon, who has been trained in this field.

Rationale

The aim is to begin to restore control to the traumatized person whose normal sense of security and control has been shattered. Many traumatized people have been questioned by the police, health and safety officers and their employer, seeking specific information for a criminal investigation or a disciplinary enquiry. People will often protect family and friends from some of the most horrific aspects of their experience. The traumatized person is then left with many partly-told tales, but never having been through the whole experience to meet their own needs. Debriefing is a structured process. The facilitator provides a safe structure in which the whole experience can be explored. The skill is in remaining person-centred within such a structure. The given agenda is the experience the person has had, and so the debriefer is careful to help them explore this carefully and methodically, but also gently and sensitively. No-one should be forced to examine in detail any parts of the experience which at that moment they find too distressing.

The preparation

It is essential that the debriefer fully explains the process to the traumatized individual to ensure they understand it, and obtains their informed consent before beginning. I explain that the process will involve going through the event three times. This can be set out as a written agenda as:

- ◆ Preparation and agreed groundrules
- ◆ Facts
- ◆ Thoughts
- ◆ Feelings
- ◆ Now
- ◆ Next.

Facts

I invite the individual to describe the context of the trauma before it happened. This is 'setting the scene' when things were normal. Aspects to note include time, weather, what was happening, general conditions, and any unusual aspects, who was there, and where they were. Then I take them through the facts—what happened, what they saw, heard, said and did, smelled, touched or tasted. I invite them to concentrate their attention at this stage on what actually happened, leaving their thoughts and feelings to the next two stages.

I go through the facts in as much detail as possible, but never push on parts they are unable at that time to talk about. Tiny details can have great significance. It is often helpful to get people to draw a plan or diagram of the situation to show where people were, and how things changed. When working with a single individual I may (and this involves sensitive judgement in each case) invite them to describe even horrific things in detail rather than generalities. Being able to articulate them, when they are ready to do so, in a calm accepting environment can be liberating, but forcing someone to speak about aspects they are not yet ready to can retraumatize them.

I encourage them to stay with the facts right through the trauma to some appropriate stage beyond. This may be when they reached hospital, or recovered consciousness, or when people gathered in a rest room to recover. Many significant happenings occur both before and after the key trauma. These may be within the same day, or even the next day.

Thoughts

Having gone through their account once, I take them through it again, inviting them to say what they were thinking during significant events. My aim is to keep thoughts separate from feelings. Many people find it difficult to distinguish between the two. Being helped to do so in the debriefing can often have important and helpful consequences later.

Feelings

Coming to the story for the third time might seem excessive, but experience of using the technique shows how helpful it is. The total amount of information that will emerge from going through it three times is an important part of the healing process. Those who tell their story unearth bits of information they have forgotten. This process of putting all the pieces of jigsaw into place is very important.

When people are helped to layer their story out in this way, they are normally able to describe their feelings without being overwhelmed by them. When facts, thoughts and feelings are all jumbled up together, the telling of the story is often more distressing.

Feelings of anger, guilt, revenge or blame are common, as are questioning your own actions and omissions—the debriefer should accept them at this stage. They can be worked with later in counselling. The debriefing may be just one part of the therapeutic process. For some it may be all they want or need. Negative emotions need to be heard before they are challenged. The woman who blamed the ambulance driver for the death of her child because of the time taken for the ambulance to arrive, needed to know that her cry of anguish had been really heard and understood before anyone asked her to be reasonable.

There is a lot of material to remember in most traumas. However, the material makes such an impact that the facilitator will usually have no difficulty in keeping all the salient points in mind without writing notes, which distract from the listening.

Now

Having been through the story three times, the next stage is to enquire what effects this trauma is having on them. Common effects include flashbacks, dreams, vivid memories, intense distress and the sudden feeling that the trauma is occurring again. Other features are likely to include some (but not all) of the following: depression, anxiety, mental confusion, guilt, anger, frustration, despair, under- or overactivity, mood changes and abnormal behaviour.

Common reactions include deliberate avoidance of associations with the trauma, memory blocks, a feeling of detachment or estrangement from others, a sense of vulnerability and insecurity, and feeling very conscious of how fragile life is. There may be an increased reliance on sleeping pills or other medication, drugs, alcohol or nicotine. Other reactions may include irritability or anger, sleep disturbance, hypervigilance, loss of concentration and memory, exaggerated reactions to noise or to stimuli associated with the trauma, and physiological reactions to an experience that resembles the trauma.

Traumatized people need to understand that most of them can expect to experience some or all of these reactions, and a variety of other common ones, in the immediate weeks after the trauma. However, some do not do so for weeks or months, whilst others never do. Often the patience of those closest to the traumatized person is quite limited. There is frequent pressure to 'pull yourself together', or 'put it behind you' or 'get back to normal working'.

Enabling people to recognize that their reactions are normal reactions to an abnormal experience helps them begin to gain control of their churned-up thoughts and feelings. The British Red Cross has produced a helpful leaflet 'Coping with a personal crisis' that gives details of common reactions. At this stage it is good to offer suggestions for behavioural techniques that people can use to tackle some of their current difficulties. One common need is for some methods to get to sleep when their mind is churning.

In most cases, symptoms of PTSD seem to substantially diminish or disappear by about 18 months after the event, although some events, particularly those involving many deaths, may have long-lasting effects. Prolonged exposures to trauma, as in an abusive relationship, can result in considerable personality changes, and a plea has been made for this to be identified separately as 'complex post-traumatic stress disorder' (CPTSD) (Herman 1992). This is addressed in Chapter 15.

Next

The final stage is to help the individual identify what they want next. It may focus around a funeral or an inquest, or a return to work or to the place where the incident occurred. It may be exploring ways of expressing things the individual wished they had said to a person before s/he died. This is the important rounding off of the debriefing. The work may be complete in itself, or a step towards counselling and further support or therapy. If the debrief has gone well, there is frequently a visible difference in those who have participated. It can be a very satisfying, if sometimes, gruelling form of work.

It is important to get good counselling supervision for this work, which can be traumatic for the counsellor. Anyone dealing with the intensity of these emotions, and sometimes horrific details, needs to off-load, reflect and receive support. A supervisor experienced in trauma work can help the practitioner to keep a sense of proportion about this work, especially at times when many people are caught up in the aftermath of a large-scale disaster.

Assessment for PTSD

There are a number of tools for assessing PTSD. The impact of events scale (IES) is one that is widely used. This is a self-assessment report that looks for intrusive experiences and avoidance of situations, ideas and feelings (Horowitz *et al.* 1979). Another which is widely used is the general health questionnaire (GHQ) developed by Goldberg and Hillier (1979) which looks for somatic symptoms, anxiety and insomnia, social dysfunction and severe depression. The key issues in assessment are examined in Joseph *et al.* (1997).

Although there have been various descriptions of treatment methods for PTSD since it was first included in DSM-III, there has been only a limited amount of empirical research on the effectiveness of them. All that can be provided here is a brief description of the principal methods that are being used, to encourage practitioners dealing with trauma to explore the field in more depth.

Methods of counselling for trauma

Cognitive therapy

The majority of counselling for trauma appears to use mainly cognitive therapy. Cognitive restructuring focuses on challenging the interpretation and meaning which traumatized people draw from their experiences, which lead to negative emotional reactions. Cognitive behavioural counselling aims to challenge negative thinking, and help the client focus on realistic thinking. Scott and Stradling (1992) and Richards and Lovell (1999) explore a cognitive approach with case examples. Tedeschi and Calhoun (1995) use a cognitive approach to explore the potential for personal growth, drawing together material from psychology, philosophy and religion. Rosenbloom *et al.* (1999) have produced a self-help workbook for healing after trauma. It is well stocked with a wide range of exercises from which counsellors can select, to offer ideas for working through beliefs about safety, control and many other factors.

Systematic desensitization

Systematic desensitization (Lyons & Keane 1989) begins by teaching the client a formal method of relaxation. The next step is to practice this whilst gradually engaging with visual images, artefacts or reminders, or visiting the scene of an event related to the trauma. Stimuli involving gradually increasing levels of anxiety are employed, until at each stage the client can tolerate the image or the actual situation and remain relaxed rather than anxious. This method may be used with teaching breathing control and panic management. Richards and Lovell (1999) include a couple of case examples, in one of which the client engaged daily in more detail with her experience by writing and reading what she had written, until she could engage with violent TV reminders of these experiences without anxiety.

Implosive therapy

Implosive therapy requires the client to be exposed to prolonged trauma-related stimuli until the anxiety associated with them is reduced (Richards & Lovell 1999). There is a review of some case histories and results in Joseph *et al.* (1997, pp. 120–123). Lyons and Keane (1989) conclude that implosive therapy needs to be combined with a supportive therapeutic relationship, and with teaching the client to develop their own coping skills.

Drama therapy

Linda Winn describes a number of creative approaches to working with traumatized people in groups (Winn 1994). These include exploring literature, painting, collage, drama, mime, group exercises, role-play, story-telling and poetry. She makes imaginative use of metaphor, a collection of small dolls and other objects to 'sculpt' relationships and explore closeness or distance.

Working with refugees

Work with victims of trauma who are also refugees is well explored by van der Veer (1998). They have often experienced repression, trauma and then expulsion from their familiar surroundings and have to adapt to a new culture and language. Van der Veer helps the therapist look at cultural differences and the additional factor of working with an interpreter. He provides a very readable text to help the counsellor understand and work effectively with such refugees, who may have experienced detention, torture, rape, exile and culture shock.

Brief therapy

Traumatic incident reduction is a structured approach which is used to treat PTSD and which its advocates suggest is best done with short-term intensive treatment, after an in-depth history-taking as part of the assessment process. The sessions are normally 90 minutes, but can take as long as they need. An important aspect of this work is to allow the client to engage with the trauma until it loses some of its emotional intensity. The method is fully described in Bisbey and Bisbey (1998).

Eye movement desensitization and reprocessing

Eye movement desensitization and reprocessing is a form of therapy discovered quite by chance, as a treatment for intrusive thoughts. The client is asked to picture in their mind the scenes which distress them, and is then asked to watch the therapist's moving finger as it moves quickly backwards and forwards for 20 or more times. The therapist asks the client about any changes in the images, and often asks the client to rate their feelings of stress or anxiety on a 10-point scale. Frequently, clients report that the images have changed, sometimes more detail is reported. This is often followed by reports that both the distress and the image have faded (Shapiro 1995). The procedure is also described and evaluated in Smith and Yule (1999).

Understanding and training

All of these methods require a thorough understanding of the therapeutic principles which underlie them, a thorough training from an experienced practitioner, and participation in an experiential training course which provides the opportunity to practice the concepts taught with fellow students before embarking on work with traumatized people.

Cultural aspects

The cultural aspects of PTSD have not been widely studied. Those few studies that exist show that people tend to experience common post-traumatic stress reactions whatever their culture. The majority of these have been of those who have been traumatized in wars. Many of them identify soldiers of different ethnic groups who all experience common symptoms; PTSD is not culturally limited (de Silva 1999).

Cultural differences are identified in some of the interpretations people make of their traumatic experiences, and in the varieties of reactions or social support traumatized individuals have received in different cultures. For example, a study by Williams (1950) compared Indian and British soldiers fighting against the Japanese in 1944. He found a higher incidence of recorded psychiatric illness among all the British troops than among all the Indian troops. He noted that for the Indian soldiers to show anxiety involved loss of face, so a number of them who were perceived to be experiencing anxiety gave themselves self-inflicted wounds as a legitimate way to get medical attention.

Other examples of cultural differences were provided from Afghan War victims, where certain physical reactions were similar to those observed in studies made in Western countries, but symptoms such as crying and, particularly, suicidal thoughts or acts were inhibited by their culture. Suicide is a criminal act in Islam. Rape victims may face social ostracism in some communities if they report the crime (de Silva 1999).

In treating victims of trauma, issues of religious, cultural and personal convictions should be given careful attention. It can be helpful, with the agreement of the client, to consult a person who comes from the same cultural group and/or faith community, for help in understanding the norms of culture and belief that are not familiar to the counsellor, and to identify what social support or pressures there are, or can be expected. However, it is also always important to explore sensitively with the client how far she or he shares the norms of their family and community.

There is now a considerable diversity in our population. Across most racial groups, including white Anglo-Saxons, there is a range of cultural practice and beliefs. In religious matters the range can be from strong convictions and social norms to indifference. These can have a significant effect on clients' views about the meaning of life and death. In moral matters the range can be from high principles to amoral attitudes, which can influence feelings such as responsibility and guilt. There can be tightly controlled family and extended family groups, or nuclear families of parents and their children, with varying degrees of openness to talking, feeling and dealing sensitively with traumas experienced by one or more members of the family. Some individuals may look outside the household circle for their primary support. Individuals who live alone can easily become isolated. All these factors are germane to the healing task in dealing with trauma.

Work with children

Finally, I would like to briefly discuss work with children who have suffered as a result of trauma. It is only since about 1985 that traumatic stress reactions in children have been systematically studied. One thing that has emerged from those studies is that often parents and teachers do not adequately recognize the child's anxiety symptoms. Sometimes they deny them; often children protect their parents, other adults and siblings, by not talking about what they are really experiencing, thinking or feeling. There are a number of evaluation studies of treatment methods working with an individual child, but no randomized controlled studies. Treatments on the whole are cognitive behavioural and seem to be adaptations of methods used with adults (Yule *et al.* 1999).

At present the principal method of assessment is to conduct thorough clinical interviews first with the parent, and then with the child. The interview with the parent should include the family history, the child's development up to the trauma, and how the child has changed since. A detailed account of what the adult believes happened is essential. This then needs to be checked very carefully and tentatively in the interview with the child to establish the facts from the child's experience. This account might include details not known, or not significant, to the parent but significant to the child.

The interview with the child needs a patient, unhurried detailed exploration of 'facts, thoughts and feelings', including the sensory memory (heard, felt, smelt, saw, tasted). Afterwards, in co-operation with the parent, the last two elements are addressed—the 'now', normalizing the child's reactions to an abnormal event, and the 'next', identifying what the child would like in the near future in terms of help, support, safety or information.

Further work will be indicated by what levels of anxiety and depression are identified in the child. If the trauma includes a bereavement, then work by Pynoos and Nader (1988) indicates the need to help the child or children to distinguish their responses to the trauma from their grief. They suggest that where several children are bereaved, small groups can be beneficial in the early stages.

The work will vary according to the age and development of the child. It can be helpful to invite a child to paint or draw a picture about the incident, and then to explain the completed picture in considerable detail with the therapist. With older children it may be more appropriate to invite them to draw a plan which details the position and movement of significant people and objects of the trauma.

Work in this field is in its early stages, but there are a number of assessment questionnaires for PTSD and for anxiety and depression in children (Pynoos & Nader 1988, pp. 40–41).

References

Bisbey, S. and Bisbey, L.B. (1998) *Brief Therapy for Post Traumatic Stress Disorder.* Wiley, Chichester.

Canterbury, R. and Yule, W. (1999) Debriefing and crisis intervention. In *Post Traumatic Stress Disorders: Concepts and Therapy* (Yule, W., ed.). Wiley, Chichester, pp. 221–238.

De Silva, P. (1999) Cultural aspects of post-traumatic stress disorder. In *Post Traumatic Stress Disorders: Concepts and Therapy* (Yule, W., ed.). Wiley, Chichester, pp. 116–138.

Dyregrov, A. (1989) Caring for helpers in disaster situations: psychological debriefing. *Disaster Management,* 2 (1), 25–30.

Figley, C.R. (1999) *Traumatology of Grieving.* Brunner/Mazel, Philadelphia.

Goldberg, D.P. and Hillier, V.F. (1979) A scaled version of the general health questionnaire. *Psychological Medicine,* 9, 139–145.

Herman, J.L. (1992) *Trauma and Recovery: from Domestic Abuse to Political Terror.* Harper-Collins, London.

Horowitz, M.J., Wilner, N. and Alvarez, W. (1979) Impact of event scale: a measure of subjective stress. *Psychosomatic Medicine,* 41, 209–218.

Joseph, S., Williams, R. and Yule, W. (1997) *Understanding Post-traumatic Stress.* Wiley, Chichester.

Lyons, J.A. and Keane, T.M. (1989) Strategies for assessing the potential for positive adjustment following trauma. *Journal of Traumatic Stress,* 4, 93–112.

Mitchell, J.T. (1983) *When disaster strikes ...* The critical incident stress debriefing process. *Journal of Emergency Medical Services,* 8, 36–39.

Mitchell, J.T. and Everly, G.S. (1993) *Critical Incident Stress Debriefing: an Operations Manual for the Prevention of Traumatic Stress among Emergency Service and Disaster Workers.* Chevron Publishing, Ellicot City.

Pynoos, R.S. and Nader, K. (1988) Psychological first aid and treatment approach for children exposed to community violence: research implications. *Journal of Traumatic Stress,* 1, 243–267.

Raphael, B. (1986) *When Disaster Strikes—a Handbook for the Caring Professions.* Unwin Hyman, London.

Richards, D. and Lovell, K. (1999) Behavioural and cognitive behavioural interventions in the treatment of PTSD. In *Post Traumatic Stress Disorders: Concepts and Therapy* (Yule, W., ed.). Wiley, Chichester, pp. 239–266.

Rosenbloom, D., Williams, M.B. and Watkins, B.E. (1999) *Life after Trauma*. Guilford Press, New York.

Scott, M.J. and Stradling, S.G. (1992) *Counselling for Post-traumatic Stress Disorder*. Sage, London.

Shapiro, F. (1995) *Eye Movement Desensitisation and Reprocessing: Basic Principles, Protocols and Procedures*. Guilford Press, New York.

Smith, R. and Yule, W. (1999) Eye movement desensitisation and reprocessing. In *Post Traumatic Stress Disorders: Concepts and Therapy* (Yule, W., ed.). Wiley, Chichester, pp. 267–284.

Tedeschi, R.G. and Calhoun, L.G. (1995) *Trauma and Transformation—Growing in the Aftermath of Suffering*. Sage, London.

Van der Veer, G. (1998) *Counselling and Therapy with Refugees and Victims of Trauma*. Wiley, Chichester.

Watson, P.B. (1987) Post-traumatic stress disorder in Australia and New Zealand: a critical review of the consequences of inescapable horror. *Medical Journal of Australia*, **147**, 443–446.

Williams, A.C.H. (1950) Psychiatric study of Indian soldiers in the Arakan. *British Journal of Medical Psychology*, **24**, 130–181.

Winn, L. (1994) *Post Traumatic Stress Disorder and Dramatherapy*. Jessica Kingsley, London.

Yule, W., Perrin, S. and Smith, P. (1999) Post-traumatic stress reactions in children and adolescents. In *Post Traumatic Stress Disorders: Concepts and Therapy* (Yule, W., ed.). Wiley, Chichester, pp. 25–50.

Chapter 15

Physical and sexual abuse

Kim Etherington

Introduction

The topic of childhood sexual and physical abuse has been the subject of many research reports and literature over the last 10 or 15 years. In attempting to write this chapter I find myself asking: How on earth can I deal with such a vast topic? What would be most useful? Will it be like opening up Pandora's box and leave me wishing I had left it where it was, under the bed and out of sight? What are the reader's expectations of me—will I be considered the expert and then judged negatively when I do not have all the answers?

If any of the above questions feel familiar to you, then I expect you have faced the problem of trying to work with physical and sexual abuse in a primary care setting. The parallels between my questions as I thought about writing this chapter and actually 'doing the work' are obvious. There may also be parallels with how clients think and feel as they come to ask for help.

So I do not intend to attempt to address the whole topic; I do not intend to provide definitions, lists of symptoms, long-term effects, etc.—all of which can be found elsewhere (Sanderson 1995; Etherington 1995, 2000; Freyd 1996; Hunter 1995; Bear 1999). My focus will be on working in a primary care setting with adults who have experienced childhood abuse and the context-based issues that may be related. The additional focus is that of working with the concept of trauma and somatic presentation in primary care.

Where do we begin?

Historically the enormity of the subject of child abuse created such overwhelming feelings that society turned away from knowing the unknowable. Nowadays this is less often the case. We are made aware, almost every day, of violations upon children, whether on our own doorstep or in the wider world. We hear of children in Belgium who have been sexually assaulted, locked in a cellar and left to die, we hear of children in Bosnia or Kosovo and other places who have undergone or witnessed appalling atrocities; children maimed by landmines, raped and tortured. Closer to home we hear of children in schools, in 'care' in local authority homes, or in the family, who are beaten, neglected and sexually abused, buried beneath concrete floors—we can no longer deny these events. Our eyes have been opened—even when we sometimes want them to remain closed.

In the 1960s and 1970s the women's movement was instrumental in lifting the veil of secrecy and silence as women were encouraged to speak out about their physical and sexual abuse. A few refuges for battered women opened up in response to emerging voices (Pizzey 1974) and links were made between the abuse of women and child abuse; 'refuges for battered women were among the first institutions in this country to recognise the prevalence of the sexual abuse of children' (O'Hara 1992, p. 4).

In the 1980s and 1990s technology exposed the global scale of the problem by bringing it into our homes through TV and the internet. Further information about how societal changes have created a situation in which it is more likely today that patients, both male and female, will disclose their experiences of childhood abuse to counsellors in general practice can be found elsewhere (Etherington 1995; Sanderson 1995; Freyd 1996; Bear 1999).

Acknowledging and disclosing

Researchers and clinicians now accept the reality of childhood abuse, although clinicians may still prefer to 'let sleeping dogs lie' for fear of stirring up material that they may feel unwilling to deal with, perhaps stemming from their own denial, lack of information and knowledge, but maybe also related to inadequate resources for referral. When asked if he would ever consider asking patients about the occurrence of abuse in their childhood, one GP replied 'it would be like opening a can of worms'; another explained 'I would be worried about putting thoughts into someone's head which weren't there before' (Santi-Ireson 1996). However, research (Frawley 1988; Courtois 1993; Etherington 2000) suggests that disclosure is experienced by the patient as ultimately relieving and crucial to healing. Physicians have been urged to risk asking questions about abuse in the same way that they might ask about other important life events that might affect their patients' health and well-being (Felitti 1998). It may be that clients will initially deny such events (if they are not ready to acknowledge or disclose), but at least they will know that their GP is open to such discussions when and if they should want to talk about it in the future.

However, the impact on the client of how those disclosures are received can also be crucial—when disclosure is dismissed, denied or disbelieved, clients can feel reabused and withdraw, perhaps never to risk disclosure again. Some GPs do not recognize the ways that abuse survivors present within the practice. Judith Herman (1992) says:

> All too commonly chronically traumatised people suffer in silence, but if they complain at all, their complaints are not well understood. They may collect a virtual pharmacopoeia of remedies: one for headaches, another for insomnia, another for anxiety, another for depression. None of these tend to work very well, since the underlying issues of trauma are not addressed. As caregivers tire of these chronically unhappy people who do not seem to improve, the temptations to apply pejorative diagnostic labels becomes overwhelming. (p. 119)

The GP's response can mirror the feelings of helplessness, rage and confusion of the abused 'child' that may be trapped within the adult who has not found a way of telling their story (Etherington 2000). Some GPs still believe that sexual and physical abuse is not something that occurs on their patch—maybe on the one next door—but certainly not on theirs. A small study undertaken by a counsellor working in general practice showed that this was the belief of the doctors with whom she was working, even whilst she was regularly dealing with these issues a few doors down the corridor in the counselling room (Santi-Ireson 1996). Needless to say, these attitudes and beliefs will not be conducive to enabling clients to disclose and subsequently, heal.

Hooper (1990), a GP in a 13 000 patient practice, sent a questionnaire to all 615 women on his personal list of 2500 patients between the ages of 20 and 60 years. There were 418 responses (65%) from 60 abused (almost 14%) and 129 non-abused women; there were 197 non-respondents. Because of the sensitive nature of the information being sought, no follow up of the non-respondents was made. Thirty three per cent of abused women in Hooper's study had some kind of psychological morbidity (including multiple consultations over many years for non-organic complaints) recorded in their notes compared with 14% of the non-abused controls. Physical morbidity was not explored. Sexual abuse was defined as experiences ranging from exposure to penetration and ranged from 'constant' to 'once only'. This sample excluded men because Hooper, although recognizing that males are sexually abused, decided it is more common in women. More recent research reports that incidence in males is less frequently reported for a variety of psychosocial reasons (Etherington 1995) and because they are not researched as frequently as women.

Statistics do not adequately inform us about the incidence of childhood abuse for many reasons. It has been recognized that in order to gather such statistics abuse needs to be reported; for abuse to be reported it needs to be defined; it also has to be acknowledged and remembered. All of these requirements create problems. There are numerous ways that people experience abuse that would be denied in those terms by others. One GP was reported as saying 'children themselves can be the abusers of adults—acting very seductively and then crying when something happens' (Santi-Ireson 1996).

Until very recently, physical abuse was accepted as a way of disciplining children—in the home and in institutions. Abuse was normalized in a patriarchal society that valued control and discipline. Acknowledgement of sexual and physical abuse requires the victim to overcome shame, fear and guilt. Some victims cope with their abuse by denial or by repressing the memories that threaten to overwhelm them if they should emerge (Whitfield 1995; Mollon 1998).

How can we help?

Counselling in primary care is, in part, a manifestation of the changing culture that I have mentioned briefly above. Part of that change has come about as the 'biopsychosocial model' has challenged the superiority of the 'medical model'; we now understand people as functioning biologically, psychologically, physically and spiritually, and the growth of alternative and complementary approaches available to the patients has reflected that change. Counselling has become part of that holistic approach. Child abuse affects every aspect of a person's being, body, mind and spirit and thus the idea of working with abuse survivors holistically, in a general practice setting, seems fitting.

The GP's role

Traditionally the doctor has been the first port of call for people who feel threatened in any aspect of their health and welfare. Many patients say that they would prefer to talk to their GP, given the choice, but the reality is that GPs do not have the time required to work psychologically in-depth with matters related to childhood abuse. GPs may be the first person that survivors use to 'test' another person's response to their disclosure; the nature of that response could very well determine whether or not the patient seeks further help. The GP's best option is to listen and reflect, empathize and support the disclosure without probing further. It may be that he/she could invite the patient to think about what kind of support they would like and how they might work together to find suitable help. People frequently fear that they will lose control of their information if they disclose it to another—it is important that the patient maintains control until they choose to share it. If there is no counsellor within the practice then GPs need to know what local resources are available and check out the qualifications of the helpers and what provisions are made for supervision. If there is a counsellor in the practice with appropriate expertise, the patient can be given information about them and about how a referral can be made.

GP counsellors

Traditionally, counsellors working in primary care are expected to offer a limited numbers of sessions. The rationale for this is an oft-quoted (and challenged) statistic that indicates that the greatest degree of improvement has been seen to occur during the first eight sessions (Barkham *et al.* 1996). The other rationale is that of limited resources.

I come into contact with counsellors working in primary care through my work as a supervisor and as a trainer on a postgraduate diploma in counselling in primary care/health settings. Through these contacts I have discovered that in reality very few counsellors work in practices where there is absolute rigidity about the limit of sessions offered to clients (see also Mearns 1998; Weller 1999). Most GPs who employ counsellors have come to recognize them as professionals with integrity and skills, who are able to make their own assessments of the needs of the client. Many GPs are also aware of the lack of suitable resources for working with this client group in the secondary care system and in voluntary agencies.

Secondary care

Patients who present with child abuse issues are frequently passed on to the secondary care services—often with little success. The pressure on secondary services has meant that people who are diagnosed as having 'problems in life', rather than 'mental illness', are deemed unsuitable for services offered within the mental health system. Patients may wait for many months only to be told that they cannot be allocated the help they seek (Hudson-Allez 1997). Secondary care psychotherapy services are being cut and waiting lists are growing.

An additional problem is that few community psychiatric nurses (CPNs) are trained counsellors, and the issues concerning abuse are rarely addressed in their training. In a recent article (Holley 1999), a clinical nurse specialist, comments on how the growing public awareness about the damaging effects of abuse has increased the number of referrals to the service. She states:

> I would like to be able to report that our awareness has also grown and that patients are receiving a quality service from practitioners who are skilled with dealing with the issues they present. Unfortunately, this is not the case. While there are many skilled mental health practitioners providing an excellent service to adult survivors, there are many more who are uncomfortable with sexual abuse for a variety of reasons. Mainly, problems arising from a lack of training'. (p. 6)

The honesty and non-defensiveness of this statement is encouraging; I am even more encouraged when the writer goes on to state that there are measures afoot to provide training and support to practitioners who are willing to do this work. However, the role of the nurse will always differ from the role of counsellor, as will the training they receive.

People working in the field have commented on the strong link between childhood abuse and subsequent mental illness. Judith Herman (1992) argued, for example, that 'many, or even most, psychiatric patients are survivors of child abuse' (p. 122). Marjorie Orr (1999) also draws our attention to similar statements made by a psychologist (Read 1997) in his international literature review which focused on the implications for practice of the links between child abuse and psychosis. The same author proposes that it is not only mild or moderate adult dysfunction that is related to childhood abuse, but also some of the most severe dysfunctions (Read 1998). One of the studies he quoted found that among patients with 'severe mental illness', 76% of women and 72% of men had been sexually or physically abused in childhood (Read 1998, p. 360).

So if there are few suitably trained and willing practitioners within the mental health system—as Holley (1999) suggests—and few that can access psychotherapy services within the NHS, where can patients go for help? Many survivors recognize that they are *not* 'mentally ill' and are unwilling to place themselves within that category anyway, even if such help were offered and available. A further consideration is that of relative costs. Secondary care services are vastly more expensive than the cost of in-house counselling, and the longer term savings in helping a patient to recover from the effects of childhood abuse are immeasurable.

Costs of not dealing with the problem in primary care

Abuse survivors tell of repeated visits to their doctor with a variety of symptoms, many of which they recognize during therapy as their unconscious way of trying to tell their story. My own experience of working with abuse survivors over many years shows evidence of repeated patterns of symptom presentation, e.g. genitourinary symptoms, unexplained abdominal pain, neurological disorders, etc. GPs often respond to the symptoms rather than the underlying disorder, resulting sometimes in costly and unnecessary interventions and surgical procedures, causing additional suffering without addressing the real problem. Symptoms that are labelled as 'psychosis', e.g. hallucinations, can turn out to be perceptual disturbances that often accompany post-traumatic stress disorder.

A study by Smith *et al.* (1995) evaluated a specialist pilot service for sexual abuse survivors. In gathering the previous medical history of a subgroup of 18 cases, it was found they had had a higher rate of contact with their GP than a non-abused control group prior to using the service (15.5% vs. 4.2%). This part of the study showed increased weight problems (56% vs. 4.2%), misuse of drugs or alcohol (28% vs. 6%), asthma (39% vs. 17%) and irritable bowel syndrome (33% vs. 14%). There were also significant increases in: prescriptions issued per year (5.2% vs. 1.7%); use of psychiatric teams (2.9% vs. 0.2%); non-psychiatric secondary care (8.3% vs. 3.5%); and psychiatric admissions (3.4% vs. 0.2%). Surgical operations performed with negative findings averaged 33% versus 10%. The cases studied were eight times more likely to have attempted suicide than controls.

A recent study of 9000 people in the USA (Felitti 1998) found that those who had been exposed to four or more episodes of childhood abuse had between a fourfold and 12-fold increased health risk for alcoholism, drug abuse, depression and suicide attempts. Such people were between two and four times more likely to smoke, to be generally ill, to have more than 50 sex partners and thus to have sexually transmitted diseases, and up to 1.6 times more likely to be obese.

A study of women who had been raped during childhood (Arnold *et al.* 1990) noted that patients had had an average of eight operations with a high rate (66–70%) of normal findings. History of childhood sexual abuse was recognized only after the use of medical and surgical interventions. It is clear from this that the cost of in-house counselling, at an earlier stage of the process, could possibly save the NHS time and money—as well as a lot of unnecessary suffering for people who have usually suffered enough already.

If I can't deal with all of it fully and to my satisfaction, is it worth starting at all?

Many counsellors working in primary care have been trained to work long term and therefore have a different set of attitudes to those who take into consideration the potential benefits of short-term, time-conscious approaches (Dolan 1994; Elton-Wilson 1996; Hudson-Allez 1997). These attitudes, which often include a belief that only clients who work uninterruptedly over several years can heal from the effects of childhood abuse, may become detrimental to their ability to help the client.

Clients who have been abused may experience an exacerbation of symptoms at different stages of life. For example, many women remember their abuse after the birth of a child, after a hysterectomy or when their child reaches the age at which their own abuse occurred. When counselling is offered in their GP surgery they may feel able to return to counselling whenever these issues are current.

Counsellors sometimes feel that once the work has begun it would be harmful or inappropriate for them to discontinue with clients. This, I believe to some degree, depends upon the contract we make as we begin to build our relationship. It is important that clients who have suffered rejection and damaged trust should not be made false promises. Clarity about what is on offer is essential to the development of trust. Trust does not mean the counsellor will always be there, any more than their ability to trust their GP depends on him/her always being available, but rather that the counsellor behaves in a consistent and trustworthy manner. Honesty and openness are essential elements of trust building, which is part of the recovery process (Sgroi & Bunk 1988). The context may also enable the client to develop trust *more* quickly or readily. A trusted doctor who recommends that his patient should see the counsellor in the practice is in a powerful position to influence the degree of trust the client places in the counsellor–client relationship. Of course the opposite can also be true.

How does the counsellor begin to find a focus?

Survivors have often kept their childhood abuse secret for many years, so when they decide to tell their story the effect of the sudden release may be like a pressure cooker exploding. Without an outlet valve through which the pressure can escape as it builds up, disclosure can seem overwhelming both to the storyteller and the listener. Some clients think that all they need to do is tell somebody and then they will be 'cured'. Some counsellors have been known to think likewise.

In the first telling of the story the counsellor needs to monitor carefully how the client is managing the unfolding disclosure. The counsellor also needs to monitor how they, as listener, are managing their own feelings. The counsellor needs to be a safe container and if the container is full of their own unresolved issues related to power and abuse, then there will be little internal space in which to contain the client's story. Clients may think they want to 'tell all', but afterwards they may go away and feel they have told too much. The sense of overexposure may replicate the feelings related to the abuse and the client might feel angry with the counsellor.

As clients begin to tell their story, gradually a focus may emerge. The counsellor may usefully ask 'why now?' What has brought the client, at this point in his/her life, to ask for help? Budman and Gurman (1988) propose a useful model for clarifying this question for abuse survivors. Their I-D-E model asks:

- Is the client experiencing a problem in interpersonal relationships? (I)
- Is the client's problem developmental? (D)
- Is the client's problem existential in its nature? (E).

Adult survivors of childhood abuse may well have problems within all three of these aspects of their lives. A fourth question concerns 'symptomatic' presentation. The symptoms should have been explored for organic cause before referral to the counsellor:

- 'Is the client focusing on a somatic complaint, bodily symptoms or physical expressions of emotional disturbance such as psychosomatic disorders, abuse of alcohol, drugs, sex, etc.?'

Trauma model

It is this latter category of symptomatic presentation that I have chosen to focus on in this chapter. It was only in 1980 that post-traumatic stress disorder was officially classified in the American Psychiatric Association's (1980) manual *Diagnostic and Statistical Manual of Mental Disorders*, 3rd edn (DSM-III). What had previously been referred to as 'gross stress reactions' and 'transient situational disturbance' was reclassified as post-traumatic stress disorder, and 12 symptoms were listed providing diagnostic criteria for acute, chronic and delayed manifestations of this psychopatho-logical response to an extreme stressor. The updated version (DSM-IV) (American Psychiatric Association 1994) reflects an increasingly sophisticated understanding of the condition, particularly in relation to its occurrence as a normal part of the after-math of childhood physical and sexual abuse. It has been recognized that the condi-tion exists along a continuum and that not every child who has been abused experiences it; and that the effects of chronic abuse are not the same as a discrete one-off occurrence. Terr (1991) suggests a type I and a type II. The former is a discrete traumatic experience, whereas type II, reflecting prolonged, repeated trauma, includes denial, psychic numbing, self-hypnosis and dissociation, and alternating between extreme passivity and rage. In DSM-IV, additional manifestations such as survivor guilt, a narrowing of social interaction, a heightened sense of ineffectiveness, and impairment of affect regulation are listed (Friedrich 1995). Whitfield (1995) suggests that, although this is certainly an improvement in understanding on previous edi-tions, the emphasis on 'the physical integrity' of the person rather limits its usefulness for abuse survivors, although the document does go on to include disturbances that cause 'clinically significant distress or impairment on social, occupational or other important areas of functioning' (American Psychiatric Association 1994, item F).

People who have suffered the terror of physical torture and sexual abuse have been studied to enable neuroscientists to develop an understanding of the biological impact of *uncontrollable* stress on human beings. Goleman (1996) states that the operative word is 'uncontrollable':

> If people feel there is something they can do in a catastrophic situation, some control they can exert, no matter how minor, they fare far better emotionally than do those who feel utterly helpless. The element of helplessness is what makes a given event *subjectively* over-whelming. (p. 204)

Childhood abuse is a form of *chronic* trauma, in which the abuser overstimulates the child's bodily senses and emotions and the child may be overwhelmed. When this hap-pens it is likely that part of the child's development will be affected, delayed or arrested. Herman (1992) argues that 'repeated trauma in childhood forms and deforms the per-sonality' (p. 96). A child faced with an uncontrollable situation in which they are repeatedly beaten, sexually assaulted, terrified or humiliated has to adapt in order to survive. The child has to find a way of developing an ability to trust those who are untrustworthy, to find some degree of safety in an unsafe environment, to have a sense of control in an unpredictable situation and power where they are powerless.

One of the ways a child may cope is to develop an abnormal state of consciousness. Whilst in a state of dissociation, day-dreaming, fantasy or amnesia, the child produces symptoms—psychological, somatic and/or social—that both conceal and reveal, to those who are capable of reading those symptoms, truths about the child's life that they cannot manifest in other ways.

Young children depend, not only on their own ego capacities, but also on the auxil-lary capacities of their primary caregivers. However, when the abuser is a close family member the child loses any ability to depend on them too. Van der Kolk (1988) sees the loss of the 'secure base' normally provided by the parents as 'the earliest and possibly most damaging psychological trauma' (p. 32). The parents who fail to protect the child, as well as the abuser, are guilty of primary betrayal. Any attempt to reveal the abuse would threaten the entire family structure upon which the child depends for its survival; to a small child this represents a threat to his very existence. In his efforts to preserve any degree of ability to depend upon the parents for emotional and physical care, the child separates his ego into two parts. One part represents:

> ... business as usual, the daytime self, the part that responds to the parent's denial by imposing its own denial. No one speaks of the other, the nightime self. It exists only as part of a dreamlike state whose very existence assumes an air of vague unreality in the light of day' (Davies & Frawley 1994, p. 54).

The 'night-time' self refers to the part that becomes split off by dissociation. Because the child cannot speak of these experiences, no verbal link exists between the two dissociated aspects of the self. Without language to represent these experiences, there can be no communication between the separate experiences of self. However, the body speaks it own language, and that is often the way to begin to open up the communication.

Somatization

Brian Broom (1997) suggests that: 'The focus is on the person as a whole. ... The bodily symptoms are considered carefully, along with the 'story' of the whole person, and a working hypothesis is developed as to the meaning of the symptoms'. He goes on to advocate that the patient and the helper then go on a 'collaborative journey of discovery and healing' (p. 4). Broom cautions that the concept of 'symptom-as-language' must not be carried too far, and that a patient's symptoms need to be taken seriously and explored for organic cause prior to working psychologically.

Over the years I have met a variety of clients who present with physical symptoms when no organic cause has been found. I have sometimes found it very difficult to 'reach' them and at times have noticed myself feeling bored, angry, frustrated and deskilled in their presence. I now recognize these feelings as countertransference and, as such, they can help me to have a sense of the clients' experience of themselves. If I am able to notice my own feelings as the client tells his/her story and mirror them back to my clients, in time, they may begin to reconnect with their own feelings and begin to create a 'self-story' that includes dissociated aspects of past experiences.

In helping clients to reconstruct (or maybe construct) their life stories, I may need to provide them with a language of emotions—teach them to make connections between words like fear and the fluttering sensation in their stomach or bowels. I might notice red marks appear on their necks that might link with the word 'anger', or blushing that might link with the word 'shame'. However, it is important to *offer* these words tentatively and not to impose them, because our assumptions may not be correct. Eventually the client will find their own words to describe their very personal feelings. Clients sometimes struggle to recognize that descriptions such as 'let down', 'pissed off' or 'fed up' might represent anger; that 'rejected', 'isolated' or 'wobbly' might represent fear; that 'hurt', 'choked up' or 'heavy' might represent sadness; and that 'over the moon', 'on the up' or 'buzzing' might represent joy. These words indicate that they might be experiencing feelings in a bodily sense; if we can track back and back to find the emotion that connects with the felt sense, they might begin to integrate the unassimilated parts of their experience (Etherington 2000).

Gendlin (1978, 1996) taught his clients to tune into this 'felt sense' through a technique he called 'focusing', using a six step model. He asked clients to identify a word, image or phrase that was connected with the felt sense and to then ask questions of what arises. A client might identify the flutterings in his guts as fear, and might ask, 'What is it about this that makes me so fearful?' Further exploration may reveal understandings that bring physical and psychological changes by connecting them with knowledge stored within the body.

Narrative and attachment styles

If clients' stories are coherent and they are able to speak about the past in ways that acknowledge and link feelings, beliefs and events, this may indicate a 'secure attachment' (Bowlby 1969, 1973) in early life. 'Insecure attachment' may come over in the form of a narrative style that is dismissive of the past, or one that may reveal that the client has little memory of past events, or an idealized version of childhood without being able to provide examples of what it was that made it a 'wonderful childhood'. Others may tell their story in a manner that indicates 'insecure enmeshed narrative' (Holmes 1998), which are the equivalent in Bowlby's terms of 'ambivalent attachment' styles; these clients seem swamped by their pasts, rambling and incoherent as if the pain of the past was still alive in the present. Holmes refers to an 'unresolved' style of narrative, which may coexist with any of the other styles mentioned above, but refers to points in their life story where the flow of logic is interrupted or disjointed, perhaps indicating the emergence of repressed memories or a manifestation of dissociation. Marjorie Orr (1999), founder of the organization Accuracy About Abuse, writes 'Buried memories, if they exist, will surface of their own accord, given time and trust, though not always accurately or coherently' (p. 59). Premature diagnosis is not helpful, but the creation of a safe space for exploration of these memories as they emerge, without the therapist using intrusive techniques or reaching conclusions, will allow the gradual reintegration of those aspects of self that will, in time, enable the client's healing. For those interested in the debate about so-called 'false memories' I would highly recommend the excellent service provided by Accuracy About Abuse that provides comprehensive information and research evidence concerning the debate. A major contribution to the debate has been made by an article in the *Journal of Psychiatry and Law* (Brown *et al.* 1999).

Clients may bring only a symptom—an incomplete or incomprehensible story—and that might be the beginning of an opportunity to create a narrative that pieces together, almost like a jigsaw, the missing parts of their life that may help free them from the past.

Case example

Becky, a single and successful business woman, came to see me when she was 27. She told me that she found it impossible to eat in public places, thus creating difficulties in social and business aspects of her life. I noted that she talked of being 'fed up' with this and wanted to 'understand' what it was all about. We began to explore—I had no idea what it might be about but I asked her what actually happened when she tried to eat in public. She said she was unable to swallow anything and that she thought she might choke to death. I asked how long she had experienced this difficulty. She remembered it starting at the age of eight. I wondered out loud if she had she found anything 'hard to swallow' when she was eight years old. She dismissed this, saying that she had had a good childhood with lots of freedom and opportunities for play.

The following session she told me that when she was eight, she had been orally raped by a 15-year-old boy who was her brother's friend, and that this had continued until she was about 11. She remembered this clearly but felt it could not have any connection with her present feelings. That was all in the past.

As Becky's story unfolded it emerged that her mother had left her father (taking Becky with her) and set up home with her lover when Becky was 13. Becky began to stay out late, smoking and drinking, having sex with much older married men. Her mother was so wrapped up in her own life that she neglected to care for her daughter. Her father was not in the picture at all and had remarried.

Becky had clearly been traumatized; her sexual abuse had been uncontrollable and had terrified her at the time. She had coped with the threat of being overwhelmed by dissociating the emotional aspects of the experience. The terror of choking to death, the shame and disgust she felt, the fear of being 'found out' and the sense of betrayal (she believed her brother knew what his friend was doing to her) had been dissociated and unassimilated into her experience of self.

Her body and her behaviour (re-enacting the abuse in adulthood through promiscuous behaviour) carried her memories for her. Over time she was able to reclaim her feelings and beliefs about the events, change her thinking about her behaviour (which she judged negatively) and her view of herself (that *she* was shameful, disgusting and bad). Quite early on in the process she changed her promiscuous behaviour—however, letting go of her fear of true sexual and emotional intimacy, her mourning for her lost childhood innocence, her sexuality, her relationships with her family, went on for much longer.

I found the model of dissociation proposed by Braun (1988a, 1988b) helpful in working with Becky. The model is conceptualized along four dimensions of experience: behaviour, affect (emotion), sensation (body feeling) and knowledge (BASK). As I listened to her story I attempted to discover which of these aspects of experience were missing. For example, she described her oral rape very calmly; there was no emotion in her telling. Her body carried the sensation of choking. Her behaviour was both avoidant (not eating in public—thereby unconsciously avoiding possible restimulation of the unassimilated feelings) and a re-enactment of the abuse through further abusive relationships.

Becky did have knowledge (a memory) of what had happened. But knowledge is multistranded; we can know and not know about betrayal at the same time—it is part of the human condition (Freyd 1996). A survivor of childhood sexual abuse who does not 'know' or forgets about the abuse, may simultaneously have memory and knowledge of events that surface in other ways such as specific phobias, learned behaviours or self-perceptions of 'being bad'. Behavioural components may intrude upon a client's life and become frightening. Sometimes sensory and body clues (such as choking) occur without knowledge of the source and are referred to as 'body memories'. The task was to help Becky to connect up all aspects of her experience, making links between her past experiences and her present problems, so that she could freely make more conscious choices in her present life.

Recovery from trauma

Clients may present in very different ways. If they are suddenly and uncontrollably put into a situation where they have to face the memories of abuse, perhaps because another family member discloses (Etherington 2000), the client may react with symptoms of acute post-traumatic stress. This has been dealt with by Michael Wright in Chapter 14. If the trauma is of type ll (Terr 1991), they may present with denial, psychic numbing, dissociation, perhaps causing depression, a sense of alienation from 'self', interpersonal problems or somatic complaints (such as in Becky's case).

Herman (1992) suggests that memories can be transformed, both in emotional meaning and in the effects in the emotional brain. She sees the conditions necessary for healing being:

1 Enabling clients to regain a sense of safety by calming their fears (perhaps by giving information about post-traumatic stress disorder that explains they are not going mad). This may be particularly needed if the client is in an acute stage, suffering flashbacks or other perceptual disturbances.

2 Helping clients to regain some control over their lives (perhaps by teaching relaxation techniques); sometimes medication helps the client to find a 'window' of calm that allows them to regain some sense of security and control until such time as re-learning can occur.

3 Helping clients to re-tell their stories in the harbour of a safe relationship.

4 Enabling clients to mourn the losses created by the trauma.

Timing and pacing of these stories is crucial—if we go too quickly, the amygdala may flood the brain and clients may be retraumatized (Goleman 1996). However, clients generally seem to have the ability to go at the pace that suits them, and—providing we do not push them into facing memories before they are ready—they will reach a point of recovery in their own time. There may be periods when flashbacks and memories are frequent or even non-stop, followed by periods when none appear for months at a time.

The counsellor encourages the client to tell the story in as much detail as possible, including smells, tactile sensations, sounds, what they saw and heard, as well as their reactions of disgust, horror or nausea. The *entire* memory needs to be put into words or pictures in order to capture parts of the experiences that may be unassimilated.

Some trauma researchers speculate that in states of high arousal of the sympathetic nervous system, which would be the case during childhood abuse, the linguistic encoding of memory is deactivated, causing the central nervous system to revert to sensory forms of memory (Raine 1999). Sensory details bring the memories more under the control of the neocortex, the thinking brain, where the reactions can be made more understandable and therefore more manageable:

> ... [the neocortex] contains the centres that put together and comprehend what the senses perceive. It adds to a feeling what we think about it—and allows us to have feelings about ideas, art, symbols and imaginings (Goleman 1996, p. 11).

Connecting sensation, feeling and thinking allows the brain to re-learn that such events can be remembered without the extreme fear response that has held the client captive in the past.

Finally, clients need to mourn the losses created by the trauma. The client is helped to let go of the past and can begin to look to the future. Sometimes a few symptoms persist, as described by Becky—some things can still trigger off memories and feelings of being abused:

> When I take my car in for repair or an MOT—smelling the oil—seeing men with dirt under their fingernails—all that triggers my fear. My abuse took place in the garage and my abuser always had dirty fingernails. It sends a shudder through me.

However, they no longer have the same power to control the present for the client. Clients may still have the emotional responses, but they have a way of dealing with those emotions that was not available to them before. LeDoux (1996), the first neuro-scientist to discover the key role of the amygdala in the emotional brain, explained that when our emotional system learns something, it never lets us let go. In therapy we can learn to control it by training our neocortex how to inhibit our amygdala. This suppresses our propensity to act and the basic emotion remains in a less intense form.

So clients may not be able to decide *when* they have strong emotions, but they can have more control over *how* they respond to them, and how quickly they recover, which may be said to be a sign of emotional maturity.

Supervision

Working with this client group is potentially fraught with a variety of countertrans-ference responses. Counsellors may find themselves caught up in the conflicts between other members of the primary care team, particularly where clients/patients have been referred to specialist services in an attempt to treat the symptoms without treating the underlying cause. The potential for further harm to patients is noted by Judith Herman (1992):

> In institutional settings the problem of staff splitting or intense conflict over the treat-ment of difficult patients frequently arises. Almost always the subject of the dispute turns out to have a history of trauma. The quarrel among colleagues reflects the unwitting re-enactment of the dialectic of trauma. (p. 152)

Splitting can be avoided when all members of the team share a common under-standing of how it might occur. Counsellors can educate other members of the team about these issues without talking about individual clients or their work. However, there can be a good case made for contracting with the client that confidentiality will be held between the counsellor and the GP, when it might be in the client's best interest. We need to be clear about the purpose of confidentiality and not to follow blindly a set of rules and regulations. Confidentiality is about creating a safe space for our clients—a container for the work. The safety of the client might well be improved by allowing the GP into the space. Having another person involved might also ensure the safety of the counsellor, which in turn adds to the safety of the client. What is most important is that our contracting about confidentiality is negotiated and understood by all parties.

Listening to our patients/clients telling their stories of devastating physical and sexual abuse can leave us with feelings of helplessness, impotent rage and despair; we may be deeply challenged to hold on to a benign view of mankind in general. Clients need us to resist being sucked into the mire, to have our feet firmly planted on the edge of the bog as they struggle to find a foothold that will enable them to find their own way out. Frequent supervision is essential if we are to maintain clear boundaries, clarify our transference and countertransference responses and notice when our own material intrudes. We need a safe place to cry and scream when we are outraged, to admit our temptations to rescue or punish our clients—and a place in which our own psychological health can be maintained.

References

American Psychiatric Association (1980) *Diagnostic and Statistical Manual of Mental Disorders*, 3rd edn (DSM-III). American Psychiatric Association, Washington, DC.

American Psychiatric Association (1994) *Diagnostic and Statistical Manual of Mental Disorders*, 4th edn (DSM-IV). American Psychiatric Association, Washington, DC.

Arnold, R.P., Rogers, D. and Cook, D.A.G. (1990) Medical problems of adults who were sexually abused in childhood. *British Medical Journal*, **300**, 705–708.

Barkham, M., Rees, A., Shapiro, D. and Hardy, G.E. (1996) Dose-effect relations in time limited psychotherapy for depression. *Journal of Consulting and Clinical Psychology*, **64** (5), 927–935.

Bear, Z. (ed.) (1999) *Good Practice in Working with Adults Abused in Childhood*. Jessica Kingsley, London.

Bowlby, J. (1969) *Attachment and Loss: Vol. 1. Attachment*. Basic Books, New York.

Bowlby, J. (1973) *Attachment and Loss: Vol. 2. Separation*. Basic Books, New York.

Braun, B.G. (1988a) The BASK model of dissociation, Part 1. *Dissociation*, **1** (1): 4–23.

Braun, B.G. (1988b) The BASK model of dissociation, Part 2. Clinical applications. *Dissociation*, **1** (2): 16–23.

Broom, B. (1997) *Somatic Illness and the Patient's Other Story*. Free Association Books, London.

Brown, D., Scheflin, J.D. and Whitfield, M.D. (1999) Recovered memories: the current weight of the evidence in science and in the courts. *Journal of Psychiatry and Law*, **27**/Spring, 5–156.

Budman, S.H. and Gurman, A.S. (1988) *Theory and Practice of Brief Therapy*. Guilford Press, New York.

Courtois, C.A. (1993) Adult survivors of sexual abuse. *Primary Care*, **20** (2): 443–446.

Davies, J.M. and Frawley, M.G. (1994) *Treating the Adult Survivor of Childhood Sexual Abuse: a Psychoanalytical Perspective*. Basic Books, New York.

Dolan, Y. (1994) On the treatment of sexual abuse. In *Ericksonian Methods: the Essence of the Story* (Zeig, J.K., ed.). Brunner/Mazel, New York.

Elton-Wilson, J. (1996) *Time Conscious Psychological Therapy*. Routledge, London.

Etherington, K. (1995) *Adult Male Survivors of Childhood Sexual Abuse*. Pavilion Publishing, Brighton.

Etherington, K. (2000) *Narrative Approaches to Working with Male Survivors of Sexual Abuse; the Client's, the Counsellor's and the Researcher's Story*. Jessica Kingsley, London.

Felitti, V. (1998) Childhood trauma tied to adult illness. *American Journal of Preventative Medicine*, **14** (6), 245–258.

Frawley, M.G. (1988) The sexual lives of adult survivors of father–daughter incest. *Dissertation Abstracts International*, **49**. (University Microfilms No. 88-06, 457.)

Freyd, J.J. (1996) *Betrayal Trauma: the Logic of Forgetting Childhood Abuse*. Harvard University Press, London.

Friedrich, W.N. (1995) *Psychotherapy with Sexually Abused Boys: an Integrated Approach*. Sage, London.

Gendlin, E. (1978) *Focusing*. Everest House, New York.

Gendlin, E. (1996) *Focusing-oriented Psychotherapy. A Manual of the Experiential Method*. Guilford, New York.

Goleman, D. (1996) *Emotional Intelligence*. Bloomsbury Publishing, London.

Herman, J. (1992) *Trauma and Recovery*. Basic Books, New York.

Holley, C. (1999) Adults who've been abused: should there be training for all nurses? *Mental Health Bulletin*, **Autumn**, 6.

Holmes, J. (1998) Narrative in psychotherapy. In *Narrative Based Medicine* (Greenhalgh, T. and Hurwitz, B., eds). BMJ Books, London, pp. 176–184.

Hooper, P.D. (1990) Psychological sequelae of sexual abuse in childhood. *British Journal of General Practice*, **40**, 29–31.

Hudson-Allez, G. (1997) *Time-Limited Therapy in a General Practice Setting*. Sage, London.

Hunter, M. (1995) *Adult Survivors of Sexual Abuse: Treatment Innovations*. Sage, London.

LeDoux, J. (1996) *The Emotional Brain*. Simon & Schuster, New York.

Mearns, D. (1998) Managing a primary care service. *Counselling in Medical Settings Journal*, **57**, 1–5.

Mollon, P. (1998) *Remembering Trauma: a Psychotherapist Guide to Memory and Illusion*. Wiley, New York.

O'Hara, M. (1992) Domestic violence and child abuse—making the links. *Childright*, **88**, 4–5.

Orr, M. (1999) Believing patients. In *Controversies in Psychotherapy and Counselling* (Feltham, C., ed.). Sage, London, pp. 53–63.

Pizzey, E. (1974) *Scream Quietly or the Neighbours Will Hear*. Penguin Books, Harmondsworth.

Raine, N.V. (1999) *After Silence: Rape and My Journey Back*. Virago, London.

Read, J. (1997) Child abuse and psychosis: a literature review and implications for professional practice. *Professional Psychology: Research and Practice*, **28** (1), 448–456.

Read, J. (1998) Child abuse and severity of disturbance among adult psychiatric inpatients. *Child Abuse and Neglect*, **22** (5), 359–368.

Sanderson, C. (1995) *Counselling Adult Survivors of Child Sexual Abuse*. Jessica Kingsley, London.

Santi-Ireson, S. (1996) *The Silent Scream*. Prize winning unpublished essay, University of Bristol, Bristol.

Sgroi, S.M. and Bunk, B.S. (1988) A clinical approach to adult survivors of child sexual abuse. In *Vulnerable Populations*, Vol. 1 (Sgroi, S., ed.). Lexington Books, Lexington, pp. 137–186.

Smith, D., Pearce, L., Pringle, M. and Caplan, R. (1995) Adults with a history of child sexual abuse: an evaluation of a pilot therapy service. *British Medical Journal*, **310**, 1175–1178.

Terr, L.C. (1991) Childhood traumas: an outline and overview. *American Journal of Psychiatry*, **148** (1), 10–20.

Van der Kolk, B.A. (1988) The trauma spectrum: the interaction of biological and social events in the genesis of the trauma response. *Journal of Traumatic Stress*, **1** (5), 273–290.

Weller, C. (1999) Has time-limited counselling had its day? *Counselling in Medical Settings Journal*, **61**, 4–8.

Whitfield, C.L. (1995) *Memory and Abuse: Remembering and Healing the Effects of Trauma*. Health Communications Inc., Deerfield Beach, FL.

Chapter 16

Sexual problems

Glyn Hudson-Allez

Introduction

In primary care, patients are presenting daily with a sexual dysfunction that they feel is affecting their relationship and their lives (Duffy 1999). Although some of these dysfunctions may have a physical aetiology, there is an inevitable psychogenic component to them also. It is, therefore, just as important for the counsellor to understand some of the physical implications and interventions of psychosexual therapy, as it is for the GP to understand the psychological consequences (Hudson-Allez 1998). Yet counselling training may not address the specifics of sexual dysfunction. Similarly, medical schools do not routinely include courses on sexual behaviour, and even sexual anatomy is considered a difficult subject to teach medical students with live patients (Leiblum 1999). So GPs are not specifically trained for dealing with sexual dysfunction, and many are not interested or are too embarrassed to do so. Maurice (1999) contends, however, that professionals who bypass sex-related questions may be considered negligent or even unethical. It is, therefore, important that GPs and counsellors in primary care have a clear understanding of the issues involved to help couples and individuals deal with the problems presented. Although a referral to a specialist who has trained in psychosexual therapy or medicine would be ideal, and may be necessary for more entrenched problems, this chapter aims to overview some of the general principles that will help the primary health care team to help their clients. In particular it will discuss both the physical and psychological interventions for the more common male dysfunctions of erectile insufficiency, premature ejaculation and retarded ejaculation, and the female dysfunctions of dyspareunia, vaginismus and anorgasmia. It will end with an overview of how both men and women lose their sexual desire.

Erectile insufficiency

Erectile insufficiency is the inability to obtain an erection sufficient for sexual penetration on more than 25% of opportunities, and total erectile failure is where a man gets no penile engorgement at all. The incidence is about 10% of all men, and 30–40% of men over 80 years old (Holmes *et al.* 1997). The reasons for erectile problems may be due to physical problems, like vascular disease or diabetes, iatrogenic causes from prescribed medication, or psychological problems like performance anxiety. It used to be considered that up to 90% of erectile failure had a psychogenic causation (Brindley 1996). Now it is thought that between 75% and 90% of all erectile problems are organic (Brindley 1996; Costa *et al.* 1997), and that pure psychological difficulties only account for the remainder. It is essential, therefore, that the client has a medical check up to determine the cause, usually by taking blood tests to monitor prolactin, testosterone and glucose levels. A medical examination may reveal signs of hormonal difficulties like testicular atrophy, sparse body hair or signs of thyroid abnormality. Weak pulses in the legs or ankles, or an unusually cold penis or lower legs may indicate vascular problems, or weak or absent genital reflexes may indicate neurological factors. However, the loss of an erection inevitably leads the client to have feelings of inadequacy and failure. So, even if the cause is primarily physical, the man may well need help to work through with a counsellor how he feels about his loss.

In assessment, the GP or the counsellor needs to question the client carefully about what happens when he loses his erection. Can he get an erection at any time or does he only lose it under certain circumstances? When he first started to lose his erection, did it have a gradual or sudden onset? Can he achieve a partial erection or is it always flaccid? Does he have spontaneous nocturnal or morning erections? What happens when he masturbates? Are there any abnormalities in the shape of his penis, or does he experience any pain in the foreskin area or upon ejaculation? If the client does report an irregular shape to his penis, it is most likely to be Peyronie's disease. This is where plaque builds up on the side of the penis shaft and pulls it out of shape. This can be rectified by surgical procedures, but it usually has a consequence of shortening the penis. If the client reports that he has no spontaneous erections, that the onset was gradual and he cannot achieve an erection to masturbate, then one is probably looking at a physical cause. If the man does have morning erections, has intermittent erectile failure with sudden onset, then the cause is more likely to be psychological. But it is important to acknowledge that, in many cases, it is probably a combination of the two.

When the counsellor is working with a man with psychogenic erectile failure that is primary, that is he has never experienced an erection, then they need to examine issues around sexual trauma, fear of penetration or sexual orientation. If the erectile failure is secondary, and occurs following prior successful sexual encounters, then the counsellor needs to look at issues around inadequacy and loss. Also, for men who are depressed or highly stressed, the loss of libido is often the first presenting symptom and the hardest to regain. Guidance on relaxation is a valuable process that the counsellor can offer. Often when a man is worried about losing his erection, he will tense his muscles to prevent that happening. That tension will make the penis go flaccid, so what he needs to do is relax. Also discourage the use of substances like tobacco, alcohol and drugs, all of which have a long-term effect on erectile tissue.

There have been several new medical developments* in the treatment of erectile insufficiency in recent years:

♦ Oral medications: Viagra™, Yohimbine™

♦ Penile injections: Caverject™, Viridal™ and Invicorp™

* GPs are no longer able to prescribe these medical interventions to patients presenting with psychogenic erectile insufficiency on the NHS. However, GPs are able to give these patients a private prescription without charge.

+ Transurethral: manual urethral system for erection (MUSE)
+ Vacuum pumps
+ Prostheses.

Viagra was not the first oral preparation to be offered to men with erectile insufficiency. Yohimbine, made from the bark of the yohimbe tree, was already a well-
established preparation, but only effective in about 33% of cases (Sonda 1990).
Viagra, on the other hand, is effective in 80% of cases (Gingell *et al.* 1996) so it is the
oral medication of choice. However, Viagra is contraindicated for all clients who take
nitroglycerine or organic nitrates for heart defects. There was an initial concern that
Viagra would increase the incidence of rapes, but actually this preparation does not
increase sexual desire at all. Indeed it cannot work without a man having the sexual
desire in the first place. The advantage of oral methods is that a tablet can be taken an
hour before sexual intercourse is desired, and then natural arousal will do the rest.
The disadvantage is that intercourse still has to be planned in advance.

Penile injections are still the most common method of help prescribed by GPs and
urologists at the present time. A small needle injected by the client into the shaft of his
penis sends a dose of prostaglandin directly into the corpus cavernosum, the two
spongy tubes that expand when engorged with blood flow. This drug will allow the
client to have an erection within 10 minutes of injection. The advantage of this
method is that the drug is localized to the penile area, rather than being in the whole
system. The disadvantages are that many men have a fear of placing a needle in their
penis (understandably) and a side effect of priapism may occur. This is when an
engorged penis fails to turn flaccid after intercourse. It is extremely painful and can
cause irreparable damage to the penile tissue if not dealt with within eight hours.

Prostaglandin is also the drug used in MUSE, which is compacted into a pellet and
inserted into the urethral tube by means of an applicator. Erection takes longer with
this method, maybe 20 to 30 minutes, and requires the user to walk around for a while
after application to help the pellet to dissolve and to enhance the blood flow. This
inevitably interferes with any foreplay. It is not so effective as penile injections, but has
the advantage of not causing any trauma to the penile area.

Vacuum pumps have been available for a long time. These consist of a tube placed
over the penis with a pump at one end that allows the blood to be drawn into the penis
as the vacuum is created. When the enlargement reaches the required size, the blood is
held in place by means of a tight rubber ring at the base of the penis. It has the advantage of being a very localized intervention, and is just a one-off cost, but the erection
only occurs from the rubber ring so the enlarged penis has an unnatural swing to it.

Penile prostheses are considered the final solution for a man with permanent erectile failure. There are two types. One comprises two malleable rods inserted through
the corpus cavernosum, which give a permanent erection. A more expensive version
has a pump inserted into the testicle, which allows the man to pump up, and later
pump down, his penis. Once prostheses are inserted, they tend to cause irreparable
damage to the penile tissue if later removed.

As medical advances can now offer this wide range of interventions for men
suffering with erectile insufficiency, clinical experience has indicated a tendency
amongst urologists to disregard the psychological perspective of erectile dysfunction

(Hudson-Allez 1998). So long as the penis can be made erect sufficient for sexual inter-course to take place, then they feel their job is done. However, clients have confided that they have still had difficulty in translating their newly acquired erectile capabilities into successful sexual intercourse. This is predominantly because the partner is often not included in the medical consultations with the man. The feelings of the partner have not been considered when discussing the appropriate medical intervention. So the partner, who hitherto used to monitor the erection as a signal of his or her own attractiveness to the client, is now presented with the *fait accompli* of an artificially induced erection. And, as has already been discussed, many of these methods interfere with the spontaneity of the foreplay when making love. So there is a lot that a GP and counsellor in primary care can do, with sufficient knowledge of the medical techniques described, to help couples discuss how they can use the medical interventions to make their love-making more natural and spontaneous. GPs, especially, can ensure that even though they may have referred their patients to a urology department for physical investigations, that the couple receive the appropriate psychological help and support by ensuring that they have on-going counselling throughout the treatment.

It should also be mentioned that even if the cause of the erectile failure is purely psychogenic, thus warranting referral to the counsellor or psychosexual therapist, that does not mean that medical interventions should not be used. A short course of oral sildenafil or intracavernosal prostaglandin can give a man with repetitive perform-ance failure the confidence boost that he needs so that he can stop penis watching, relax and enjoy what he is doing.

Early ejaculation

One of the reasons that some men start experiencing erectile insufficiency is that they have had a prior problem of premature ejaculation. This is defined as ejaculating without sufficient erection for intercourse, or prior to, or within 15 seconds of, pene-tration (ICD-10/DCR-10 1994), with a prevalence rate of 29% (Laumann *et al.* 1994). However, some argue that early, or premature, ejaculation is any emission occurring before both partners wish it (Stephan & Richards 1982), even if it is longer than half an hour (Mohanty 1997). Premature ejaculation has been associated with trauma to the sympathetic nervous system, pelvic fracture, urethritis, prostatitis and neurologi-cal diseases like multiple sclerosis (Maurice 1999). GPs should therefore conduct a thorough medical examination as well as referring to the counsellor.

Some men will endure years of experiencing this problem without seeking help, but as they become more frustrated with their own performance, it eventually starts sap-ping away self-esteem and feelings of adequacy. It can be equally frustrating for the partner, of course, as the sexual act is over virtually as soon as it has begun. Plus, the older a man becomes, the longer his period of resolution before he can resume inter-course. Thus some men who have used the strategy of masturbation prior to penetra-tion in the hope that this will allow them to last longer have found that this, too, becomes ineffective.

Adequate assessment of this is very important, as some men who cannot last for as long as they would like (using Mohanty's example of half an hour), or for as long as it takes their partner to orgasm, may present with premature ejaculation. As Kaplan (1989) points out, around 75% of women do not experience orgasm with vaginal penetration without clitoral stimulation, so it may be that the situation is being mis-interpreted. The average man will ejaculate within two minutes of penetration (Kinsey *et al.* 1949). So it is helpful to get the man to be precise about time delay and number of thrusts between vaginal penetration and ejaculation. It is also useful to know whether there is any residue of guilt from masturbation, which causes a conflict between the normal sexual drive and the desire to get it over with quickly. Does he have any fears or worries concerning penetration? Are there any times when it is worse than others, for example when he is tired or has been drinking alcohol? And is there any association of pain with ejaculation or tightness of the foreskin?

As anxiety is known to aggravate the problem of early emission (Bancroft 1995), a personality type emerges that can be related to this sexual dysfunction, indicating the psychological component of the complaint. These men are often anxious, impetuous people who are always in a hurry and often never satisfied. Thus, counselling men experiencing premature ejaculation involves encouraging them to slow down and relax more. However, they may be impatient with the therapy and look for quick fixes. The counsellor may explore issues of guilt over sexual activity, especially related back to adolescence and religious education. The client may have built intellectual defences that detach him from sexual pleasure (Athanasiadis 1998). Masturbatory exercises where he brings himself to the point of inevitability, i.e. the moment prior to ejaculation, and then stops and allows the desire to subside, will help him build up ejaculatory control.

It has also been found that specific serotonin re-uptake inhibitors, like Seroxat™, have the side effect of slowing down ejaculation, so if the masturbatory exercises do not work then his performance anxiety can be reduced by low doses of this medication taken two to six hours before intercourse.

Retarded ejaculation

Retarded ejaculation occurs when the man is unable to ejaculate at all, so there are no feelings of climax or natural ending to the sexual act. Sometimes men will complain that ejaculation never occurs during penetration, but can occur during vigorous masturbation, others do not ejaculate at all.

Assessment will require the GP or the counsellor to determine whether the man actually experiences a sensation of orgasm in conjunction with the ejaculation. If he has the orgasm but no ejaculate, then it is more likely to be retrograde ejaculation where the ejaculate is passing through the sphincter at the bladder neck into the bladder. This can be a side effect of some medication, as most drugs used for the treatment of depression or obsessive compulsive disorder are associated with ejaculatory or orgasmic difficulties (Segraves 1995). If he does not experience orgasm yet does ejaculate, then it is ejaculatory anorgasmia. The determination that it is retarded ejaculation is that there is no ejaculation and no orgasm, even when fully aroused. However, some men will present when this occurs only when they are with their partners, but they are able to experience orgasmic ejaculation during private masturbation (or with a different partner). In these circumstances, then the origin will be psychogenic.

It has been argued that sometimes men fail to ejaculate in front of their partners because they are angry with them, and it is a subconscious withholding (Kaplan 1987). So counsellors may need to help them examine their feelings about their partner, and determine whether there are underlying problems, particularly of power, in the relationship. However, Apfelbaum (1989) argues against this proposal, suggesting the opposite. He contends that these men are unable to ejaculate because they cannot stop giving, and are unable to be selfish and have an orgasm just to please themselves. They therefore develop resentment from their compulsion to please their partner and thus sexually sabotage themselves.

Counselling a man with retarded ejaculation can be quite difficult. He does not want to give you anything, mirroring not wanting to give his partner anything. He may also fear losing control, so tends to hold himself back in the counselling session. Such men also tend to be constant spectators, watching their performance, which can increase the incidence of performance anxiety. It would also be useful to determine whether the man has any specific issues about 'sex and mess', as some men can be quite phobic about their own semen. The counsellor could also recommend reading for the client as homework. Zilbergeld (1977) in his book helps men to explore the myths about masculine sexuality and suggests tasks to help men with their own sexual dysfunctions.

Dyspareunia

Dyspareunia is painful intercourse. A few men experience dyspareunia, usually for physiological reasons. It may be due to painful retraction of the foreskin or small tears in the frenum as a result of vigorous intercourse or masturbation. Lesions or inflammation of the penis from herpetic infections will cause pain, as will hypersensitivity of the glans penis following ejaculation. Or it may be due to deformities of the penis, as in Peyronie's disease or hypospadias (incomplete development of the penis).

However, as the majority of presentations of dyspareunia are from women, this section will move on to the more common problem of vaginal discomfort during intercourse. The reasons for painful sex may be an interaction between the physical and the psychological. The pain may be caused by vestibulitis, polyps inside the vaginal wall, infections like herpes, chemicals like soaps and deodorizers, scar tissue from an episiotomy following childbirth, or even overzealous personal hygiene (Graziottin 1998). Or it may be vaginal atrophy typically found in postmenopausal women that is causing the pain. Before referral to the counsellor, the GP needs to ensure the physical possibilities have been thoroughly excluded. However, physical problems themselves can produce a fear of penetration, fear of pregnancy or be reminiscent of a history of sexual trauma. So the GP or the counsellor needs to question the patient carefully about the pain. Is it at the vaginal entrance or deep inside the vagina? Is it a sharp sting or a dull ache? Is there pain on passing water? Does the pain only occur during intercourse or does it persist? Such questions will help to determine the true nature and extent of the problem.

The counsellor also needs to investigate whether the pain serves the function of preventing intercourse for some reason. What else is painful in the woman's life?

Sometimes previous painful experiences are manifested by vaginal pain. Is there a fear following traumatic childbirth or rape? Is she ambivalent about expressing herself as a sexual person in view of previously conditioned messages or moral or religious teaching? Or maybe her partner fails to give her enough time in foreplay, so she is just not aroused and has not lubricated sufficiently for penetration. Maybe she just does not fancy her partner any longer, and is unable to say so. Goldsmith (1995) offers a comprehensive review of painful sex, which a woman could read to evaluate her own situation.

Vaginismus

Women who experience dyspareunia over a long period may develop vaginismus, which occurs when the pelvic muscles contract, preventing penetration. It is an involuntary spasm of the muscles in the lower third of the vaginal barrel, produced when genital approaches are made with a penis, finger, tampons or speculum. As the muscle spasm is not under conscious control, relaxation techniques alone will not improve it. Pain will occur if the partner persists in penetrating the contracted muscle. Often one of the triggers to women to seek help for this problem is the inability to conceive.

During assessment the counsellor should determine whether the response is consistent across all vaginal approaches. Does it happen if she inserts her own finger or a tampon? Does it occur with just one partner and not another? Does she experience it with medical vaginal examinations, and does it occur whether the doctor or nurse is a man or a woman? GPs need to be mindful of this if wishing to conduct a physical examination and question the patient carefully before doing so. If the problem originally occurred as a result of trauma during medical examination or treatment, it may be more appropriate to refer direct to the counsellor. These questions will help determine whether the problem is global or situation-specific. The counsellor needs to look for the psychological triggers that started the problem. For example, is there a fantasy that the vagina is too small? It is important to check on the dynamics between the woman and her partner. Very often it is the very nice, understanding, modern, unassertive partner that can become part of a colluding problem in vaginismus situations.

Ng (1999) has recently argued that therapists have taken too much account of the physical muscular response in this dysfunction, and ignored the fact that it is essentially a psychological difficulty. As the aim of therapy is to extinguish what is essentially a conditioned response, a cognitive behavioural approach is going to be the most appropriate method of treatment. The counsellor can review the fearful cognitions with regard to fear of penetration, or debrief past trauma. The behavioural approach of sensitizing the woman to graded insertions of fingers or vaginal trainers alongside relaxation techniques are essential to the successful outcome.

Anorgasmia

Years ago, British women were not expected to enjoy their sexuality, and if they did they were considered 'loose' or 'immoral'. There is still a considerable proportion of the Victorian legacy passed down from mother to daughter, or religious prohibitions, that inhibit some women from experiencing an orgasm today (Heiman & LoPiccolo 1988). However, modern magazine articles labour the point of clitoral versus vaginal orgasms and finding the 'G spot', whilst the television and movie media emphasize multiple orgasmic situations during rampant sex. No wonder many women become very confused and wonder what they must be missing as it is not like that for them.

As two-thirds of woman fail to achieve an orgasm during sexual penetration (Hite 1976), it is important to determine whether a woman presenting with anorgasmia is actually experiencing a personal difficulty, as opposed to a difficulty in the sexual repertoire of the partnership, that does not allow her to achieve orgasm. Equally she needs to take responsibility for her own orgasm rather than just expecting her partner to achieve it for her. So the counsellor needs to check out whether she gets aroused, and if so how much. Does she ever feel on the point of orgasm? Can she have an orgasm in any circumstances, for example during masturbation or oral sex? Check whether she is on medication, as some specific serotonin re-uptake inhibitors are known to inhibit orgasm. And, again, check whether there is a history of sexual abuse. A woman who had an orgasm as a child during an abusive situation may find herself anorgasmic as an adult in an unconscious desire to keep sex safe.

If the woman does get into a situation of high arousal, but is never quite able to tip over the edge into an orgasm, it would be useful for the counsellor to examine any fears she may have of letting go or being out of control. What does she imagine an orgasm would be like, and what fears or fantasies does that produce for her? Does she fear urinating during orgasm? How does she feel about her own sexuality? Are there any inhibiting messages from others who would prefer if she were not too overtly sexual? It is interesting, as mentioned in the section on erectile insufficiency, that there are numerous medical interventions that help men recapture their sexuality when it fails, but there is a reluctance to do the same for women. Even in the wake of Viagra where some women have found it extremely advantageous in enhancing their sexuality, there seems to be a cultural fear of allowing women total free reign in experiencing their bodies. However, the counsellor can encourage a woman to do so by suggesting she tries sensual bathing, exploring herself with mirrors, arousing herself with aromatherapy smells and erotic literature or videos, and masturbating with a vibrator. Kegel, or pelvic floor, exercises increase the blood flow to the genital area and thus increase its sensitivity. Heiman and LoPiccolo (1988) offer a really good manual for women to work through to develop their sexuality.

Loss of sexual desire

Reduced or absent sexual desire is the most frequent complaint amongst women presenting with sexual dysfunction. An increasing number of men are also able to distinguish between the loss of desire and erectile failure. It is considered that 33% of women and 16% of men report sexual disinterest (Frank *et al.* 1978), whereas Kaplan (1995) reports 38% of their sample met the criteria for sexual desire disorders. For women, especially, they seem to have a switch that they turn off when sexual desire seems inappropriate, for example within uncertain or insecure relationships, when caring for very young children or during emotional changes. Unfortunately, the desire is not so readily switched on again, and it has proved very difficult to help and generally has a poor long-term outcome.

If a couple present with one partner seen as the 'problem', having 'gone off sex', then it is wise to have some individual sessions where the counsellor can check more closely what is really going on. Is it that the person has gone off sex, or just gone off sex with this person? Are there any other symptoms like loss of energy or depression? Check out if there is a lot of stress around for that person. Have they gone off sex, or are they just too tired? Do they indulge in any intrapersonal sexual activity, like fantasizing, masturbating or nocturnal orgasm?

Kaplan (1995) described various levels of sexual arousal ranging from hypoactive (no drive), normal low, average, normal high and hyperactive 'sex addiction'. These levels are extremely important in the assessment of loss of sexual desire because if one partner has a normal high level, and the other has a normal low level, then the problem is merely one of a discrepancy between the two partners, and not a sexual dysfunction *per se*. In these situations one may find that one partner is constantly asking for (or even demanding) sex, and then feeling rejected when the other refuses. The refuser also feels under considerable pressure to 'perform' when he or she does not feel inclined, and tends to stop other forms of intimacy in case it leads to sex. This can lead to feelings of anger and resentment in the partnership. As such the counsellor needs to help with not only increasing the drive of the low partner, but also reducing the drive of the high partner. Sexual timetables (Crowe & Ridley 1986) work extremely well in these situations. Certain days of the week are timetabled for sexual activity. For the rest of the time, it is banned. This allows the partner with high desire to feel comfortable knowing it will occur on a certain day, and takes the pressure of the other partner in not having to refuse all the time, and allows intimacy to return.

Treating sexual dysfunction in the primary health care team

Sexual dysfunction is an interaction between the physical and psychological. Thus this chapter advocates that rather than having either a GP or a counsellor working with the patients/clients, the preferred method of help for couples experiencing sexual difficulties is when the GP and the counsellor work in unison as part of the primary health team. As some GPs may be reluctant to get involved in psychosexual treatments, it may be as well for the counsellor working in a GP partnership to find a GP who would be willing to work alongside the counsellor as the practice specialist in sexual problems. This allows other GPs to refer within their own practice, and the counsellor and specialist GP could work in parallel. Both the GP and the counsellor need to be open about initiating discussion about sexual behaviour. Clear questioning and giving clients appropriate words to use when discussing the genitals, helps relieve the pressure and provide for a more accurate assessment of the presenting situation. A non-judgemental attitude is essential, especially if the patient is presenting with sexually transmitted disease. Maurice (1999) offers an excellent text to highlight the appropriate physiological and psychological assessment questions. Both the GP and the counsellor need to familiarize themselves with aids for sexual enhancement, both medical interventions and sexual toys, because when the patient's confidence in the therapy grows, he or she will ask about them, as they will ask for factual information about the biology of sex.

If the sexual dysfunction is so entrenched that after, say, six counselling sessions there has been no movement forward, then a referral to a specialist in psychosexual therapy or psychosexual medicine will be appropriate. Specialist services vary from region to region, but can usually be found either based within, or attached to, urology departments or departments for genital and urinary medicine. Failing that, the private sector is another option, and the British Association for Sexual and Relationship Therapists can provide details of qualified therapists within the area. However, the majority of work can be conducted in primary care. Thus with a GP–counsellor team helping with sexual dysfunction, the patient can be assured of getting a much more holistic approach to their care in safe and familiar surroundings.

References

Apfelbaum, B. (1989) Retarded ejaculation. In *Principle and Practice of Sex Therapy. Update for the 1990s*, 2nd edn (Leiblum, S.R. and Rosen, R.C., eds). Guilford Press, New York, pp. 168–206.

Athanasiadis, L. (1998) Premature ejaculation: is it a biogenic or psychogenic disorder? *Sexual and Marital Therapy*, 13 (3), 241–255.

Bancroft, J. (1995) *Human Sexuality and its Problems*. Churchill Livingstone, New York.

Brindley, G.S. (1996) Intrapenile drug delivery systems. *International Journal of STD and AIDS*, 7 (Suppl. 3), 13–15.

Costa, P., Jaccovella, J. and Bouvet, A. (1997) Efficacy and tolerability of moxisylyte and placebo injected intracavernovously in patients with erectile dysfunction (ED): a multicentre double-blind study. Paper presented at the British Erectile Disorder Society Annual Conference, Stratford on Avon.

Crowe, M. and Ridley, J. (1986) The negotiated timetable: a new approach to marital conflicts involving male demands and female reluctance for sex. *Sexual and Marital Therapy*, 1 (2), 157–173.

Duffy, F.D. (1999) Foreword. In *Sexual Medicine in Primary Care* (Maurice, W.L.). Mosby, St Louis, p. ix–x.

Frank, E., Anderson, C. and Rubenstein, D. (1978) Frequency of sexual dysfunction in normal couples. *New England Journal of Medicine*, 299, 111–115.

Gingell, C., Jardin, A., Giuliano, F.A. *et al.* (1996) The efficacy of sildenafil (Viagra), a new oral treatment for erectile dysfunction, demonstrated by four different methods in a double-blind placebo-controlled, multinational clinic trial (Abstract). *European Urologist*, 30 (Suppl. 2), 353.

Goldsmith, M. (1995) *Painful sex. A Guide to Causes, Treatments and Prevention*. Harper Collins, London.

Graziottin, A. (1998) Organic and psychological factors in vulval pain: implications for management. *Sexual and Marital Therapy*, 13 (3), 328–338.

Heiman, J.R. and LoPiccolo, J. (1988) *Becoming Orgasmic. A Sexual and Personal Growth Programme for Women*, 2nd edn. Prentice Hall, London.

Hite, S. (1976) *The Hite Report: a Nationwide Study on Female Sexuality*. Macmillan, New York.

Holmes, S., Kirby, R. and Carson, C. (1997) *Male Erectile Dysfunction*. Health Press, Oxford.

Hudson-Allez, G. (1998) The interface between psychogenic and organic difficulties in men with erectile dysfunction. *Sexual and Marital Therapy*, 13 (3), 285–293.

ICD-10/DCR-10 (1994) *Pocket Guide to the ICD-10 Classification of Mental and Behavioural Disorders with Glossary and Diagnostic Criteria for Research*. Churchill Livingstone, Edinburgh.

Kaplan, H.S. (1987) *The Illustrated Manual of Sex Therapy*, 2nd edn. Bruner/Mazel, New York.

Kaplan, H.S. (1989) *How to Overcome Premature Ejaculation*. Bruner/Mazel, New York.

Kaplan, H.S. (1995) *The Sexual Desire Disorders*. Brunner/Mazel, New York.

Kinsey, A.C., Pomeroy, W.B. and Martin, C.E. (1949) *Sexual Behaviour in the Human Male*. W.B. Saunders, Philadelphia.

Laumann, E.O., Gagnon, J.H., Michael, R.T. and Michaels, S. (1994) *The Social Organisation of Sexuality: Sexual Practices in the United States*. University of Chicago Press, Chicago.

Leiblum, S.R. (1999) Foreword. In *Sexual Medicine in Primary Care* (Maurice, W.L.). Mosby, St Louis, pp. vii–viii.

Maurice, W.L. (1999) *Sexual Medicine in Primary Care*. Mosby, St Louis.

Mohanty, K.C. (1997) *Sexual Behaviour and Sexual Dysfunctions in Men*. KCM Academic Publications, Shipley.

Ng, M.-L. (1999) Vaginismus—a disease, symptom or culture-bound syndrome? *Sexual and Marital Therapy*, 14 (1), 9–13.

Segraves, R.T. (1995) Antidepressant-induced orgasm disorder. *Journal of Sex and Marital Therapy*, 21, 192–201.

Sonda, L.P. (1990) The role of yohimbine for the treatment of erectile impotence. *Journal of Sex and Marital Therapy*, 16, 15–21.

Stephan, P. and Richards, D. (1982) *Sexual Rejuvenation*. Frederick Muller, London.

Zilbergeld, B. (1977) *Men and Sex. A Guide to Sexual Fulfilment*. Harper Collins, London.

Chapter 17

Fertility

Sue Jennings

O wind of Tizoula, O wind of Amsoud!
Blow over the plains and over the sea,
Cary, O, carry my thoughts
To him who is so far, so far,
And who has left me without a little child.
O wind! remind him that I have no child.

O wind of Tizoula, O wind of Amsoud!
Blow away that desire for riches
That sends our young men away
And makes them forget the girls they've married,
Their mothers, and the old ones left in the village.
O wind! remind him that I have no child.

    (Berber woman's song, Ancient)

Introduction

This chapter addresses the concerns of those people who are experiencing difficulty in conceiving and the type of counselling that could be useful for the GP and the primary health care team (PHCT) to provide. Attention is also directed at those wishing to limit their fertility, and issues around teenage pregnancy. However, since subfertility affects some one in seven of the general population, I intend to devote more attention to this area.

It is a matter of individual choice whether GPs and the PHCT choose to offer the specialist advice and preliminary counselling themselves, or to use a counsellor attached to the practice. In either case there is a need for medical knowledge of recent advancements in subfertility treatments (Lee 1996; Furse 1997; Human Fertilisation and Embryology Authority 1999a, 1999c), an awareness of the complex legislation (Human Fertilisation and Embryology Authority 1998) and specialist skills in fertility counselling itself (Human Fertilisation and Embryology Authority 1998). Although fertility counselling provision must be available by law in licensed centres for fertility treatments (Human Fertilisation and Embryology Authority 1998), it is my conviction that the PHCT is in an important position to offer a considerable amount of counselling (Burnard 1989), information and advice, before decisions to refer patients are made.

Introduction to fertility counselling

The Berber woman's song at the beginning of this chapter illustrates very poignantly the deep-rooted desire and longing experienced by most people to produce their own children. In my work over many years as a fertility counsellor, I have witnessed both the very strong grief experienced by men and women if they are unable to realize their wish for children, a grief which until recently was ignored by most professionals (Jennings 1989; Penn 1985; Furse 1997), and the overwhelming confusion when that grief is discharged and the longed for infant becomes a reality. Because there is now the possibility of 'high-tech' treatment for fertility problems (what might be termed the 'reproduction revolution'), public awareness has been heightened and the demand for possible treatment has accelerated. Many people are seeking advice from their GPs at an earlier stage (some even inappropriately early), and indeed have become more knowledgeable about potential treatment on the one hand, while increasing their worry about reproductive failure on the other. I refer throughout to 'fertility' counselling rather than 'infertility' counselling; the latter already casts a sense of gloom and depression over the situation. At the London Hospital Medical College we have found that patients respond more optimistically with this change in language. Fertility counselling needs to address the uncertainty and stress of possible childlessness, as well as being able to consider the possible outcomes of treatment and their implications, particularly where there is the use of donated gametes.

There may, in some cases, be a need for more extensive therapeutic counselling or psychotherapy, when referral to another agency is more appropriate. Fertility counselling is a new specialism within counselling rather than being a discipline in its own right. I think there is a case to be argued for more development of 'counselling within reproductive medicine'—this would include fertility, psychosexual issues, hysterectomy, abortion, neonatal death and multiple miscarriages (Jennings 1994).

The central role of the primary health care team in counselling fertility problems

As someone who works at the secondary and tertiary levels of health care, I see an urgent need for both increased fertility awareness and knowledge for the PHCT on the one hand, and an endorsement of existing counselling skills and experience on the other. Generalist counselling in general practice is looked at elsewhere in this book (see Chapters 1 and 2) and many of the skills—empathy, active listening, focusing, for example—should all be part of the GP's basic repertoire. From my own experience, many GPs integrate these skills into good practice, together with up-to-date information and judicious advice. Many general practices have at least one member of the group with an obstetric/gynaecological specialism who would seem the obvious person to take responsibility for pre-referral fertility counselling.

Later in this chapter I address the requirements laid down by the Human Fertilisation and Embryology Authority (HFEA) in relation to counselling provision together with the British Infertility Counselling Association guidelines; however, this only applies to those counsellors who work in the secondary/tertiary health care sectors. GPs need to be encouraged to develop their counselling skills which, in turn, enable the client/ patient to see fertility and other counselling as a part of health care rather than as an extra 'tacked on'. Once patients are on the fertility treatment roller coaster, it is less easy to have informed reflection on their situation. Counselling by the PHCT is invaluable in reducing human stress, not to mention later anxiety and depression. It could also be argued that early counselling and advice-giving could reduce economic costs for all concerned.

Main causes of sub/infertility

Research suggests that the largest single cause (32%) of infertility is due to the male factor of poor sperm (Hull 1991; Furse 1997), either in quality or quantity. Medical treatment for sperm disorder is unproven but the 'processing' of poor sperm can assist conception success. The reduction of tobacco and alcohol use can improve sperm quality (Lee 1994, 1999). With new and developing microsurgical techniques, quantity is less of a problem providing the quality is high.

According to the HFEA (1999a), causes of female infertility are more complex and 42% is 'unexplained'. A further 33% is associated with tubal damage, and the remaining 25% is caused by endometriosis (8%) and other medical conditions.

There are also congenital causes such as the absence or maldevelopment of vas, ovaries, uterus and testes. It is important for GPs to remember that radiotherapy and laser treatment can damage reproduction. Most people these days are better informed, and some will seek to store sperm before treatment commences. However, it is important to remember that sometimes advice regarding this is not 'heard' at times of high anxiety.

GPs need to be aware that lifestyle factors such as use of alcohol, tobacco and other dependency drugs, long-haul flying and some drug treatments, contribute to some loss of fertility, even if it is temporary. Most books on fertility now recommend healthy diets and exercise as part of a positive approach to conception (see, for example, Furse 1997).

Many practitioners now agree that 'stress' is a contributory factor in conception failure but as yet we have no conclusive research to demonstrate this, especially as it is impossible to isolate the stress caused by fertility treatment in itself (Norman-Taylor 1999). However, there is no such thing as an 'infertile personality'. The results of a pilot project (Jennings 1993) suggest that certain forms of dependency could contribute to fertility problems. Issues around despair, desperation, expectations and family pressure can be addressed in early counselling and advice.

Some infertility is still a mystery and whereas many clinicians suggest that eventually all known causes will be known and individually treatable, others suggest that there are social and environmental causes which need more investigation. Some couples are just 'unlucky so far', especially if they seek help within three years. There is increasing anecdotal evidence which suggests that actually stopping treatment, adopting or deciding not to 'try for a baby', may bring about an unexpected conception.

Assisted conception techniques

Treatment methods and their terms are being updated all the time. There are two current sources for the latest information. One is the HFEA and their three excellent patient guides: *Infertility and IVF* (1999b), *IVF Clinics* (1999a) and *Donor Insemination* (1999c). The other is a new bi-annual publication (most recent edition, 1999) *Pathways to Pregnancy* which aims to provide accessible information regarding treatments and conditions from as many perspectives as possible. Perhaps GPs could have it available in the waiting rooms. In addition, *The Infertility Companion* (1997) by Anna Furse is an excellent compendium of information on all aspects of the subject. Furse herself conceived through in vitro fertilization (IVF) which makes the book additionally 'user friendly'.

Current techniques are:

1 Donor insemination (DI):
   - with husband's sperm; *or*
   - with partner's sperm; *or*
   - with donor's sperm.

2 *In vitro* fertilization and embryo transfer (IVF-ET or 'test tube method') which can include donated gametes (sperm or ovum) or embryos (surrogacy).

3 Gamete intrafallopian fertilization (GIFT)—also with donated transfer gametes (surrogacy).

4 Microsurgical epididymal sperm aspiration (MESA) for congenital absence of vas. The exudate obtained from the epididymis can be used for donor insemination (DI), GIFT or IVF.

5 Ovum donations (OD) by a volunteer for congenital absence of ovaries or premature menopause. The ova may be used for GIFT or IVF.

6 A female volunteer (historically a relative or friend) elects to receive a couple's fertilized eggs (or embryos) created by IVF, through embryo transfer.

IVF-ET is currently the most commonly practised treatment, especially where there is tubal damage. The average conception rate with IVF-ET is one in six cycles of treatment (Human Fertilisation and Embryology Authority 1999a), which translates into a 12% maternity rate (per treatment cycle). Some clinics distort this rate by counting twins as two successes and triplets as three, whereas they should all be counted as only one.

Assisted conception techniques must be undertaken in a licensed treatment centre whose work and practice is regulated by the HFEA.

Fertility counselling required by the HFEA

The recent legislation regulating medical treatments for fertility problems includes a mandatory requirement for the provision of counselling.

> People seeking licensed treatment (i.e. *in vitro* fertilisation or treatment using donated gametes) or consenting to the use or storage of embryos, or to the donation or storage of embryos, must be given 'a suitable opportunity to receive proper counselling' (Human Fertilisation and Embryology Authority 1998, p. 12, 2.10).

The HFEA, which is the statutory body empowered to enforce the recent Act, has provided a code of practice, guidelines and a consultation document to make sure that licensed centres and their staff understand their responsibilities in relation to the provision of fertility counselling. For example:

> Centres must make implications counselling [*sic*] available to everyone. They should also provide support or therapeutic counselling in appropriate cases or refer people to sources of more specialist counselling outside the centre (Human Fertilisation and Embryology Authority 1998, p. 38, 6.4).

Despite the requirement by law for licensed centres to make this counselling provision, there is still uncertainty amongst doctors about what constitutes such counselling. The code of practice states that:

> Counselling should be clearly distinguished from the normal relationship between the clinician and the person offering donation or seeking storage or treatment, which includes giving professional advice (Human Fertilisation and Embryology Authority 1998, p. 37, 6.2).

However, though highlighted by HFEA, clinicians seem unable to distinguish this, and counselling appears to be confused with the giving of advice and information on the one hand, and the practice of psychotherapy on the other. The definitions and practice of counselling in its several forms are clarified elsewhere in this book (see Chapter 1).

The HFEA (1998, pp. 37–38) have identified the following types of counselling which must be available through licensed clinics for people contemplating assisted conception:

1 *Implications counselling*: this aims to enable the person concerned to understand the implications of the proposed course of action for themselves, for their family and for any children born as a result. It may include genetic counselling.

2 *Support counselling*: this aims to give emotional support at times of particular stress, e.g. when there is a failure to achieve a pregnancy.

3 *Therapeutic counselling*: this aims to help people to cope with the consequences of infertility and treatment, and to help them resolve the problems which these may cause. It includes helping people to adjust their expectations and accept their situation.

The HFEA *Code of Practice* (1998) obviously considers that implications counselling, especially in the case of donated gametes, is most important as it devotes considerably more detail to its practice. It emphasizes that both existing and unborn children's needs must be considered. Clients and prospective donors need implications counselling in relation to both treatment decisions and gamete donation in itself. They need to consider their feelings about not being the biological parents of their child, and what they will decide to tell the child as well as their extended family.

It is generally assumed that openness with existing and future children is preferred, rather than keeping secrets for life that might be guessed at anyway. Children born from assisted conception have a right to know their biological origins if they ask, although anonymity is preserved for donors of gametes. However, this difficult ground rule is currently under review. Counsellors have sometimes to deal with the situation where a couple request the use of a known donor, and the implications counselling reveals that it is not in the best interest of all concerned. The following case history illustrates such a situation.

Case history 1

Mr and Mrs J attended for 'implications counselling' before making treatment decisions. Mrs J had no ovaries and wanted to accept her sister's offer of donated eggs. The couple insisted that they wanted known donorship within the family, and Mrs J said, darkly: 'and she owes me something anyway'. I suggested a session with the sisters together, which Mrs J refused, but said that her sister would come to see me. Ms W, the sister, came to see me in a very distressed state, saying that she wanted 'everything to be all right', and that this was why she was offering her eggs. She was a single woman with no ideas at the time of having a family. When asked about 'everything being all right', she burst into tears and said that her father had abused her and that she felt so bad that perhaps this was something good she could do. Patently more counselling was necessary to explore the different issues that were emerging before final decisions could be taken.

My own view is that more emphasis should be placed on the variations between the presenting problems of people who attend fertility clinics and assisted conception units. For example, there are a significant number of people who have a psychosexual problem and turn to fertility clinics for assistance. This, of course, raises the whole issue of whether assisted conception treatments should be used for social and psychological problems rather than medical ones. There are those who suggest that if people choose to have assisted conception rather than sexual intercourse, then it is their decision; however, with the people that I counsel, there are usually feelings of guilt and distress concerning the psychosexual problem and a lack of knowledge of where to turn for help, illustrated by case history 2.

Case history 2

Mr and Mrs S appeared to be suffering from unexplained infertility, as preliminary investigations showed no medical problems with sperm, ovulation or tubes. Mrs S requested counselling and presented as very tense, attending with her husband who was loud and florid in his attempts to suggest that his wife had 'the problem'. Careful probing brought to light the fact that they did not have vaginal intercourse through to full orgasm as Mr S had to climax orally and his wife had hoped that some semen would spill before withdrawal to enable her to conceive. Once having disclosed 'the secret', it was then possible for them to request psychosexual help rather than assisted conception.

There may be couples who need to be referred for marital therapy because of the stress of their relationship, and there are times when the presenting behaviour is so disturbed that a psychiatric referral is necessary rather than a gynaecological one. The following are considerations for the GP before making a referral:

1 How long have the couple been trying to conceive? Up to three years may be within the normal range. However, most clinics have waiting lists of at least two years which may affect the timing of referral.

2 Are the couple having regular vaginal intercourse? Could this be a psychosexual problem in disguise?

3 Has organic disease in either partner been excluded by referring to previous history and by appropriate examination and tests (including gynaecological examination, examination of male genitalia, and tests for example for thyroid deficiency)?

4 Are there any eating disorders? In the case of anorexia, bulimia or obesity, the Ponderal Index should be calculated to indicate the likelihood of ovulatory disorder, and an appropriate referral made.

5 Is there an assumption that it must be 'the woman's problem' and, therefore, she must have the investigation? Fertility clinics will not usually proceed with invasive investigation until there has been a sperm test.

6 What is the presenting level of distress? Anger, depression and guilt are the most common feelings.

7 How much pressure is on the couple from their families or towards each other? What support is available to the couple before and during treatment?

8 Has the couple considered the possibilities of childlessness? The loss of the 'dream child' that never was can be as acute as losing a child that lived.

9 What is your response to single women seeking treatment? Having taken into account the HFEA's requirement for consideration of the welfare of the child, especially a child's need for a father, do you have your own personal stance?

10 How do you respond to a lesbian couple seeking assisted conception, given that some prefer to attend an assisted conception unit rather than undertake self-conception (see also the previous point).

Summary for GPs considering giving fertility counselling

There is a strong case for GPs, or members of their PHCT, to undertake fertility counselling with patients prior to referral to a fertility clinic. By this I mean something more than the advice and information needed for people to address the complex issues involved in considering 'high-tech' treatments.

GPs can provide information packs on the problems of fertility and their management (see 'Useful contacts' below). They are well placed to explore the varied reasons for fertility problems, as well as providing support for patients embarking on a lengthy, stressful period of treatment with uncertain results.

Currently, the British Infertility Counselling Association (BICA 1992, 1999) and the British Fertility Society (1999) are trying to establish guidelines for approved training in fertility counselling skills. There is more literature on the practice of fertility counselling (Lee 1994; Read 1995; Furse 1997), with more recognition of the need for a specialized knowledge base within counselling practice. For those GPs with access to a drama therapist or art therapist, increasing expertise in fertility work is being developed within these specialisms (Jennings 1999, 2001; Lee and Gilling-Smith 2000).

However, in the new 'commissioner/provider' milieu, many health authorities are not willing to fund assisted conception treatment. It is important for GPs to be aware of the policy of their health authority, thus avoiding undue disappointment.

Even where treatment is provided, GPs and other PHCT members will need to support those for whom this is unsuccessful through the period of subsequent mourning.

Counselling to limit fertility

There seems a certain irony in the contrast between people who are desperate to have children and those who are desperate not to. There is also the painful reality that many hospitals run their antenatal clinic and their fertility clinic in the same space and at the same time.

With the reduction in resources for well-women centres and family planning clinics, it is inevitable that the PHCT members will give more advice and provide more information, as well as counselling when required.

Community Health Councils and the Family Planning Association provide up-to-date information leaflets and posters. There is now a wide choice of methods to be used before and after childbearing. Why then, are so many conceptions in some sense unwanted or unintended? Patently not all of these result in unwanted children; nevertheless there has been a drive from government to provide better access to family planning (Department of Health 1992).

Prompted by the spread of HIV, the government has emphasized the importance of re-education regarding unprotected sexual intercourse and the spread of AIDS-related and other sexually transmitted diseases. However, sexual health includes not only the control of disease, but also family planning. Family planning services play an important part in the health of children and families.

One of the targets set in the early 1990s was to reduce the conception rate amongst under-16s by at least 50% by 2000, from 9.5 per 1000 girls aged 13–15 years in 1989, to no more than 4.8 (Department of Health 1992). It is now recommended that boys should be targeted as well as girls. There is some indication that 'condom consciousness raising' is having some effect, both girls and boys being more likely to carry condoms.

Although the National Curriculum requires pupils aged 11–14 years to understand the processes of conception in human beings as well as the physical and emotional changes of adolescence and the responsibilities of sexual behaviour, it is left to schools' governing bodies to decide whether any further sex education should be provided.

Government targets for reducing teenage pregnancy are not being met. Primary care could be the pivotal point through which teenage pregnancy issues can be channelled. As well as providing family planning information and counselling, the PHCT could develop more outreach work with schools, colleges and youth groups.

Some innovatory work is being developed. For example, theatre in education (TIE) companies are now trying to address these issues. TIE Tours take teen pregnancy programmes into inner London schools with participation by pupils.

Reflections for GPs and the PHCT in family planning/contraceptive counselling

GPs are responsible for providing comprehensive information and advice on all forms of contraception (leaflets are available in several languages). However, the attitudes of some GPs towards, for example, underage sex or homosexual behaviour, can discourage people and so limit the contribution that primary care can make. Within the PHCT there needs to be one identified specialist to co-ordinate practice initiatives and policy. None the less, the whole team should be aware of what people need to know about contraception, and how they can be helped to take responsibility for their choices. For example:

- Are people aware of the wide range of choices of contraception, including the advances made in 'natural methods'?
- Is contraception or 'safe sex' the prime reason for consultation?
- Within the couple relationship, is one person taking responsibility for avoiding pregnancy?
- How can people's autonomy be encouraged in family planning?
- What are the team's assumptions about homosexuals and regular drug users?
- What are the team's attitudes towards underage intercourse and how far are young people encouraged to discuss contraception?
- Is contraception seen as the woman's or the man's responsibility?
- Is it possible that more explicit sex education is required in order for people to understand contraception?

Family planning and fertility care—the PHCT

Even if there is an individual within the practice who specializes in fertility counselling and advice, the PHCT as a whole should integrate the 'womb to tomb' life journey, through all the stages of birth, menstruation and puberty, fertility and family planning, psychosexuality, mid-life changes and ageing. The team's counselling expertise should include the GPs, the practice family planning nurse, the health visitors and the midwives. Patients of all ages and cultural backgrounds should be able to find sensitive responses to any lack of information, anxiety, distress and confusion.

The PHCT knows people within their social, cultural and domestic setting in a way that is impossible for secondary and tertiary agencies. Good counsel can be based on local knowledge and understanding of family circumstances. Young people especially need to be encouraged to use primary care and, as previously mentioned, there is a strong case for the PHCT doing outreach work in schools and communities. Some PHCTs already have counsellors attached to them who take on complementary roles to the other specialists involved. Some are also able to avail themselves of interpreters and nursing and midwifery aides who are able to discuss in greater depth both the symptoms and cultural practice in a person's first language. Orientation courses for practice receptionists can also enhance good practice.

PHCTs will have greater demands put upon them in the future as other clinics close down, and it is vital that sufficient resources are allocated for additional personnel and specialist training.

Conclusions

GPs and their team have a key role in relation to fertility treatment as well as fertility regulation, and in helping, wherever possible, all pregnancies to be welcome ones and all to become parents who wish to do so. A fertility counsellor supports people at any stage of the procedures—before, during or after treatment. Perhaps most importantly, the counsellor is there to assist people to come to terms with the likelihood of treatment not resulting in a take-home baby. At times, this will be akin to bereavement counselling, as people grieve for the loss of the child they never had. I have suggested some issues for consideration in relation to this and to family planning, including access to information, as well as a confrontation of our own prejudices and assumptions. I hope that the complexity of this field is now clearer to GPs, who are often the first port of call.

Acknowledgement

I am indebted to Dr Sammy Lee's help with the technical aspects of this chapter.

References

British Infertility Counselling Association (1999) *Guidance on the Inspection and Provision of Counselling in Assisted Conception Units*. British Infertility Counselling Association, Sheffield.

British Infertility Counselling Association (1992) *Infertility Counselling: Guidelines for Practice*. British Infertility Counselling Association, Sheffield.

British Infertility Counselling Association and British Fertility Society (1999) *Training and Accreditation for Infertility Counselling*. University of Sheffield, Sheffield.

Burnard, P. (1989) *Counselling Skills for Health Professionals*. Chapman & Hall, London.

Department of Health (1992) *The Health of the Nation*. Cm 1986. HMSO, London.

Furse, A. (1997) *The Infertility Companion: a User's Guide to Tests, Technology and Therapies*. Thorsons, London.

Hull, M. (1991) *Infertility Treatment: Needs and Effectiveness*. Department of Obstetrics and Gynaecology, University of Bristol, Bristol.

Human Fertilisation and Embryology Authority (1998) *Code of Practice*. Human Fertilisation and Embryology Authority, London.

Human Fertilisation and Embryology Authority (1999a) *The Patients Guide to IVF Clinics*. Human Fertilisation and Embryology Authority, London.

Human Fertilisation and Embryology Authority (1999b) *The Patients Guide to Infertility and IVF*. Human Fertilisation and Embryology Authority, London.

Human Fertilisation and Embryology Authority (1999c) *The Patients Guide to Donor Insemination*. Human Fertilisation and Embryology Authority, London.

Jennings, S. (1989) Legitimate grieving? Working with infertility. In *Children and Death* (Papatou, D. and Papadatos, C., eds). Hemisphere, New York, pp. 277–282.

Jennings, S. (1993) The drama in counsel: the counsel in drama. *Counselling*, 4, 3.

Jennings, S. (1994) *Infertility Counselling*. Blackwell Scientific Publications, Oxford.

Jennings, S. (1999) *Introduction to Dramatherapy*. Jessica Kingsley, London.

Jennings, S. (2001) *The Fertile Path*. Capall Bann, Chieveley.

Lee, S. (1994) Male factor infertility. In *Infertility Counselling* (Jennings, S.). Blackwell Scientific Publications, Oxford, pp. 66–78.

Lee, S. (1996) *Counselling in Male Infertility*. Blackwell Science, Oxford.

Lee, S. (1999) Sperm counts. *Pathways to Pregnancy*, 1, 00.

Lee, S. and Gilling-Smith, C. (2000) Art and ART, the healing of infertility. In *Pathways to Pregnancy*, 2, 80.

Norman-Taylor, J. (1999) The stress factor. *Pathways to pregnancy*, 1, 62.

Read, J. (1995) *Counselling for Fertility Problems*. Sage, London.

Useful contacts

British Agency for Adoption and Fostering, Skyline House, 200 Union Street, London SE1 0LX. Telephone: (020) 7593 2000.

British Infertility Counselling Association (BICA), 69 Division Street, Sheffield S1 4GE. Information line: 01342 843880. *BICA aims to promote high quality, accessible counselling services for people with fertility problems. The Association offers information to patients who are seeking details of counsellors specialising in infertility.*

British Pregnancy Advisory Service, Austy Manor, Wootten Wawen, Solihull, West Midlands B95 6DA. Telephone: 015642 3225.

Child (support and information for those with infertility problems), PO Box 154, Hounslow, Middlesex TW3 0EZ. Telephone/fax: (020) 8571 4376.

Child (The National Infertility Support Network), Charter House, 43 St Leonards Road, Bexhill-on-Sea, East Sussex TN40 1JA. Telephone: 01424 732361; fax: 01424 731858; e-mail: office@email2.child.org.uk; website: http://www.child.org.uk. *Provides fact sheets, a quarterly magazine, publications, medical advice and emotional support including helplines, local groups and local and national meetings.*

COTS (Childlessness Overcome Through Surrogacy), Loandhu Cottage, Guids, Lairg, Sutherland IV27 4EF, Scotland. Telephone/fax: 01549 402401.

Council for Complementary and Alternative Medicine, 179 Gloucester Place, London NW1 6DX. Telephone: (020) 7724 9103. *Information on all forms of alternative medicine.*

Daisy Network (Premature Menopause Support Group), PO Box 392, High Wycombe, Bucks HP15 7SH. Telephone: 01628 473446 (Monique Francis, evenings) or (020) 8569 1234 ext 2648 (Monday, Wednesday or Friday during office hours). *Support group for girls and women who suffer early ovarian failure. Exchange information on IVF, HRT and on ways to have a family through egg donation, surrogacy or adoption. Provides informal telephone counselling by members and quarterly newletter.*

DI Network, PO Box 265, Sheffield S3 7YX. Telephone/fax: (020) 8245 4369. *Provides support for those considering the use of donated gametes through donor insemination and IVF with donor sperm or donated eggs.*

Family Planning Association, 2-12 Pentonville Road, London N1 9FP. Telephone: (020) 7837 5432. *Information on sexual and reproductive health.*

Human Fertilisation and Embryology Authority (HFEA), Paxton House, 30 Artillery Lane, London E1 7LS. Telephone: (020) 7377 5077.

Issue (The National Fertility Association), Lichfield Street, Walsall WS1 1SZ. Telephone: 01922 722888; fax: 01922 640070; e-mail: webmaster@issue.co.uk; website: http://www.issue.co.uk. *Members receive independent individual support and information. Members and non-members alike can telephone for help. Callers are answered personally 24 hours a day. Confidential telephone counselling by qualified counsellors is available to all every weekday evening.*

Life, Life House, Newbold Terrace, Leamington Spa, Warwickshire CV32 4EA. Telephone: 01926 421587. *Information and advice on pregnancy, abortion, miscarriage and stillbirth.*

London Lesbian Health Care, c/o London Women's Centre, Wesley House, 4 Wild Court, London WC2.

Marie Stopes Clinic, 108 Whitfield Stree, London W1P 6BE. Telephone: (020) 7388 2585. *Advice and counselling on vasectomy, infertility, sperm bank facilities and well man screening.*

Miscarriage Association, c/o Clayton Hospital, Northgate, Wakefield, W. Yorks WF1 3JS. Telephone: 01924 200799; fax: 01924 298834. *Provides support and information on the subject of pregnancy loss.*

Multiple Births Foundation, Queen Charlotte's and Chelsea Hospital, Goldhawk Road, London W6 0XG. Telephone: (020) 8383 3519; fax: (020) 8383 3041. *Provides professional support and information about all aspects of multiple births.*

National Childbirth Trust (NCT), Alexandra House, Oldham Terrace, London W3 6NH. Telephone: (020) 8992 8637 (9.30 am–4.30 pm Monday to Friday); fax: (020) 8992 5929.

National Egg and Embryo Donation Society, Regional IVF Unit, St Mary's Hospital, Whitworth Park, Manchester M13 0JH. Telephone: 01706 829428.

National Endometriosis Society, 50 Westminster Palace Gardens, Artillery Row, London SW1P 1RL. Telephone: (020) 7222 2776; fax: (020) 7222 2786. *Provides a helpline, local groups and clubs, a newsletter and other publications, workshops and conferences.*

National Infertility Awareness Campaign (NIAC), PO Box 2106, London W1A 2DZ. Telephone: freephone 0800 716345. *A lobbying organization campaigning for NHS funding for all infertility treatment on an equal basis across the UK. Gives advice on the current situation with regard to NHS funding and on campaigning/lobbying activities.*

Overseas Adoption Helpline, PO Box 13899, London N6 4WB. Telephone: 0990 168742.

Parentline, Endway House, The Endway, Hadley, Benfleet, Essex SS7 2AN. Telephone: 01702 554782. *Offers confidential support to parents under stress.*

Planned Parenthood Federation of America, 810 Seventh Avenue, New York, NY, USA. Telephone: 212 841 8962.

Pregnancy Advisory Service, 11-13 Charlotte Street, London W1P 1HD. Telephone: (020) 7637 8962.

Progress Educational Trust, 140 Gray's Inn Road, London WC1X 8AX. Telephone: (020) 7278 7870; fax: (020) 7278 7862; e-mail: admin@progress.org.uk; website: http://www.progress.org.uk. *Provides information on fertility and genetics, and promotes discussion on their ethical and legal implications. Publishes a news journal, 'Progress in Reproduction'.*

Resolve (counselling, referral and support for infertile couples), 1310 Broadway, Somerville, Massachusetts 02144, USA. Telephone: 617 623 0744.

Twins and Multiple Births Association (TAMBA), PO Box 30, Little Sutton, South Wirall L66 1TH. Confidential helpline: 01732 868000 (open 7–11 pm weekdays, 10 am–11 pm weekends). *Provides support for families with twins, triplets or more, and for professionals involved with their care. Network of local twins clubs, specialist support groups, publications and an information pack.*

Women's Health and Reproductive Rights Information Centre, 52-54 Featherstone Street, London EC1Y. Telephone: (020) 7251 6332.

Chapter 18

Terminal illness

Dorothy Poingdestre

Introduction

In this chapter I discuss the range of issues and feelings that are likely to be important in relation to care for those with a terminal illness (see also Spilling 1986; Buckman 2000; Macleod 2000; Peberdy 2000), in an attempt to demonstrate the contribution which counselling can make to that care. Much of what I say is relevant to terminal illness at any stage of life, but particular attention is paid to those who are seen as dying 'before their time', as it is often in these circumstances that the most difficult issues arise and specialist counselling can be of most evident help.

In my view, counselling is the act of helping people to look comprehensively at their situation and empowering them to make their own decisions for their own future. Working with the terminally ill requires of the counsellor the ability to stand where they are standing, on the threshold of death.

Death is the only unavoidable event that confronts us all. The aim of counselling is to enable patients to face death as a reality and to lead them forwards positively, comfortably and peacefully; enabling them to do what needs to be done, both emotionally and practically, before death.

Time is the most precious gift that can be offered to the dying. Through time spent in counselling, dying patients are enabled to see their worth as people in their own right. Dame Cicely Saunders has said, 'You learn the care of the dying from the dying themselves'. Most people are afraid of dying. Talking about death and working with the dying faces counsellors with fundamental questions about life and death, and their own limited lifespan. This requires a certain maturity, which only comes from experience of life. Only then can empathy be shown to patients, families and friends.

Counsellors have to take a serious look at their own attitude towards death and dying before they can sit quietly and without anxiety next to terminally ill people; letting them know by their words and actions that they are not going to run away if dying is mentioned. Counsellors need to have the ability to maintain an attitude of concern, acceptance and tolerance; to enable patients and carers to express their inner feelings and to feel safe doing so.

Responding to loss

When people realize that something valuable is about to be lost, there is a sense of shock and the usual activities of life are disrupted. Severe trauma produces a protective emotional numbness, which, together with denial, allows time to adjust to the new situation. Once the truth is faced, questions come: 'Why me?', 'What have I done to deserve this?' or 'I've lived a long life, I suppose I've got to die of something'. Anger may come if others can be blamed, even to the point of reacting violently against them. If patients think it is their own fault, guilt or a feeling of retribution for past deeds may be felt, as well as grief and sadness; a longing to turn back the clock; self-blame and regret followed by a sense of emptiness and despair.

Dr Elisabeth Kubler-Ross, one of the pioneers of the 'dignity in death' movement in the USA has listed five stages faced by terminally ill patients (Kubler-Ross 1969):

1 Denial and isolation, when patients select the facts they want to accept.

2 Anger, often directed to those nearest to the patient, who find such a response confusing.

3 Bargaining, when patients attempt to prolong their lives by promising to be better people if only God will let them live a while longer.

4 Depression, when patients may turn their face to the wall, not wanting to communicate their feelings, and are difficult to help.

5 Acceptance, when patients admit the truth of what is happening to them.

Patients rarely pass through stages 1–5 in that order, but these can serve as guidelines. Counsellors need to discover what the loss of function, loss of independence and loss of life mean to each terminally ill patient.

The dying patient: to tell or not to tell

All people who know they have a terminal illness will go through, at their own pace, some of the emotions explained above. If depression or communication difficulties are inhibiting their functioning, counselling intervention may be helpful.

If patients want to know the truth, they will ask someone they trust. If they are not answered truthfully, trust disappears. Patients are the counsellor's best guide regarding how and when to tell. Never collude with fantasy. First, discover how much is known already. What is understood from what the individual knows? Would he/she like any further explanation? Is he/she asking to be told? If the answer to any of these questions is met with hesitation, the truth must not be forced upon the patient, but an opportunity must remain open to learn more when he/she is ready. Confronting reluctant patients with the truth will be unhelpful and may seriously damage the counselling relationship. Attentive listening, once the function of neighbours and church, may be sufficient to allay feelings of distress and isolation.

Unlike sufferers from a fatal heart attack, patients with a progressive illness have time to realize what is happening to them, and to prepare for death. Not all patients think this is such a bonus! Many experience a feeling of helplessness or of events taking over. It is hard to be assertive when one's life is in the hands of a hospital team. Counsellors can rebuild the patients' confidence and help them regain the control they may have lost.

Shock and denial

Patients and carers are numbed with shock when first told there is no more that can be done. They need space and time to accept the news. Counsellors can help by going over their reactions with them. Tears may not have been shed yet. Encourage them to cry, as tears are part of the healing process. Talk about their plans for the future which may not now be fulfilled. Most people need help to express suppressed anger and fears. There is nothing wrong in being worried about what is happening to them; we would all be upset and anxious in their situation.

Some fears, however, are unrealistic and can disappear after discussion. Most people are not so much afraid of death as of dying in pain. Counsellors can be sounding boards for such fears and provide a trustworthy and safe environment for the open exploration of feelings, which helps to relieve anxiety.

Anger

Displaced anger can cause problems. We all believe we should live into old age, and find the concept of dying before then unbelievable. Once permitted to do so, younger dying patients are likely to express a flood of hurt feelings, together with past feelings which re-emerge with force. They may be angry with the world in general, or with the general practitioner who did not send them to the hospital early enough, or with themselves for ignoring the first signs of illness.

Some are resentful at having to leave a loving family, which they have worked so hard to achieve. They may feel cheated, angry and bitter at having to die. Counsellors can allow patients to express such feelings, without saying too much at this time. Being able to tolerate such remarks, while showing that it is natural for patients to have such strong negative feelings is sufficient at this stage. Counsellors understand where the anger is coming from and where it needs to be directed. Once patients realize their anger is against the disease itself, they can be at peace with those around them.

Counsellors can explain that it is difficult for carers to tolerate anger because they themselves are worried, feeling vulnerable and concerned to say the 'right thing'. Nobody knows instinctively how the patient feels. Everyone deals with trauma differently. They are the one who is dying. Counsellors represent what patients are losing— health, emotional and physical strength, control, confidence, the ability to fulfil a role in society and plan for the future. While patients want to talk to people who are sufficiently sure of their own identity not to be overwhelmed, these very characteristics reflect their own forthcoming losses.

Grief

In his foreword to Elisabeth Kubler-Ross's (1969) book *On Death and Dying*, Colin Murray Parkes writes: 'Whatever we believe is to come after death, the loss of so many of the things that we prize must be painful, and since our own death gives grief to others it is natural that we feel sad on their behalf.'

Grief takes us through varying emotions: confusion, turmoil, sadness. At this time patients may well wish to review what has happened during their lives—the lost opportunities or the things they regret having done, but cannot change. These can be relatively small incidents which seemed unimportant at the time, but which assume significance in the face of terminal illness. In stressful situations, the negative aspects of life are dwelt on. By careful listening, the counsellor can confirm the individual's value as a person and help them remember the positive experiences, relationships and achievements which may be lost amid the regrets, assuring them that everyone's life is a mixture of success and failure. With a counsellor, they can be sad without being told to stop being morbid, or made to feel that their sadness is upsetting everyone else. A conflict of emotions may be experienced—the hope that carers will not be distressed by their death, but also the fear that they have not made a lasting impact on the carers' lives and will soon be forgotten.

Resignation and acceptance

Not all patients want to accept that they are dying. Seeing their distress and fight against death right up until the end is painful to watch. It is always easier to see someone slip away peacefully. Some patients only reach a stage of resignation; they seem hopeless and give up, turn their face to the wall, withdraw from life and wait for death. Some go a little further, into a more positive attitude, determining to live as much as possible in the time they have left or to rethink their priorities. As the illness progresses, reassurance is sometimes needed that acceptance of care is not a failure, but is a yielding to the love of others who want to make their last days as easy as possible.

Dying patients who are depressed or anxious are not usually suffering from a depressive illness or an anxiety state in the psychiatric sense. They are likely to be facing difficulties in coming to terms with their own mortality, in communication with professionals and carers, in coping with the effects of the disease or treatment, or in adjustments in their role as the illness progresses.

Patients may become despondent when, having accepted their impending death, they do not die as quickly as they would wish. 'It's like a death sentence, without knowing the date it's going to happen', one said. Some patients scan the newspapers for news of any breakthrough treatment for their illness. They would rather be a guinea-pig in testing, than lie back and accept their fate. Counsellors need to recognize what stage patients have reached in adapting to their illness. Are they facing and accepting the reality of their own death? Are they giving up the hard work of staying alive? Has social interaction become less important? They may not want to joke or take responsibility for maintaining social exchanges. Withdrawal is understandable. It is distressing for patients who are tired and who have had enough, to be reminded that they have in some way a duty to keep fighting; not to let down their family and to be chivvied back into a social world which they are ready to give up.

Communication

Counsellors aim to answer any questions from patients and carers with honesty and to deal with the issues such honesty produces. Some patients do not know much about their diagnosis and prognosis. This can be because they have not asked, or they have not been offered the information, or they have not heard what they have been told. They are sometimes dissatisfied with the information given by medical staff either because it was insufficient, or they did not understand the terminology, or they were confused and felt too diffident to seek further clarification. There is also the fear of taking up too much of the doctor's valuable time. Counsellors need to ensure that there is effective communication about what they know, the proposed action and the likely outcome.

Different patients react differently to the news of having a terminal illness, depending on their personality and past coping strategies. People who use denial as their main defence will use denial more extensively now. People who faced past stressful situations with open confrontation similarly will do so in their present stressful situation. They may not want to discuss their terminal illness, but may want reassurance that counsellors are available should they want to do so later. Counsellors need to let patients know that they are ready and willing to share their concerns, however painful they may be. By stating: 'This is a difficult time for you', counsellors are expressing their willingness to see things from the patient's point of view. Alternatively, they may just wish to talk about their feelings of anger, confusion and fear. They may be concerned about upsetting others, causing embarrassment, worrying about protecting their carers from distressing experiences, and feeling socially and emotionally isolated. There should be no false attempts at cheerfulness, though humour can be found in most situations. They should be allowed the relief of being sad without being alone. The opportunity of simply expressing themselves to someone who is perceived as being reliable and trustworthy is often a great relief in itself.

Some carers insist that the patients are not told their diagnosis, but this can leave them thinking their condition is even worse than it is. Terminally ill patients have special needs, which can be fulfilled if time is taken to sit and listen to what these needs are for that patient. In the hospice movement, highly trained doctors, nurses and social workers are there to acknowledge the forthcoming death, to concentrate on easing physical pain and to give true emotional support to patients and carers. This enables patients to come through the shadow of death and be calm, up to the moment when they simply and acceptingly cease to live. The skilled application of common sense, human sympathy and honesty helps to ease physical, emotional and spiritual pain. Once such pain has been conquered, patients are freed to be themselves again.

Dying patients and their carers

Most dying patients have a suspicion of how ill they are. The carers have their own suspicions, but neither side is able to be open for fear of upsetting the other. This makes for tension when they meet, with everyone avoiding that which is uppermost in their minds—questions as to how long the patient has to live. There is the conflict between the wish to confide and be comforted and the wish to protect each other from the distress of the truth. Children and elderly parents, though vulnerable, still need time to talk and be prepared for a death in the family, giving them the opportunity to say those special things that are not often put into words. Counsellors can help people understand what is happening to them; arranging to see carers on their own, with a partner or within the whole family group to facilitate open discussion.

Relationships can change under the stress of dying. A fiancé may break off the engagement, or a divorced spouse may return to be the carer. Difficulties can arise when one partner is naturally outgoing and open about problems and feelings, while the other likes to keep thoughts and feelings bottled up. Patients are likely to feel trapped and frustrated as they become more housebound. This personal pain may lead to social isolation and further relationship breakdown. Counsellors can enable each to express these feelings by acknowledging that they exist; making direct statements about patients and carers looking tense, angry, sad; saying that many people feel like this in these situations and that it is natural both to have such feelings and to talk about them together. Counsellors can provide an element of safety and control for such talking to happen. Counsellors may feel ruffled, but need to be perceived as calm, reliable, tolerant, unshockable and concerned in threatening situations.

Counsellors must be able to act in a way which cannot be expected of friends or family, and to provide some continuity and stability which is missing from life at that time.

Overwhelming tiredness can make some patients withdraw from family life. Even visits from friends can seem too tiring. Patients living alone may wish to die at home alone. Some dying patients in a close relationship may wish to marry before they die. The registrar will conduct the wedding ceremony at the bedside or at home. Some carers try to protect patients from the daily problems they are facing in their own lives, but being left out of ordinary discussions only makes patients feel worse—as though they may as well be dead already. Counsellors need to show that their carers are not trying to deprive them of their role, but are trying to protect them, and in some sense themselves, from having to make the changes which are required.

Some carers want to know what to expect at the end. Many will never have seen a dead person. Counsellors can give practical advice as to who to contact when death occurs—the general practitioner, the ambulance, the hospice home care team, etc. Carers often experience helplessness, watching the patient die. It can be some comfort to be informed about the process of dying. There is a time in a patient's life when the mind slips off into a dreamless state, when the need for food becomes minimal, and the awareness of the environment all but disappears into darkness. Carers who have the strength and the compassion to sit with a dying patient in the silence will know that this moment is neither frightening nor painful, but a peaceful cessation of life.

Carers do learn to cope and gain much in return. Counsellors can help partners and other carers explore their feelings about having to give up work to look after the patient, as well as the regrets associated, for example, with this happening on the threshold of retirement, just when time could have been spent together. Some carers turn away from the truth, and do not want to discuss a future without their partner. It would be cruel to make them face the truth, if they are not ready to do so.

Various issues need to be addressed, for example, have the roles changed within the relationship? Who paid the bills and wrote the cheques and shopped and cooked? The remaining partner may not be equipped with the knowledge and resources to take on these tasks. The terminally ill partner may be well enough to instruct the other while there is time. Some carers cannot cope with toileting, medication or washing, and may need support in finding appropriate help in these tasks. Having a lower threshold of coping does not make a person less of a human being or less caring.

Counsellors need to gain a general overview of possible problem areas and assess at what stage carers are in relation to their own grief prior to the death. Often carers cannot understand that someone can stop fighting to stay alive and may interpret their readiness to die as personal abandonment. Counsellors can explain that this is a common reaction and not a personal rejection.

Common patient–carer problems are:

1 Coping with patients' illness at home; fear of causing unnecessary suffering; fear of finding them dead.

2 How to answer patients' questions about deterioration; wanting to protect them from the truth.

3 What to tell children and other family members.

4 How to live with anticipated loss; the disruption of life and the struggle to see meaning in what is happening.

Carers and patients sometimes need to shelve their anticipation of loss in order to keep on living. It is hard for most people to be expected always to talk of their death in a deep, meaningful way. Sometimes they need encouragement to enjoy the time they have left. It does not have to be doom and gloom. However, difficulties can arise as time goes on. The caring can become quite a strain; the patient is on the carer's mind all day long. Carers may become physically tired. Counsellors may have to help the carers sort out what they can realistically expect of themselves and of the patient during this terminal stage, thus helping to alleviate any feelings of guilt, frustration and helplessness.

Problems related to the disease and treatment

Patients often fear that, as their disease progresses and they change their physical appearance in some way, they will become less acceptable to their carers. Many issues need to be explored—body image: feeling infected, mutilated, unclean; becoming emaciated or being bloated; coping with a colostomy or hair loss; becoming housebound; loss of interest in sex; the effects of the various treatments; the lack of a cure and the disappointment at hearing there are no more treatments to try. Do they feel loved, cherished and cared for? Is having to depend on others difficult after a lifetime of independence? Are they worrying that their previous lifestyle has contributed to this illness? Do they understand what is and is not contagious?

Some treatments aimed at cure may have severe side effects. The time may come when a decision has to be made about whether such treatment should continue. Perhaps it is no longer effective, or the distress it causes outweighs the possible benefits. Some patients find it difficult to discuss this with their physician. A few may want to give up prematurely because they have become tired of the struggle to live. Others, perhaps because they are so afraid of death or of accepting defeat, may want to persist with treatment when it is clear that they would be better off with palliative treatment, giving a few weeks of comfort and tranquility with their carers before death. Counsellors are not in charge of treatment, so they may be in a good position to explore these issues with patients and help them make the best decision for themselves. If they work closely with the doctors and nurses, for example, as members of a primary health care team, then they can make themselves well informed with regard to the value or otherwise of persisting with treatment.

Problems in role adjustment

Terminal illness brings with it a series of role changes, from, for instance, an active, care-giving, wage-earning parent to a weak, helpless, dependent patient. Counsellors can help patients and their carers to adjust appropriately to these changes. Some patients give up too soon, or are pushed into the sick role by overanxious carers when there is much they can still do. For many hours, patients have to be in bed or sitting in a chair, with time on their hands to think about their illness. They then become bored and upset because they feel useless and a burden. They are less in control of their lives than before: less in control of their timetables; less in control physically and financially; less in control of the ordinary activities of daily living—washing, cooking, cleaning.

Some patients give their carers undue distress because they are unable to accept the care they really need. They exhaust themselves trying to prove that the illness is not that serious. They find it hard to watch someone else take over jobs around the house that they once did. Resentment and jealousy about this can turn relationships sour at the time when they need to be a source of strength. Some patients and carers become 'out of step' in the adjustments they each have to make. The patient may feel ready to stop fighting and rest, while the carer cannot bear to see this happen, encouraging them to get up when they are too weak to do so. One carer feared that the patient would become even weaker through staying in bed.

Many carers want to see the patient eat when they are no longer hungry. Counsellors can help carers see that in trying to keep their loved one with them a few days more, they are making those days even harder for them.

Religious beliefs or lack of them

Counsellors seeking to help dying patients should be aware of their own prejudices concerning the role of religion and their attitude towards clergymen as sources of help. Some patients find comfort in religion, or may have become more aware of a need for religion in their lives since becoming terminally ill. Awareness of the spiritual aspects of dying may produce questions about what will happen following death. Clergymen may well provide a source of reassurance, clarification and spiritual comfort which some counsellors may find difficult to convey. Counselling which takes religious problems seriously, and which is informed by the counsellors' concern for ultimate value and meaning, is religion in its widest sense.

It is important to find words which patients would use to discover where they stand concerning their faith. Most people have a faith or a philosophy of life, even if they would not call themselves religious. Do they think life has a meaning? People who have had a near-death experience state that they are more accepting of death the next time. Some patients turn to healers and find comfort and strength. Dying need not be the dread experience most of us imagine it to be. One patient, not a church-goer, was realistic about her death although she still did not want to leave her loved ones. She was convinced she would meet her mother and her first child again. During a church service, she felt all her worries slip away and was at peace, for the first time in years. Her newly formed belief in an afterlife brought her comfort. While on holiday, she bought a painting of an open doorway, leading into a distant garden, which symbolized for her what would happen to her in death. She was glad her family would have that painting to see after her death. When nearer to death, she found novels too shallow, finding comfort in the Bible instead.

It is important to discover if patients' beliefs have changed since becoming ill. Is their faith still important to them? Are they still practising their faith? Would a visit by their chaplain be helpful? In what way has their faith been challenged by this illness? Do they believe their illness is God's will? They may need help in looking at their fear that God is punishing them through this illness. They may be guilt-ridden about some real or imagined 'sins' and may be greatly relieved when offered an opportunity to share these thoughts. All human beings are vulnerable and make mistakes. They sometimes lose touch with God and need to know that God has never lost touch with them. Patients' anxieties can then be relieved, allowing them to die without a struggle.

Children of dying parents

When a parent is dying, the child needs to know that the parent loves him and that the death is not his responsibility. One parent was able to share all that was happening to her with her children, but did find difficulty acknowledging their anxiety about her illness. Some parents find it difficult to tell their children that a family member is dying, and are confused about how and what to say. Some of the concern is the fear of coping with the children's reaction to such news. Who is there to listen to the children in a family when each is concerned with their own grief and fear? Counsellors can see children on their own, or assist relatives to tell the children. If parents have been ill for a while, the children will understand that they are not getting better. Older children often tell younger siblings, but all may still need emotional support from carers and/or counsellors.

Any emotional problem at home can cause major behavioural problems at school. One boy, playing up at school, did not want to be there, but with his dying parent at home. Teachers should be kept informed of such major life-crises in the homes of their pupils. Children are imaginative creatures and it is better to tell them the truth gently than to let them imagine what is happening for themselves.

Children are also startlingly frank with their questions, which may upset carers. On being told, 'Mummy is very ill', a child is likely to ask, 'Will she die?' This can be answered truthfully by saying that the doctors are doing all they can for her, but they may not be able to make her better. Counsellors can prepare carers with such possible dialogue before they speak to the children. Parents can only be advised to tell their children. If they are adamantly opposed to this, there is nothing else to be done, except to be available if needed.

Conclusions

Not all counsellors have the temperament to stay alongside the dying, sharing the feeling of helplessness felt in the face of death. Poignant counselling situations are those where the dying patient is the age of one's spouse, child, parent or friend. It is a reminder of how precious are one's own relationships; how no one knows when death will come; how every day must be lived fully as if the last. Counsellors have to travel along a tightrope of avoiding not only overinvolvement, but also cold detachment, for to see a patient only as a sickness and not as a person who happens to be sick is dehumanizing. People never lose the need for warmth and affection, the need to care about others and be cared about. As in all counselling, some patients may feel better able to face what is happening to them after a short counselling intervention, others may need more support, right up until the moment of death. Experience will show the counsellor what is right in each circumstance, but much will depend on the strength of the patient's own support system.

Even though death is seen by many to be a sad subject, giving cause for wonder at how anyone could work with the dying all day, every day, it has much to give counsellors. It is a privilege to be entrusted with patients' inner feelings, fears and hopes, and to be allowed to offer guidance and support at this time; helping them maintain some sense of their own value and individuality. This reinforces that they are valued for themselves and for their unique contribution to the life they have made for themselves and for those connected with them.

References

Buckman, R. (2000) Communication in palliative care: a practical guide. In *Death, Dying and Bereavement* (Dickinson, D., Johnson, M. and Katz, J.S., eds). Sage, London.

Dryden, W., Charles-Edwards, D. and Woolfe, R. (eds) (1989) *Handbook of Counselling in Britain.* Tavistock/Routledge, London.

Kubler-Ross, E. (1969) *On Death and Dying.* Tavistock Publications, London.

Macleod, R. (2000) Learning to care: a medical perspective. *Palliative Medicine*, 114, 209–216.

Peberdy, A. (2000) Spiritual care of dying people. In *Death, Dying and Bereavement* (Dickinson, D., Johnson, M. and Katz, J.S., eds). Sage, London.

Smith, C.R. (1990) *Social Work with the Dying and Bereaved.* Macmillan Education, London.

Spilling, R. (ed.) (1986) *Terminal Care at Home.* Oxford University Press, Oxford.

Chapter 19

Bereavement

Sheila Thompson

A hazard not an illness, bereavement comes to us all

Attachment and loss are paired together. Bowlby (1967, 1980), drawing widely upon animal ethnology as well as upon a range of studies of human development, has shown that as strong attachments between mother figure and infant, and also between mating couples, have been necessary for the evolution and preservation of human and more evolved animal life, so threats to these bonds produce intense anxiety and there are strong and painful reactions to their severance. However, parents and offspring do eventually have to separate and in almost every attached couple one survivor is left. As we have the capacity, vital to our survival, to make attachments, so we have the capacity to survive when they come to an end.

But on the other hand, and it is a big 'other hand', unresolved bereavement is now recognized as a major health hazard. Although it is difficult to demonstrate a clear and direct link between an illness or disturbance and any one precipitating factor, considerable evidence has been accumulated about the risks bereavement can bring to mental and physical health. It has been shown to lead to psychiatric illness (Bowlby 1980) and also to impaired physical health (Parkes *et al.* 1969; Stroebe *et al.* 1993) and, at every age, to higher mortality and suicide rates (Smith 1978). It was Caplan (1964) who first brought bereavement within the area of primary preventive care, including it among the crises which come to disrupt established coping mechanisms and force change not only in outer circumstances but throughout the inner worlds of the people involved.

There is also an accumulating body of evidence, despite the difficulty of precise measurement, that skilled bereavement counselling can significantly improve the outcome, in particular if introduced early and promptly for individuals considered at high risk (see Raphael 1984; Parkes 1988; Stroebe *et al.* 1993). It so happens that widows have been the group most investigated and, specifically, it has been found that widows receiving counselling show a significantly lower incidence of such symptoms as sleeplessness, back pain, panic, poor appetite, excessive tiredness and weight loss, as well as less smoking, drinking, tablet taking and depression, and fewer visits to the doctor's surgery (Raphael 1977). There are therefore clear implications for primary health services.

Assessing the risk

Many people come through bereavement safely with no wish or need for counselling help. The support and understanding they require comes through the responses of friends and family and such members of the health and community services with whom they are already in contact. Some of the factors that help or hinder this process can be identified through the following questions that draw attention to those likely to be at greater risk.

What social support network is available?

Are there close family ties, family members near at hand and supportive friends and neighbours? The dispersal and geographical separation of the extended family can leave many people isolated.

The support a family provides may be insufficient. People grieve at different rates, and even if there is a family presence the slow mourner may find that other family members who are through their mourning become impatient. Social networks can also fail to respond; friends and neighbours may withdraw, or may even stay to hinder the grief work because of their own incompletely resolved losses.

Was the death timely and generationally appropriate?

Deaths of old people are anticipated and adult children expect to have to mourn their parents. Problems are compounded when the death seems untimely, if a young marriage partner dies or if parents lose a child.

Was the death expected, providing an opportunity to prepare for it?

If death is anticipated and the survivors are prepared, much of the grief work can be done in advance. Deaths that are sudden, violent or unanticipated can leave behind an additional legacy of fear, blaming, regrets and greater existential insecurity, with a stronger feeling of vulnerability and of the fragility of life.

What was the nature of the relationship with the dead person?

An unequal relationship with exceptional dependence on one side, or an ambivalent relationship, are among the pointers to a difficult bereavement. The more mature and better founded the relationship and the fewer regrets about unfinished business that remain, the easier it is to let go.

How open was communication at the end?

Experience in terminal care teams has shown that if family members are able to share with the dying person the knowledge that the situation is serious and death a likely or inevitable outcome, they will find it easier to let him or her go after death. The fears and fantasies about death itself, about what the dying person may have been experiencing, and any guilt at being the survivor, seem to be reduced. Counselling can with advantage begin at this stage.

What losses has the bereaved person sustained in the past, and how were they resolved?

Poorly resolved losses from the past will be recalled to add their load on top of the grief of the present and interfere with its expression. Losses encountered early in life, losses that brought deprivation and losses inadequately mourned, make people less resilient and less able to trust in the help that others can offer.

Is there any history of depressive episodes?

Depression is an expected feature of bereavement but a feature that is expected to pass. It can become intractable if loaded onto a more chronic depression from the past.

Are there any concurrent stresses?

Illness, another recent bereavement, financial worries perhaps caused by the death of the breadwinner, or any other difficult circumstances, can further deplete reduced resources and delay the completion of mourning.

Is this a death by suicide?

The stigma and taboo of suicide can cut off survivors from their community and the usual sources of help and leave them particularly isolated and at risk. There is also the possibility of pre-existing family disturbance requiring more specialist treatment.

Bringing together many of the above pointers, Parkes (1972) has identified as being at particular risk the young widow with dependent children and without other relatives nearby, now financially insecure and ill-equipped to manage on her own, with a strained marital relationship in the past, difficulty in expressing her feelings and a history of depressive episodes.

In contrast, Skynner (1976) quotes research into so-called 'exceptionally healthy families' characterized by open communication and flexible relationships, showing that such families have an enhanced ability to cope with change and loss of all kinds, including even the death of close family members.

Counselling the bereaved

The way in which grief is experienced, expressed and resolved depends upon the social context. Mourning is shaped by cultural and social expectations, and the process is promoted or hindered by the feedback and reactions received. With bereavement counselling we enter the social context in order to influence and augment it, introducing feedback and reactions that are deliberate, focused and skilled.

Care needs to be taken to ensure that this intervention is not allowed to replace or discourage other existing relationships. The risk of this was brought home by the comment of one family member: 'We are so glad that the bereavement counsellor has taken on mother. We were all finding it a strain to have to do so much visiting ourselves'.

Bereavement counselling requires an understanding of the circumstances of the loss, of the nature of the relationship that has been lost, and of the sources of the bereaved person's response. It includes the following factors: the provision of a safe relationship; the concept of normality; facilitation of the mourning process; and monitoring of the progress.

The safe relationship is a relationship with someone not personally caught up in the grief, who will not withdraw or criticize or try to cut short the mourning process, with whom all the overwhelming, conflicting and perhaps seemingly unacceptable feelings can find expression and be safely contained. It is a relationship with someone familiar with the grief process who accepts its normality among the apparent abnormality and who understands that mourning is a process of recovery. Like adolescence, another time when bonds are being severed, apparently abnormal patterns of behaviour can be accepted as transient phenomena within this framework.

Facilitation supports and eases the bereaved person through the tasks and difficulties of each stage of mourning. Monitoring identifies any areas where more intensive help may be needed.

The bereavement process

Process implies progression, and this progression can for our convenience be divided into stages. But this framework has to be used with great caution—it is an artificial simplification of a complex and confused experience. And we should, as Feifel (1988) has warned, 'beware of promulgating a coercive orthodoxy of how to mourn'.

Following Worden (1991), four developmental phases or stages can be postulated. There is the stage of taking in what has happened; of experiencing all the pain of the loss; of adjusting to the changed circumstances; and finally of taking up life again without the person who has died. The grieving process can become arrested at any of these stages.

According to this model, there are tasks for the bereaved person at each stage which have to be mastered in an approximate order and which in turn indicate tasks for the bereavement counsellor.

The first stage

First there may be feelings of numbness, disorganization and helplessness, and then of disbelief and denial. Even with an expected death, the reality of the dead person's presence can be felt so strongly that it over-rides the knowledge of the death. There may be an apparent searching for the lost person, in the way that migrant birds have been observed to search for a lost mate. This activity appears to be a biological response, necessary when the loss is assumed to be retrievable. It can also be understood as an attempt to make the unmanageable manageable, to force a postponement of the full realization of what has happened. It is a delaying tactic, a managing tactic, a brake that some survivors need to apply in order to slow down the process and bring it within their capacity to absorb shock and change.

Occasionally, the survivor may find it hard to accept that the loss has occurred at all, particularly if there has been no opportunity to view the body and dispose of it with funeral rituals.

The task of the counsellor is to support and help the bereaved person through this process of becoming aware of the loss, representing reality and discouraging evasion, but always keeping within the bereaved person's current capacity. The counsellor may need to ask specific and detailed questions about the death and the funeral, avoiding euphemisms, helping the survivor to recall and understand that the dead person has gone and can never return. Bereaved people, particularly if they perceive themselves abandoned and unsupported, may try to remain at this stage, resisting the realization of what has happened and its consequences for fear of a full understanding of the loss from which there is no going back.

During this time the presence of two contradictory ideas competing in the survivor's mind, that X is dead and that X cannot be dead, can bring instability and a fear of madness. The counsellor may have to provide reassurance that the bereaved person is not going mad.

The second stage

Stage two begins with the full realization of the loss and its permanence. X is dead and will never return. The depressed feelings that are a feature throughout the mourning process are at their most acute now. This can be a period of intense despair and pining. The survivor may withdraw his or her energy from daily life and devote it to the contemplation of the loss. There may be a persistent preoccupation with memories of the dead person and their life together in which each segment of this life has to be retrieved and recollected.

The grief has a purpose. Only through this activity can the bereaved person achieve sufficient mastery of what has happened to make it possible to let the acute grief go and regain personal autonomy and independence. Before this can happen, the internal mental image of the dead person and of their relationship has to be reformed to include the fact that he or she has died.

Where the identification has been close, the survivor may struggle to preserve the continuing presence of the dead person within. This may lead to attempts to replicate outward characteristics, sometimes even symptoms of the last illness. What is feared is the extinction of the parts of the self that were invested in the dead person. The survivor may need help to go over the past and identify all the aims and ideals that were shared so that they can now be freed from any exclusive attachment to the dead person and can be retained to become part of the life ahead.

With the pining comes other complex feelings: anger, guilt, anxiety, fear and self-reproach. These feelings may be less acceptable than grief and difficult to express and share with others. But if they not identified and acknowledged they are likely to persevere to delay the mourning process and go on to interfere and distort relationships in the future. Any irrational components of these feelings need to be recognized and discarded as more accurate perceptions of reality return.

Anger appears to be felt by a majority of bereaved people, sometimes in intense outbursts, sometimes as a more prolonged bitterness. Anger as a response to feeling abandoned by the dead person may be too painful to be experienced directly and so is turned into anger towards others, towards medical staff for instance. It can also be directed towards the self as self-blaming, bringing lowered self-esteem, depression or even suicidal thoughts.

Acute anxiety and fear may also be felt. When a major component of personal safety and security is lost there can be a heightened awareness of personal mortality and fears for other members of the family. Memories of being lost and unsupported as a child may be revived. If bereaved people can now find access to the sources of these feelings they may be able to reduce their impact through talking them over with a counsellor.

Guilt is also a feature of mourning. Even being the survivor can be a source of guilt. Reproaches, with the memory of things said and done, or not said and done, are left as a residue even when relationships have been happy. A long illness, the burden of caring, may have brought a wish that it could soon be over. The counsellor needs to emphasize the inevitability of such wishes, representing reality and bringing back reminders of care that was given and efforts that were made, acknowledging the fact that all relationships have their ambivalence and that not everything that has been lost will be missed.

Some counsellors may encourage their patients to say or write all the things that they wished they could have said to the dead person if the pressure of unfinished business is making it hard to move on. However, it is important to avoid ending such activities on a new negative note, to maintain a balance and to recognize that good and bad feelings are a part of all relationships.

If feelings of guilt and depression remain at an intense level, the counsellor may need to ask if the survivor has ever thought of harming him or herself, enquiring about thoughts rather than intentions. When such thoughts can be shared and accepted they lose some of their force and the sense of isolation is reduced.

The grief may never be given up altogether, sadness may continue, but there comes a time when the sadness no longer dominates and the establishment of a new equilibrium becomes possible.

How long does this stage last? One answer is 'as long as it takes', and it is important that the bereaved person be allowed the time required. But even so there comes a point when this stage needs to end.

The third stage

Even though some sadness remains, the emotional energy that has been absorbed in dealing with the grief needs to be released now to tackle the more practical tasks of readjustment. The woman who has been X's wife has to establish her new position as X's widow with a new role and a different place in society and in her family. There may have to be a reallocation of roles and responsibilities. The spouse who has gone may have been breadwinner, tennis partner, chauffeur, gardener, cook, family disciplinarian, etc. and adjustments will have to be made to fill the gaps.

The bereaved person may have been permitted or encouraged to regress during the period of intense grieving and now the task of the counsellor is to ease return to daily living. The loss may have depleted existing resources and help may be needed in regaining confidence, negotiating a new reality, acquiring new skills and taking on new responsibilities. Where grieving is seen as a duty to the dead, the counsellor may have to support the idea that the duty has been completed.

Difficulties at this stage appear in a failure to adjust to the new circumstances and in a prolongation of helplessness and dependency after the period of acute grief has passed.

The fourth stage

Now comes the stage when the bereaved person takes up life again, with energy available once more to be reinvested in other activities and other relationships. Patterns of sleep, appetite and energy should have been restored, and sexual feelings, if lost, return. Help may still be needed to support this new life and provide confirmation that it is acceptable to find enjoyment and fulfilment in relationships and activities that the dead person will never know.

In the recent past there has been much stress on the need to abandon relationships with the dead in order to move on, perhaps in a reaction against Victorian models of perpetual mourning, perhaps in response to social changes that place a greater value upon personal autonomy and economic efficiency. Now new shifts in thinking are acknowledging once more the existence of continuing bonds between the living and the dead that can be integrated into the new life and, given sufficient progress through earlier stages of the grieving process, can play a rich and valuable part in it. The purpose of the grieving process, then, becomes not so much the severance of bonds with the dead person as their absorption into the life that lies ahead (Walter 1999).

Family counselling

Most discussions of bereavement counselling focus upon the needs of the single individual. However, bereavement is a family event and often plays an important part in family development. Even when bereavement counselling is sought for one family member there may well be others at risk. The bereavement counsellor needs to have an awareness of the family as a system in which the different members interact and in which the loss of one influences each of the others through its impact upon the system as a whole. Who has gone? What gap has been left within the family? How are the family members communicating with each other about the loss?

Different family members grieve and recover at different speeds. There may be frustrations with the ones left behind who threaten the recovery of the whole. There may be anxiety about the health of other family members as security has been shaken and personal vulnerabilities exposed.

Families appear to deal best with crises if there is open communication and flexible boundaries, if members can move towards each other and change and adapt their roles within the family. Families, like individuals, that are more rigid and struggle to remain unchanged, tend to deny the loss and fail to grieve adequately. An attempt to preserve those qualities of the dead person that were important to the family may bring unrealistic and burdensome expectations of others; a junior family member, for example, may be expected to show some of the characteristics of a dead parent or sibling; a surviving parent may impose unrealistic tasks upon him or herself, or have them imposed by others.

The counsellor who is seeing one family member needs to make a point of enquiring about the others, noting who is, and who is not, being mentioned, and looking to see if there is need and opportunity to bring them all together and facilitate a discussion in which they can share their feelings about the loss and mobilize additional family resources.

Children

Children need special consideration. Studies of the effects of bereavements in childhood were summarized by Black (1978) and the importance of informed adult responses has been underlined by Smith and Pennells (1996).

Bereavement counsellors are frequently asked what the children should be told and when and how this should be done. All the considerations that apply to helping the adult bereaved apply with equal force to children. Children also need to comprehend what has happened and to have opportunities to express all the complex feelings involved, even though their intellectual understanding of death and finality may not be complete.

There are, however, added considerations. With less maturity and experience, children have less capacity to bear concentrated pain and the younger they are the longer it will take for them to absorb what has happened and to realize that it is irreversible. The process may not be completed for years, perhaps not until they are grown up themselves. Adults responsible for children can help by keeping memories and feelings alive and accessible, so that the children can continue to work on them as and when they are able to. This does not always happen. The bereavement may be complicated by concealment or evasion, as adults strive to protect the children, or to protect themselves from exposure to the children's grief. It is in these circumstances that adults will sometimes report that the children do not seem to have been very affected, even by the loss of a parent or sibling.

On one such occasion a counsellor, told by the adults that the children were unaffected by a family tragedy and going to check this out, found them repeatedly playing funerals. When this was pointed out to the parents they began to talk to the children for the first time about the death of their baby. Through this they were able to start expressing their own feelings which had been blocked by the efforts they had been making to shield the children from awareness of their grief.

It seems desirable for the adults to be as open and frank with the children as they can, not excluding them from family discussions and explanations, offering them— with appropriate preparation—an opportunity to go to the funeral. Children too need to say goodbye.

Secrets in the family are considered to do more harm than the truth can ever do; and when children are supported by adults whom they trust they are better able to deal with reality, however upsetting, than with the misconceptions and misunderstandings that may otherwise remain (Pincus & Dare 1978).

Help for children should come, if possible, from those adults who are close to them rather than from a stranger. The adults, involved in their own grief, may have difficulties in finding the words to use and it may be helpful for a counsellor to talk to the adults about the event, using simple words and images that they can then use themselves with their children.

Teenagers

Teenagers also need special consideration. The death of a parent may come at a time of great ambivalence when teenagers are beginning to pull away from the family.

One 15-year-old boy avoided his mother's sick room because he found the details of her last illness intolerable and took little part in her care. After her death he was blamed for being uncaring and his isolation from the rest of the family intensified. Only after the counsellor had made a prolonged and ultimately successful effort to have him included in family discussions was he able to reveal and share his grief.

How long should bereavement counselling last?

Concentrated work may be needed for a few weeks or a few months. Less concentrated involvement may then need to continue, with the contact being kept open. There are identifiable landmarks—the first Christmas, the anniversary of the death, birthdays and important family events—when vulnerability may temporarily increase and it may be necessary to counsel in advance that these may be difficult times.

Other significant losses

Bereavement does not always involve loss by death. The process of loss is the same whether the loss is of parent or spouse, cat or dog, breast or limb, a loss of abilities and valued functions, or any other loss that impinges upon the security of the person and their conception of self.

The intensity and duration, the significance and impact, of these events may vary greatly but the process still passes from loss through recognizable stages to recovery. The amputee has to realize what has happened and then identify and mourn what has been lost, experiencing a complicated range of emotions before he or she can find the inner resources to adjust. Any counsellor involved will have to bear in mind all the considerations already discussed.

There are also the losses where accident or illness drastically alters a relationship although the loved one survives physically. The relatives of a head-injured patient, for example, also need to 'know and name and express the pain' (Raphael 1984). To do this they have to separate out what has been lost from what still survives so that they can mourn those aspects of the relationship and of their future hopes that have been taken away while they continue to hold on to what remains. This complicated process may have to take place surrounded by medical staff who are maintaining an atmosphere of bright optimism at every tiny gain and inviting the family to share in this, leaving little room for expression of the intense grief the family is feeling. 'For the family there is no final resolution. The person, as they knew him or her before, is no longer there ... There is a paradox of coping with the horrors of head injury and at the same time being grateful that the person is alive' (Williams & Kay 1991).

Grief that fails to resolve

If a survivor is not responding to bereavement counselling, then the counsellor will need to identify the stage at which he or she remains fixed and focus more narrowly and more intently. If the grieving still persists, the problem may extend beyond the immediate circumstances of the bereavement. Bereavement is a receptacle for disturbances of all kinds and other difficulties may have become attached to it. Caplan (1964) noted that during crises old problems in some way linked to the present problem can be reactivated to constitute an additional burden if not satisfactorily dealt with in the past.

Case history 1

Mrs A was still in black two years after her husband's death and making a three-hour bus journey every week to visit the grave. Enquiry revealed that Mr A had been an only child, and that his widowed mother was still actively grieving too. It gradually became clear in counselling that the two women had always competed for Mr A's attention and that now neither was prepared to relinquish the role of principal mourner. After they were seen together and the counselling shifted to the relationship between the two of them, the older woman was able to take the lead in moving on.

Case history 2

Mrs C was overwhelmed with anxiety and phobic fears after her husband's death and after some months was still unable to leave her flat. In counselling she recalled the mysterious disappearance and death of her twin sister when she was six, never explained, and the panic attacks she had suffered prior to her marriage. These symptoms had now returned in an acute form. In this case bereavement counselling was not considered sufficient to address deep-seated problems now brought back into the open and she was referred for psychiatric help.

Case history 3

Mrs F asked for help more than a year after the death of her mother, complaining of restlessness, inability to concentrate, and pains in her hands and wrists. It transpired that she had had an acute grief reaction to the death of her father 12 years earlier and her family had arranged for her to see a psychiatrist at that time. Prescribed tranquillizers by the psychiatrist, she subsequently had a difficult time weaning herself from them, and she considered that they had done her a lot of harm. After her mother's death she was afraid to express her grief directly for fear that her family would once more treat her as mad. In counselling it was necessary to go back through the mourning process for both her parents, but it was equally important to work through her anger with her family and her fears of madness or of being perceived as mad. After eight one-hour sessions she reported that the immediate symptoms were much reduced and family relationships had improved. The way was left open for her to return if she needed to.

Who provides bereavement counselling?

Bereavement counselling is now offered by specialist hospice and terminal care teams, by some hospitals, and also by community-based bereavement services. The counsellors may be specialist bereavement counsellors or trained volunteers. Increasingly, bereavement counselling is being provided by the traditional caring professions who have extended their work to include this area.

The primary health care services

The question for the family doctor and the practice team is not so much whether to become involved in bereavement care as how far the involvement should go. Should formal bereavement counselling be included within the work of the team, and at what stage should there be a hand-over to specialist services? The case for keeping bereavement counselling within the traditional professions, for not treating it as a pathology requiring a specialist service, has been argued by Reilly (1978) and endorsed by Worden (1991). If the first need of the bereaved is for a supportive network, including a broadly based facilitating response, then the caring professions have a responsibility not only to respond themselves in an informed way but also to promote this response in the community at large. They are the pace setters. The message given when bereavement is passed over to others by the primary services could be seen as a counterpart to the message given by the neighbour who crosses the road to avoid talking to someone recently bereaved. Moreover, bereavement is a time when consistency, familiarity and continuity of past, present and future life is important, when a known and trusted source of help is likely to be preferred to an unknown specialist service. The counselling should be readily accessible at any point during a bereavement process which may be of long duration, difficult to fit within a timeframe, and in which symptoms may appear or reappear after an interval or be activated or reactivated by subsequent events.

Bereavement is a time when general health may deteriorate and more frequent visits made to doctor's surgeries. The symptoms identified by Parkes and Raphael as responding to counselling were largely physical symptoms. The ability to eliminate specific disease, or access to those who can, may be important. The counselling should take place in a context that makes it possible to include other family members where this seems appropriate.

If counselling is to be offered within the general practitioner services, who should provide it? There are several possibilities. A specialist counsellor may be recruited to join the team and work within its shared experience and authority. Alternatively, or in addition, an existing member of the team could be designated to provide counselling as their primary function, or one or more team members could undertake it as an extension of existing practice. Alternatively, counselling could be a shared responsibility of the team as a whole with a specialist counsellor available for consultation.

Additional training may be needed. Bereavement counselling has its own knowledge and skills and brings us into an area in which we are required to make use of the self in a disciplined way, dismantling or reducing the defences that we all (professionals and non-professionals alike) use to protect ourselves against the misery of others. Training sessions in bereavement counselling habitually have a large experiential content in which participants are given the opportunity to explore personal attitudes to loss.

Some of the implications of extending the practice of counselling was considered by a home care team attached to a hospice. Bereavement counselling was at first undertaken by social workers, who had had specific training. This was then extended at the team's request to include nurses and doctors as well so that the bereavement counselling could be seen as an extension of the terminal care in which all were involved, continuity could be preserved, and opportunities for professional and team development increased. Consultation with colleagues was always available and resources shared, and all bereavement cases were regularly reviewed at meetings of the whole team.

This change brought the question of professional boundaries to the fore. Some knowledge is specific to a particular profession, but in addition each professional worker also draws upon a wide area of knowledge that is shared with others and in which some other profession may have primacy.

To carry work deliberately into this shared area, and to learn from colleagues of other disciplines, requires a confidence from each worker in his or her own professional identity and area of exclusive knowledge. It is only when secure within one's own traditional boundaries, and secure in the knowledge that colleagues of other disciplines know and respect these boundaries, that one can risk 'crossing the frontiers of professional practice' (Thompson 1999).

Such developments within and between disciplines, including the growth of multidisciplinary teams, can be related to the adoption of open systems concepts in the place of the static closed systems thinking of the past. Formerly, as Skynner (1976) has described, training was considered to have been completed when 'enough' knowledge had been acquired, after which the worker would remain within his or her boundaries and try to protect them from disturbing change. However, we now think in terms of more open systems and more permeable boundaries that permit the constant intrusion of information from outside. The task now is to make selective use of what comes in without being swamped by it, and to preserve stability in conditions of confrontation, challenge and feedback unknown in the past.

Supervision

This leads on to the final point, the need for on-going supervision (consultation may be a preferred term for a process which need carry no hierarchical implications and which is largely concerned with the pooling of resources and the sharing of knowledge and skills). Counselling shares an area of professional work with psychotherapy and social work in which such supervision is considered a necessary and valuable resource and protection.

There are a number of models. There could be supervision with a specialist supervisor, with a senior colleague in the same discipline, or with a member of another discipline who happens to be experienced in this area. It could be group supervision or peer group supervision in which some may have more experience than others, and with or without the presence of a group facilitator.

Supervision/consultation recognizes that the observer often sees more of the game, and that it is possible to become lost in the counselling maze. As bereaved people use their counsellor not only to help them through the mourning process but also as a reference point outside it, so too the counsellors themselves gain through an opportunity to discuss the problems encountered with someone who can also provide an outside reference point.

Conclusions

We have discussed the task and process of bereavement counselling within the context of primary health care. It can be argued that this is where it most appropriately belongs. It is to the general practitioner and the primary health care team that patients in need come, and it is here that many patients find their first and only resource.

This is despite the fact that in many ways it is hard to place bereavement within the traditional medical model. We are dealing with the destabilization of interpersonal relationships with potential long-term consequences, and with the search for a new stability that can only be facilitated through interaction with others. Outcome is hard to evaluate beyond the short-term relief of symptoms.

Whatever model is used, the members of the team will continue to confront the short- and long-term consequences of bereavement and loss in their daily work. The need for an informed recognition and response remains. This response will be facilitated in teams which give bereavement a higher profile through the addition of structured bereavement counselling and the availability of a trained counsellor. The additional facility for patients can also be a resource for the whole team.

References

Black, D. (1978) The bereaved child. *Journal of Child Psychology and Psychiatry*, **19**, 287–292.

Bowlby, J. (1967) *Attachment and Loss. 1. Attachment.* Hogarth Press, London.

Bowly, J. (1980) *Attachment and Loss. 3. Sadness and Depression.* Hogarth Press, London.

Caplan, G. (1964) *Principles of Preventive Psychiatry.* Tavistock, London.

Feifel, H. (1988) Grief and bereavement: overview and perspective. In *Grief and Bereavement in Contemporary Society*, Vol. 1 (Chigier, E., ed.). Freund Publishing House, London, p. 5.

Parkes, C.M. (1972) *Bereavement Studies of Grief in Adult Life.* Penguin, Harmondsworth.

Parkes, C.M. (1988) Can we predict outcome after bereavement? In *Grief and Bereavement in Contemporary Society*, Vol. 1 (Chigier, E., ed.). Freund Publishing House, London, pp. 125–133.

Parkes, C.M., Benjamin, B. and Fitzgerald, R.G. (1969) Broken hearts, a statistical study of increased mortality among widowers. *British Medical Journal*, **1**, 240–243.

Pincus, L. and Dare, C. (1978) *Secrets in the Family.* Faber & Faber, London.

Raphael, B. (1977) Preventive intervention with the bereaved. *Archives of General Psychiatry*, **34**, 1450–1454.

Raphael, B. (1984) *The Anatomy of Bereavement.* Hutchinson, London.

Reilly, D. (1978) Death propensity, dying and bereavement: a family system perspective. *Family Therapy*, **5**, 35–55.

Skynner, A.C.R. (1976) *One Flesh: Separate Persons.* Constable, London.

Smith, K. (1978) *Help for the Bereaved.* Duckworth, London.

Smith, S. and Pennells, M. (eds) (1996) *Interventions with Bereaved Children.* Jessica Kingsley, London.

Stroebe, M., Stroebe, W. and Hansson, R.O. (eds) (1993) *Handbook of Bereavement.* Cambridge University Press, New York.

Thompson, S. (1999) *The Group Context.* Jessica Kingsley, London.

Walter, T. (1999) *On Bereavement: the Culture of Grief.* Open University Press, Buckingham.

Williams, J.M. and Kay, T. (1991) *Head Injury: a Family Matter.* Paul H. Brooker, Baltimore.

Worden, J.W. (1991) *Grief Counselling and Grief Therapy.* Routledge, London.

Part 4

Conclusions

Chapter 20

Conclusions

Jane Keithley, Tim Bond, and Geoffrey Marsh

Introduction

Primary care is at the forefront of health care provision in the UK. It is primary care that responds to the vast majority of health problems that individuals bring to the NHS. It follows that as counselling plays a larger role in health care, one of the key locations of counselling services will be in general practices. As more and more of the counselling workforce is employed in the NHS, many of the central counselling debates have become debates about counselling in primary care. A recent issue of the *British Journal of Guidance and Counselling* (edited by Mellor-Clark 2000) was devoted to discussing aspects of this counselling 'specialism'. The medical profession has also demonstrated a continuing interest in the relationships between counselling and health care, with a steady stream of articles and editorials in the major journals, including the recent articles in the *British Medical Journal* referred to below (Bower *et al.* 2000; Ward *et al.* 2000).

Our aim in this book has been to inform, to encourage reflection and to stimulate debate in this field. As readers will have recognized, we do not attempt to produce simple answers, nor even a consensus of opinion; none exist. The commissioners of primary care services are faced with difficult decisions about the allocation of scarce resources to counselling. Those who are at the forefront of providing such care face dilemmas about the best way to respond to the many individuals who seek help from the primary health care team (PHCT) with their psychological and relationship problems. Both need to be aware of the current range of thinking in this field.

We have produced a book that is intentionally diverse in style and content, intending to convey the variety of views and perspectives that exist. Our authors have discussed the range of contributions that counsellors can make to primary health care and the practical and philosophical issues that can arise and need attention. Many of our authors are actively involved in this field and most are supportive of such services, but we have also included some with substantial reservations. It is thus not an easy task to summarize our conclusions. However, we shall attempt to draw out some of the themes that run through many of the separate chapters of the book, relating to the current state of counselling in primary care, together with some of the factors that are likely to shape its future development.

In the early years of the twenty-first century, counselling in primary care finds itself at a watershed. It is more widely available than ever before, yet more challenged, perceived as under threat in a number of ways and insecure about its future. In line with developments in counselling more generally, its practitioners are becoming more 'professionalized', yet in primary care they are also more 'managed' and fearful of losing their autonomy. Some of the major questions that face primary care counselling are about coping with the seemingly infinite demand; deciding what works; how to ensure the quality of counsellors; and the implications of the new structures for delivering primary care.

Coping with the 'bottomless pit'

As this book makes clear, the potential demand for counselling is huge. The 1999 National Service Framework for Mental Health recognized that nine out of 10 of the large number of individuals with mental health problems are treated by GPs and other PHCT members (Department of Health 1999). Our authors have indicated the wide range of other problems of living for which counselling help could be appropriate, ranging from substance misuse to relationship problems, fertility to bereavement. No wonder some GPs talk anxiously about 'Pandora's box' and 'bottomless pits'!

GPs are the main gatekeepers to counselling in primary care, as well as to other specialist counselling services. During the 1990s, while some practices have expanded their counselling provision, others have had none at all. The increased emphasis on equity and on the elimination of 'postcode medicine' in recent years is likely to mean access for more patients to primary care counselling. A scarce resource will become even more thinly stretched. GPs will thus have to consider even more carefully who needs that resource and how much of it they need. Effective 'filtering' by GPs and others who can refer to counselling has two requirements. Firstly, there is a need for adequate knowledge on the part of the PHCT of what counselling might be able to offer for whom, in what circumstances and, just as importantly, when it unlikely to be helpful. This understanding of counselling also needs to be effectively communicated to patients. Secondly, GPs and their primary care colleagues need to make maximum use of the counselling or 'listening' skills they have, or could acquire. We would suggest that they can provide help and support to a large number of patients with emotional, psychological and/or relationship difficulties for whom counselling is unavailable and/or unnecessary, even within the confines of a short consultation. The value of this to patients is emphasized in a recent 'endpiece' in the *British Medical Journal*:

> Because the doctors cared, and because one of them still believed in me when I believed in nothing, I have survived to tell the tale ... To sit quietly in a consulting room and talk to someone would not appear to the general public as a heroic or dramatic thing to do. In medicine there are many different ways of saving lives. This is one of them (Coate 1964, cited in *British Medical Journal* 2001).

Just being there and listening, whilst someone for whom they care struggles to express their difficulties—frequently not of a 'medical' nature, but of great significance for their health—is what a sensitive GP can provide. It is all that many patients need and it is not unreasonable for them to expect this from their own doctor.

It may be helpful in this respect to think of counsellors in primary care as a secondary, specialist service. As is the case in relation to other aspects of health care, the

PHCT itself does and should have the ability and confidence to respond to all but a very small proportion of problems.

Does counselling work?

Perhaps the most long-standing of the challenges to counselling relates to the effectiveness of counselling. The answer to the question of whether it works is still fiercely contested. Historically, as we have seen, the tendency has been for more qualitative studies and those that focus on user views to produce favourable results, while studies that have used more controlled, experimental research designs, such as randomized controlled trials (RCTs), have often had more negative findings. In an era when evidence-based health care is founded on the assumption that the RCT is the 'gold standard', this poses difficulties for counselling. In relation to primary care, it has been suggested that a combination of scepticism about the effectiveness of counselling with an increasing emphasis on the acquisition of counselling skills by GPs and nurses could lead to the disappearance of specific counselling services in this setting altogether (Eatock 2000). This may be an unduly pessimistic speculation. There is early evidence that the trend in research findings about counselling effectiveness are becoming more positive. In some cases this may be due to refinements in the research design as experience accumulates in addressing the difficulties of researching this subject. Early studies were often vulnerable to the criticism that they were undiscriminating in what they considered to be counselling. The professionalization of counselling has made it easier for researchers to focus their studies on practitioners who are credibly identifiable as counsellors. The improvement in identification of the provision of counselling has enabled comparative studies between the efficacy of different types of service provision. King and his colleagues have done a great deal to refine the application of RCTs to this kind of research question. One of the findings from this process is a recognition of how hard it is to evaluate whether counselling is more effective than other interventions such as cognitive behaviour therapy, GP care or antidepressants prescribed to treat depression (Friedl *et al.* 1997).

One response has been to suggest that more complicated questions need to be asked about what works, for whom, in what circumstances. However, a recent study (too recent to be taken into account by our authors) published in the *British Medical Journal* (Bower *et al.* 2000; Ward *et al.* 2000) also draws some interesting conclusions and deserves attention. Based on an RCT of non-directive counselling, cognitive behaviour therapy and usual GP care for depression, the authors found that the two psychological therapies were more effective than usual GP care in the short term, but after one year there was no difference in outcome. A parallel cost-effectiveness study also showed significant short-term benefits in using the psychological therapies, but no differences after one year. In addition, they concluded, unlike some other studies, that there was no significant difference between the two types of psychological therapy. Perhaps most interesting of all was the overall conclusion that the researchers drew from these results. They suggested that, on this evidence, commissioners of services, such as primary care organizations, should consider making their decisions on factors other than outcomes and costs, such as staff and patient preferences or the availability of particular kinds of staff. The future of counselling in primary care could in the end rest on how much people like it. Given the high rates of reported demand and satisfaction, this is good news for counsellors and perhaps for users too!

If one looks beyond the application of RCTs to other types of research there is compelling evidence that personal experience is consistent with claims that counselling is effective. A large-scale survey in the United States, undertaken by the equivalent to our Consumers Association, analysed the experience from 2900 respondents who had received counselling or psychotherapy services from the following: psychologists (37%), psychiatrists (22%), social workers (14%) and marriage counsellors (9%). About 1000 saw their family doctor. The respondents were evenly divided between male and female with a median age of 46 years and usually well educated and middle class. The findings have had a significant impact on service provision and research in the USA. Notwithstanding the difficulties of transferring the findings across different patterns of service provision and culture, this study deserves more attention than it usually receives in the UK. It found that most groups of professional providers were equally effective although marriage counsellors and family doctors were much less effective. The level of benefit that individuals attributed to their therapy corresponded to their degree of choice over their selection of therapist and the duration of their therapy. Freedom of choice and a lack of restrictions on length of time increased perceived effectiveness. The report concluded that patients benefited very substantially from counselling and psychotherapy. The author also argues for the value of a dual-pronged approach to studying effectiveness that takes account of both RCTs and this type of rigorously analysed survey evidence (Seligman 1995).

A systematic review of brief psychological therapies in primary care presents a convincing case for the need for great care in interpreting the evidence of the value of all psychological therapies (Hemmings 1999). The author directs this caution against oversimplistic arguments against primary care therapies.

It is still early days in the research of effectiveness of talking therapies. However, there are the first signs that the refinements in RCTs are producing more positive findings and that these findings, which if repeated and further refined, will make a significant contribution to the case for the development and delivery of these services. The evidence for the effectiveness of counselling looks even more compelling if you take the view that some of the difficulty in answering questions of effectiveness has been excessive reliance on a single research design and that researchers should be willing to countenance diverse sources of information analysed by a variety of research designs and methods, and to take an overview. Rowland and Goss carefully consider the difficulties of developing effective research and the critical evaluation of its results in an earlier chapter. A theme that runs throughout this chapter is the progressive refinement of research strategies and this is the best hope of being able to evaluate the effectiveness of counselling in ways that can usefully inform the delivery of services.

Safeguarding the client

A growing element in the critique of counselling has been the contention that it is not only ineffective, but can actually do harm. Paradoxically, this is a concern that is likely to grow as counselling is taken more seriously as a professional therapy, rather than seen as 'just talking'. For some critics, the harm induced by counselling is endemic: associated with, for example, the neglect of structural factors that impinge on the well-being of individuals, and too much focus on individual choice and responsibility. There is the danger that some identify of an undesirable professionalization of helping activities. Counselling, it is argued, risks undermining more general (and by implication more desirable) community and family sources of help. It imposes its own moral code while adopting the mantle of non-judgementalism and non-directive help.

However, for others the concern is not about all counsellors, but about the poorly qualified, unregulated counsellor. This has been a particular concern in primary care. In the mid-1990s, counselling in primary care was largely *ad hoc*. The nature and level of services varied across the country and between individual practices, due to the 'bottom-up' nature of development, based largely on individual agreements between practices and counsellors. The counsellors themselves came from a range of backgrounds, with different levels of training and professional affiliation (Sibbald *et al.* 1993). They could be quite isolated from other counsellors. Guidelines were available to help practices make appropriate appointments, but anyone could call themselves a 'counsellor'. Moves were only just beginning to bring together and standardize all the forms of training and preparation that did exist and to clearly identify those who could be 'accredited'.

One of the major trends in counselling in primary care in recent years has been towards more management and regulation, attempting to reduce the uncertainty and variety in 'who was doing what' in this field and to strengthen confidence in the quality of the counselling. A proliferation of professional bodies has sought to accredit, organize and represent counsellors in general and the 'specialism' of primary care counselling in particular. Counsellors in the future will have to possess a recognized qualification and to be accredited as a generic counsellor and also maybe as a specialist primary care counsellor. They will be expected to participate in audit and in specified continuing professional development (incorporating the regular supervision that has long been part of the counselling tradition). The pace of these developments has accelerated as various groups jostle for position ahead of imminent regulation. In 2000, a Private Members Bill was introduced into the House of Lords by Lord Alderdice to regulate psychotherapy, independently of counselling psychology and counselling. The Bill failed, but it has focused attention on issues concerning fitness to practice across all the 'talking therapies'. Participants in the debate pointed out the similarities between psychotherapy and counselling and the dangers of regulating one and not the other. It now looks likely that the regulation of these talking therapies will take place under a new Health Professions Council currently being established. The earliest possible date for this to occur is 2003 (Browne 2001). Formal regulation will be welcomed by many and is likely to be accompanied by a drive from government to make counselling more socially inclusive and more widely available. However, it is also likely to intensify the tensions between the tradition of the counsellor as autonomous practitioner and the counsellor as employee of a state-managed service.

The most recent research suggests that counsellors in primary care are reasonably placed to face the rigours of regulation. Based on the analysis of 1031 questionnaires obtained in 1997–98, the research challenges any concerns about a poorly trained workforce that barely satisfies the practice requirements of the responsible professional bodies. This has been one of the persistent interpretations of an earlier study (Sibbald *et al.* 1993) discussed above. Again, the latest study has been published too late to be taken into account by most of our contributors. It presents a picture of growing professionalism in terms of professional qualifications, length of experience and conforming to additional professional requirements. Eight seven per cent of the respondents were women with an average age of 48 years and 6.2 years of experience; 75% held diploma qualifications; 31% had additional degree qualifications; 99% were receiving regular supervision. One of the difficulties faced by these counsellors was trying to liase adequately with other members of the primary care team whist being employed on a part-time basis (Mellor-Clark *et al.* 2001). The overall impression created by this study is of a rapidly emergent profession that is both highly motivated and seeking to establish and work to agreed professional standards.

The new organization of primary care

The development of primary care groups and primary care trusts, together with a strengthened commitment to equity of access and to improved clinical governance, have encouraged more 'top-down', managerialist and evidence-based approaches to commissioning counselling services. This has a number of implications. Primary care counsellors can increasingly expect to be part of a team of counsellors, as well as part of PHCTs. In some parts of the UK, they are becoming part of the broader organizational structure for delivering mental health services. Where integrated provision develops, they will find themselves working more closely with social care providers, including social workers. Issues of professional autonomy, professional boundaries and multidisciplinary working are bound to become more important and more contentious. Some counsellors fear that the desire to become integrated into health care services brings with it the danger of 'medicalization' of counselling and the loss of the distinctive approach to health and healing that it can bring (Wiener & Sher quoted in Eatock 2000). Counsellors may also find themselves providing counselling over a number of practices, rather than identifying with one. They can expect to be subject to more standardized terms and conditions, both in relation to their employment and in relation to the kind of service they provide. Equity principles may mean that existing counselling resources are spread more thinly over a larger population, strengthening the tendency for primary care counselling to be short-term counselling (Hudson-Allez 2000).

Fears that counselling services would disappear from much of primary care as a result of primary care group and primary care trust commissioning decisions have not (so far at least) been realized, but major change is inevitable, in ways that are not universally welcomed by counsellors. For some, increased security of employment and a reduction in professional isolation will not be adequate compensation for loss of the autonomy, self-employed status and the links with a particular practice that they previously enjoyed. Individual practices and GPs also are likely to find themselves with less autonomy in relation to the level and nature of counselling services provided for their patients. Some of these patients will find a reduction in the amount of counselling available, or new constraints on the way the service operates, but others will have access to a previously unavailable source of help. All should experience a greater choice from a team of (diverse) counsellors and have confidence in their qualifications and professional competence.

Developments such as these are likely to contribute towards a formalization of the relationships between counsellors, other members of the PHCT and service users, and to a clarification of the role that the counsellor is expected to play. However, in the end, the success of counselling in contributing to the quality of primary health care will depend on less tangible and timeless factors: the degree of mutual respect and understanding between counsellors, GPs and other health professionals; the extent to which all these professionals listen to and respond to the needs and preferences of their local populations; agreement over realistic expectations and a cautious attitude to easy or universal answers; a critical appreciation of the potential and limitations of all forms of help that individuals can be given to maximize their health and well-being; and a collective commitment to looking for ways to improve. Beyond this, there is no one 'blueprint' for counselling services in primary care. Each commissioning agency and each group of providers will want to develop a service that is attuned to local needs, preferences, resources and expertise. However, we hope this book has provided both information and food for thought for all those involved in these endeavours.

References

Bower, P., Byford, S., Sibbald, B., Ward, E., King, M. and Lloyd, M. (2000) Randomised controlled trial of non-directive counselling, cognitive-behaviour therapy, and usual general practitioner care for patients with depression. II: Cost effectiveness. *British Medical Journal*, 321, 1389–1392.

Browne, S. (2001) Regulation coming soon. *Counselling and Psychotherapy Journal*, 12 (2), 4–5.

Coate, M. (1964) *Beyond all Reason*. Constable, London (cited in *British Medical Journal* (2001), 322, 653).

Department of Health (1999) *National Service Framework for Mental Health—Modern Standards and Service Models*. HMSO, London.

Eatock, J. (2000) Counselling in primary care: past and present. *British Journal of Guidance and Counselling*, 28, 161–173.

Freidli, K., King, M., Lloyd, M. and Horder, J. (1997) Randomised controlled trial assessment of non-directive psychotherapy versus routine general practitioner care. *Lancet*, 350, 1662–1665.

Hemmings, A. (1999) *A Systematic Review of Brief Psychological Therapies in Primary Health Care*. Counselling in Primary Care Trust/Association of Counsellors and Psychotherapists in Primary Care, Staines.

Hudson-Allez, G. (2000) What makes counsellors working in primary care distinct from counsellors working in other settings? *British Journal of Guidance and Counselling*, 28, 203–213.

Mellor-Clark, J. (2000) A personal foreword. *British Journal of Guidance and Counselling*, 28, 157–159.

Mellor-Clark, J., Simms-Ellis, R. and Burton, M. (2001) *National Survey of Counsellors Working in Primary Care*. Occasional Paper. Royal College of General Practitioners, London.

Seligman, M.E.P. (1995) The effectiveness of psychotherapy: the Consumer Reports Study. *American Psychologist*, 50, 965–974 (website: http://www.apa.org/journals/seligman.html).

Sibbald, B., Addington-Hall, J., Brenneman, D. and Freeling, P. (1993) Counsellors in English and Welsh general practices. *British Medical Journal*, 306, 29–33.

Ward, E., King, M., Lloyd, M. *et al*. (2000) Randomised controlled trial of non-directive counselling, cognitive-behaviour therapy, and usual general practitioner care for patients with depression. I: Clinical effectiveness. *British Medical Journal*, 321, 1383–1388.

Index

Page numbers in italic, e.g. 54, signify references to figures.
Page numbers in bold, e.g. 8, denote references to tables.